W0254339

Heparin-Induced Thrombocytopenia

FUNDAMENTAL AND CLINICAL CARDIOLOGY

1. *Drug Treatment of Hyperlipidemia*, edited by Basil M. Rifkind
2. *Cardiotonic Drugs: A Clinical Review, Second Edition, Revised and Expanded*, edited by Carl V. Leier
3. *Complications of Coronary Angioplasty*, edited by Alexander J. R. Black, H. Vernon Anderson, and Stephen G. Ellis
4. *Unstable Angina*, edited by John D. Rutherford
5. *Beta-Blockers and Cardiac Arrhythmias*, edited by Prakash C. Deedwania
6. *Exercise and the Heart in Health and Disease*, edited by Roy J. Shephard and Henry S. Miller, Jr.
7. *Cardiopulmonary Physiology in Critical Care*, edited by Steven M. Scharf
8. *Atherosclerotic Cardiovascular Disease, Hemostasis, and Endothelial Function*, edited by Robert Boyer Francis, Jr.
9. *Coronary Heart Disease Prevention*, edited by Frank G. Yanowitz
10. *Thrombolysis and Adjunctive Therapy for Acute Myocardial Infarction*, edited by Eric R. Bates
11. *Stunned Myocardium: Properties, Mechanisms, and Clinical Manifestations*, edited by Robert A. Kloner and Karin Przyklenk
12. *Prevention of Venous Thromboembolism*, edited by Samuel Z. Goldhaber
13. *Silent Myocardial Ischemia and Infarction: Third Edition*, Peter F. Cohn
14. *Congestive Cardiac Failure: Pathophysiology and Treatment*, edited by David B. Barnett, Hubert Pouleur, and Gary S. Francis
15. *Heart Failure: Basic Science and Clinical Aspects*, edited by Judith K. Gwathmey, G. Maurice Briggs, and Paul D. Allen

16. *Coronary Thrombolysis in Perspective: Principles Underlying Conjunctive and Adjunctive Therapy*, edited by Burton E. Sobel and Désiré Collen
17. *Cardiovascular Disease in the Elderly Patient*, edited by Donald D. Tresch and Wilbert S. Aronow
18. *Systemic Cardiac Embolism*, edited by Michael D. Ezekowitz
19. *Low-Molecular-Weight Heparins in Prophylaxis and Therapy of Thromboembolic Diseases*, edited by Henri Bounameaux
20. *Valvular Heart Disease*, edited by Muayed Al Zaibag and Carlos M. G. Duran
21. *Implantable Cardioverter-Defibrillators: A Comprehensive Textbook*, edited by N. A. Mark Estes III, Antonis S. Manolis, and Paul J. Wang
22. *Individualized Therapy of Hypertension*, edited by Norman M. Kaplan and C. Venkata S. Ram
23. *Atlas of Coronary Balloon Angioplasty*, Bernhard Meier and Vivek K. Mehan
24. *Lowering Cholesterol in High-Risk Individuals and Populations*, edited by Basil M. Rifkind
25. *Interventional Cardiology: New Techniques and Strategies for Diagnosis and Treatment*, edited by Christopher J. White and Stephen R. Ramee
26. *Molecular Genetics and Gene Therapy of Cardiovascular Diseases*, edited by Stephen C. Mockrin
27. *The Pericardium: A Comprehensive Textbook*, David H. Spodick
28. *Coronary Restenosis: From Genetics to Therapeutics*, edited by Giora Z. Feuerstein
29. *The Endothelium in Clinical Practice: Source and Target of Novel Therapies*, edited by Gabor M. Rubanyi and Victor J. Dzau
30. *Molecular Biology of Cardiovascular Disease*, edited by Andrew R. Marks and Mark B. Taubman
31. *Practical Critical Care in Cardiology*, edited by Zab Mohsenifar and P. K. Shah
32. *Intravascular Ultrasound Imaging in Coronary Artery Disease*, edited by Robert J. Siegel
33. *Saphenous Vein Bypass Graft Disease*, edited by Eric R. Bates and David R. Holmes, Jr.
34. *Exercise and the Heart in Health and Disease: Second Edition, Revised and Expanded,* edited by Roy J. Shephard and Henry S. Miller, Jr.
35. *Cardiovascular Drug Development: Protocol Design and Methodology,* edited by Jeffrey S. Borer and John C. Somberg
36. *Cardiovascular Disease in the Elderly Patient: Second Edition, Revised and Expanded,* edited by Donald D. Tresch and Wilbert S. Aronow
37. *Clinical Neurocardiology,* Louis R. Caplan, J. Willis Hurst, and Mark I. Chimowitz

38. *Cardiac Rehabilitation: A Guide to Practice in the 21st Century,* edited by Nanette K. Wenger, L. Kent Smith, Erika Sivarajan Froelicher, and Patricia McCall Comoss
39. *Heparin-Induced Thrombocytopenia,* edited by Theodore E. Warkentin and Andreas Greinacher

ADDITIONAL VOLUMES IN PREPARATION

Silent Myocardial Ischemia and Infarction, edited by Peter F. Cohn

Heparin-Induced Thrombocytopenia

edited by

Theodore E. Warkentin

McMaster University and Hamilton Health Sciences Corporation
Hamilton, Ontario, Canada

Andreas Greinacher

Ernst-Moritz-Arndt University
Greifswald, Germany

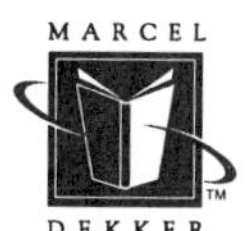

MARCEL DEKKER, INC. NEW YORK • BASEL

ISBN: 0-8247-0271-9

This book is printed on acid-free paper.

Headquarters
Marcel Dekker, Inc.
270 Madison Avenue, New York, NY 10016
tel: 212-696-9000; fax: 212-685-4540

Eastern Hemisphere Distribution
Marcel Dekker AG
Hutgasse 4, Postfach 812, CH-4001 Basel, Switzerland
tel: 41-61-261-8482; fax: 41-61-261-8896

World Wide Web
http://www.dekker.com

The publisher offers discounts on this book when ordered in bulk quantities. For more information, write to Special Sales/Professional Marketing at the headquarters address above.

Current printing (last digit):
10 9 8 7 6 5 4 3 2 1

PRINTED IN THE UNITED STATES OF AMERICA

To the late Professor Michael F. X. Glynn, for *initiating* my hemostasis interests; to Dr. John G. Kelton, for *amplifying* these through boundless opportunities; and to Erica, Andrew, Erin, and Nathan, for *downregulating* my passion, as a caring family must.

T.E.W.

To my co-workers and students for their contributions and efforts; to Sabine, Sebastian, Anja, and Jan.

A.G.

Series Introduction

Although I used to think heparin-induced thrombocytopenia (HIT) was an extraordinarily rare and elusive disease, nothing could be further from the truth. If a high level of suspicion is maintained, HIT will be diagnosed frequently. Surprisingly, it causes deep venous thrombosis and pulmonary embolism far more often than arterial thrombosis. These blood clots cannot be treated with standard anticoagulation, and routine management may yield catastrophic results. Therefore, it is imperative that clinical cardiologists, internists, hematologists, and vascular medicine and surgery specialists familiarize themselves with HIT. To achieve this objective, it is a pleasure to introduce this landmark book, *Heparin-Induced Thrombocytopenia*, edited by two of the most renowned clinical investigators in the field.

I will keep my personal copy on my closest bookshelf to help me as I consult on these perplexing patients. Nowhere else is the research from this emerging field pulled together so comprehensively and lucidly as in this scholarly and practical book.

Samuel Z. Goldhaber

Preface

An anticoagulant turns procoagulant; thus, an antithrombotic causes thrombosis. This is the fundamental paradox of heparin-induced thrombocytopenia (HIT), an antibody-mediated prothrombotic drug reaction without parallel in clinical medicine.

Heparin justifiably is listed as an ''essential'' drug by the World Health Organization (1997): with a rapid onset of action, simple laboratory monitoring, and a low cost, heparin has benefited countless patients. And yet, beginning some 40 years ago, a few physicians asserted that heparin caused unusual and sometimes catastrophic thrombi in some of their patients who received the drug for a week or more. Subsequently, two landmark studies led by a vascular surgeon, Donald Silver, identified the key elements of the HIT syndrome: thrombocytopenia, thrombosis, and heparin-dependent antibodies in the patient's blood (Rhodes et al., 1973, 1977; see Chap. 1). But key questions remained: how can heparin cause thrombosis? What is the frequency of this event? How should these patients be treated? This book summarizes a quarter-century of observation and study that has begun to provide answers to these questions.

The reader will observe several ''themes'' in this book. One is that HIT should be considered a *clinicopathologic syndrome*. This means that HIT should be diagnosed only when 1) one or more unexpected clinical events occur during heparin treatment (most commonly, thrombocytopenia with or without thrombosis), and 2) heparin-dependent antibodies can be demonstrated in the laboratory. A corollary is that the inability to demonstrate the antibodies using reliable assays means that an alternative diagnosis must be considered. Both editors view HIT through this ''filter'' of confirmatory laboratory testing. For us, the laboratory has been crucial to defining the HIT syndrome, by making it possible to distinguish patients who really have HIT from those affected by the numerous other causes of thrombocytopenia encountered in clinical medicine. Indeed, our own first studies on HIT, presented at the XIIIth Congress of the International Society on Thrombosis and Hemostasis in Amsterdam, focused on improvements and innovations in diagnostic testing using platelet activation assays (Greinacher et al., 1991; Warkentin et al., 1991). Coincidentally, this was the same scientific meeting at which Jean Amiral and colleagues (1991) announced the identity of the protein coantigen of HIT (platelet factor 4; PF4), providing another diagnostic avenue (enzyme immunoassay). Thus, when we stepped onto the patient wards, we increasingly relied on the laboratory to confirm or refute the diagnosis of HIT. Through mutually reinforcing experiences of clinic and laboratory, the nature of the HIT syndrome unfolded. And, over time, the wide spectrum of complications of HIT, and its high frequency in certain clinical settings, became apparent.

Our focus on HIT as a clinicopathologic syndrome has implications for the terminology we have used in this book. Because the causative role of heparin can generally be established—in the appropriate clinical context—by the demonstration of pathogenic, heparin-dependent antibodies, we have used the simple designation *heparin-induced thrombocytopenia* to describe this syndrome (i.e., heparin can be shown convincingly to have "induced" the platelet count fall in a particular patient). In contrast, we use the term *nonimmune heparin-associated thrombocytopenia* (nonimmune HAT) to describe patients who have developed thrombocytopenia during heparin treatment and in whom a pathogenic role for HIT antibodies cannot be shown. In our view, this term unambiguously denotes that HIT antibodies are not responsible for the thrombocytopenia, while leaving open the possibility that heparin may have played a role in the causation of the platelet count fall by nonimmune mechanisms (although coinciding thrombocytopenia from another cause is probably the most frequent explanation for this event). We have also introduced the term *pseudo-HIT* to indicate those patients with nonimmune HAT that, by virtue of associated thrombosis or the timing of onset of thrombocytopenia, closely mimics HIT (see Chap. 12).

A second theme of this book is the importance of *in vivo thrombin generation* in the pathogenesis of HIT. By virtue of antibody-mediated activation of platelets and endothelium, and the neutralization of heparin by PF4 released from activated platelets, *the HIT syndrome can be understood as a prothrombotic disorder characterized by activation of the coagulation system*. This concept of HIT helps explain its association with venous as well as arterial thrombosis (by analogy with other hypercoagulable states, such as congenital deficiency of natural anticoagulant factors), and also the occasional HIT patient with decompensated, disseminated intravascular coagulation (DIC).

Marked thrombin generation in HIT also helps explain its association with *coumarin-induced venous limb gangrene*, an unusual syndrome now recognized as a potential complication of coumarin treatment of HIT-associated deep venous thrombosis (see Chap. 3). This iatrogenic disorder represents perhaps the most striking of all the HIT treatment paradoxes (see Chap. 13): two antithrombotic agents with distinct adverse event profiles that interact to produce a profound

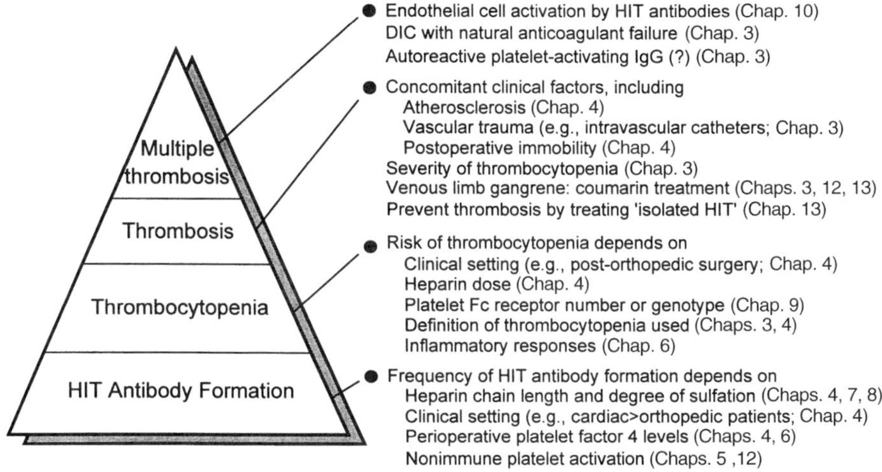

Figure 1 The iceberg model of heparin-induced thrombocytopenia as an index for this book.

disturbance in procoagulant–anticoagulant balance, i.e., increased thrombin generation (secondary to HIT) together with acquired, severe protein C deficiency (secondary to coumarin treatment). Finally, the concept of HIT as a hypercoagulable state with in vivo thrombin generation provides a rationale for understanding the efficacy of new therapies that either reduce thrombin generation by inhibition of factor Xa (e.g., danaparoid) or directly inactivate thrombin (e.g., lepirudin).

A third theme of this book is the peculiarly inconstant nature of HIT, in particular, its *variable frequency and clinical presentation among different patient populations treated with heparin*. Figure 1 depicts HIT as an iceberg within which a variety of clinical and laboratory factors interact to influence antibody formation, development of thrombocytopenia, and, finally, resulting clinical complications, such as thrombosis. A recent, novel concept is that the size and buoyancy of the HIT icebergs can vary among different patient populations who receive heparin. This concept of multiple icebergs of HIT is shown in Chapter 4, Figure 3 (p. 104). Unraveling the clinical and laboratory determinants for these differences in the icebergs among patient populations is a major challenge of current and future investigation.

Why should HIT be the subject of a book? First and foremost, HIT is common, and nonimmune HAT is very common. According to the Council for International Organization of Medical Sciences (CIOMS III), adverse drug reactions can be classified as *common* if they occur in 1–10% of patients, and *very common* if they occur in 10% or more of patients. There is convincing evidence that HIT occurs in as many as 5% of certain patient populations, such as postoperative orthopedic patients receiving unfractionated heparin. The clinical influence of HIT is substantial: about half of these patients develop HIT-associated thrombosis. Nonimmune HAT occurs in as many as 30% of certain patient populations. Thus, physicians need to be able to reliably distinguish among the various thrombocytopenic disorders that occur during heparin treatment. This will minimize the risk of inappropriate treatments, such as failing to stop heparin administration in a patient with probable HIT, or deciding to stop heparin in a patient with nonimmune HAT or pseudo-HIT. Because HIT is a life- and limb-threatening iatrogenic illness with many diagnostic and treatment pitfalls, medicolegal consequences of caregiver's action or inaction can be significant (see Chap. 18).

A second reason for the compilation of this book is that most of the pieces of the HIT puzzle are now firmly in place. Consensus has emerged on several key aspects of the syndrome, including the nature of its target antigen, the participation of platelet and endothelial cell activation in the pathogenesis of thrombosis, the frequency of HIT, and optimal laboratory testing. The publication of this book reflects this coherence in our understanding of the HIT syndrome. Yet there remain important unresolved issues: for example, what is the fundamental nature of the "autoimmune" response to the PF4–heparin neoepitope? Why is the immune response to the HIT antigen so transient? Why do only a subset of patients who form HIT antibodies develop clinical HIT?

Heparin has been, and will continue to be, one of the most important agents for the prophylaxis and treatment of venous and arterial thromboembolism. Consequently, HIT will continue to be an important management problem for some time to come. Both of us have spent a decade of our scientific careers providing, in the context of other investigators' work, a rational management approach aimed at minimizing morbidity and mortality among the many patients who develop the most common immune-mediated adverse drug reaction in clinical medicine. The importance of controlling thrombin generation in HIT is now widely appreciated. The book should help guide clinicians through the often paradoxical clinical and management problems posed by patients with HIT (see Chaps. 13–17).

The book is a tribute to our scientific mentors, John G. Kelton and Christian Mueller-Eckhardt, and the close cooperation of many of our scientific colleagues and personal friends whose efforts made this project possible.

We would also like to acknowledge the help of many individuals in this project. In North America, we thank Jo-Ann Sheppard for technical support over the years, and also for preparing many of the figures in this book; James W. Smith, for help with vexing computer problems; Katherine Bean, for able secretarial assistance; and Erica Warkentin, for checking references and manuscripts.

In Germany, we thank Uta Alpen for excellent secretarial assistance and Petra Eichler, Norbert Lubenow, Lena Carlsson, and Oliver Ranze for valuable discussion and review of manuscripts.

Theodore E. Warkentin
Andreas Greinacher

REFERENCES

Amiral J, Bridey F, Dreyfus M, Vissac AM, Fressinaud E, Meyer D. Identification of PF4 as a target for antibodies generated in heparin-induced thrombocytopenia. Development of a diagnostic test [abstr]. Thromb Haemost 65(suppl):865, 1991.

Greinacher A, Michels I, Mueller-Eckhardt C. Heparin induced platelet activation (HIPA) test: a rapid and sensitive tool for diagnosing heparin associated thrombocytopenia (HAT) and selecting a compatible heparin [abstr]. Thromb Haemost 65(suppl):795, 1991.

World Health Organization. Seventh report of the WHO Expert Committee. The use of essential drugs. WHO Technical Report Series. Geneva: World Health Organization, 1997, p. 37.

Rhodes GR, Dixon RH, Silver D. Heparin induced thrombocytopenia with thrombotic and hemorrhagic manifestations. Surg Gynecol Obstet 136:409–416, 1973.

Rhodes GR, Dixon RH, Silver D. Heparin induced thrombocytopenia: eight cases with thrombotic-hemorrhagic complications. Ann Surg 186:752–758, 1977.

Warkentin TE, Kelton JG. Determinants of platelet donor variability in diagnostic testing for heparin-induced thrombocytopenia [abstr]. Thromb Haemost 65(suppl):1036, 1991.

Contents

Contributors

Susanne Alban, Ph.D. Senior Researcher and Lecturer, Institute of Pharmacy, University of Regensburg, Regensburg, Germany

Jean Amiral, Ph.D. Scientific Director, HYPHEN BioMed, Andresy, France

Gowthami M. Arepally, M.D. Assistant Professor, Department of Medicine, University of New Mexico Health Sciences Center, Albuquerque, New Mexico

Richard H. Aster, M.D. Professor, Department of Medicine, Medical College of Wisconsin, and Senior Investigator, Blood Research Institute, The Blood Center of Southeastern Wisconsin, Milwaukee, Wisconsin

Steven G. Bacsi, Ph.D. Fellow, Blood Research Institute, The Blood Center of Southeastern Wisconsin, Milwaukee, Wisconsin

Beng Hock Chong, M.B.B.S., Ph.D., F.R.C.P.(Glasgow), F.R.A.C.P., F.R.C.P.A. Professor and Senior Consultant Hematologist, Department of Hematology, Schools of Pathology and Medicine, University of New South Wales, and Prince of Wales Hospital, Sydney, New South Wales, Australia

Douglas B. Cines, M.D. Professor, Department of Pathology and Laboratory Medicine, and Director, Hematology and Coagulation Laboratories, University of Pennsylvania School of Medicine, Philadelphia, Pennsylvania

Gregory A. Denomme, Ph.D. Assistant Professor, Department of Laboratory Medicine and Pathobiology, University of Toronto, and Staff Scientist, Department of Pathology and Laboratory Medicine, Mount Sinai Hospital, Toronto, Ontario, Canada

Karl-Georg Fischer, M.D. Division of Nephrology, Department of Medicine, University Hospital Freiburg, Freiburg, Germany

Andreas Greinacher, M.D. Professor, Institute for Immunology and Transfusion Medicine, Ernst-Moritz-Arndt University, Greifswald, Germany

McDonald K. Horne III, M.D. Senior Clinical Investigator, Hematology Service, Clinical Pathology Department, Warren G. Magnuson Clinical Center, National Institutes of Health, Bethesda, Maryland

Volker Kiefel, M.D. Professor, Institute of Transfusion Medicine, University of Rostock, Rostock, Germany

David H. Lee, M.D., F.R.C.P.(C) Assistant Professor, Department of Medicine, Queen's University, Kingston, Ontario, Canada

Katharina Madlener, M.D. Senior Physician, Department of Hemostasis and Thrombosis, Kerckhoff-Klinik, Sprudelhof II, Bad Nauheim, Germany

Dominique Meyer, M.D. Professor of Hematology, INSERM U-143, Hôpital de Bicêtre, Bicêtre, France

Mortimer Poncz, M.D. Professor, Department of Pediatrics, University of Pennsylvania School of Medicine, and Children's Hospital of Philadelphia, Philadelphia, Pennsylvania

Bernd Poetzsch, M.D. Professor, Department of Experimental Hematology and Transfusion Medicine, Rheinische Friedrich-Wilhelms-University Bonn, Bonn, Germany

Klaus Ulsenheimer, Dr.iur., Dr.rer.pol. Professor, Faculty of Law, University of Munich, Munich, Germany

Gian Paolo Visentin, M.D. Associate Investigator, Blood Research Institute, The Blood Center of Southeastern Wisconsin, Milwaukee, Wisconsin

Theodore E. Warkentin, M.D., F.R.C.P.(C), F.A.C.P. Associate Professor, Department of Pathology and Molecular Medicine and Department of Medicine, McMaster University, and Associate Head, Hamilton Regional Laboratory Medicine Program, Department of Transfusion Medicine, Hamilton Health Sciences Corporation, Hamilton, Ontario, Canada

Heparin-Induced Thrombocytopenia

1

History of Heparin-Induced Thrombocytopenia

Theodore E. Warkentin
McMaster University and Hamilton Health Sciences Corporation, Hamilton, Ontario, Canada

I. THE DISCOVERY OF HEPARIN AND ITS FIRST CLINICAL USE

The following account of the discovery and first clinical development of heparin was recorded by the physiologist, Charles H. Best (1959), a codiscoverer of insulin as well as a pioneer in studies of heparin. Incidentally, in 1916, while working at Johns Hopkins University to characterize procoagulant substances, Dr. Jay McLean (1916) identified a natural anticoagulant substance. Further studies of this material were performed by his supervisor, Dr. Howell, who coined the term, "heparin" to indicate its first extraction from animal hepatic tissues (Gr. ἧπαρ [*hēpar*], liver) (Howell and Holt, 1918). Despite its in vitro anticoagulant action, the inability of heparin to prevent platelet-mediated thrombosis (Shionoya, 1927) made it uncertain whether it had antithrombotic potential. However, animal (Mason, 1924) and human studies (Crafoord, 1937) showed that heparin could prevent thrombosis. By the 1950s, heparin was established as an important therapeutic agent in the treatment of venous and arterial thrombosis.

II. THE PARADOX OF HEPARIN AS A POSSIBLE CAUSE OF THROMBOSIS

A. Weismann and Tobin

On June 1, 1957, at the Fifth Scientific Meeting of the International Society of Angiology (North American Chapter) in New York, two physicians suggested

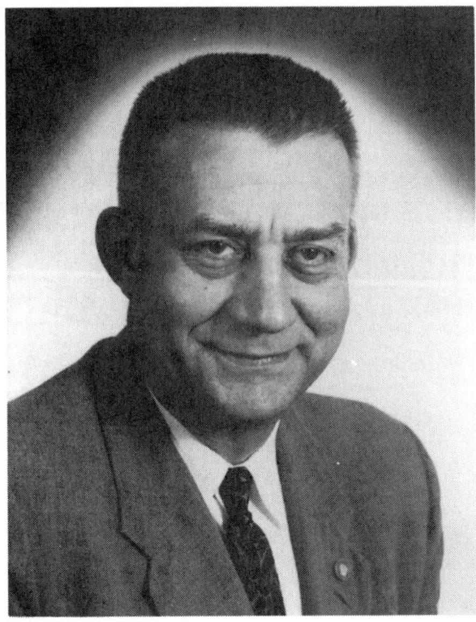

Figure 1 Photograph of Dr. Rodger Elmer Weismann, taken circa 1958.

that heparin might cause arterial embolism in some patients. Rodger E. Weismann, a 43-year-old Assistant Professor of Clinical Surgery at the Dartmouth Medical School (Fig. 1.), and his Resident in Surgery, Dr. Richard W. Tobin, presented their 3-year experience with ten patients who developed unexpected peripheral arterial embolism during systemic heparin therapy at the Mary Hitchcock Memorial Hospital, in Hanover, New Hampshire. Their first patient with this complication was reported in detail, and to this day represents a classic description of the syndrome:

> This 62-year-old white woman was admitted to the Hitchcock Hospital Feb 8, 1955, with left retinal detachment, complicating longstanding myopia. . . . Left scleral buckling was carried out on Feb. 10, and strict bed rest was required during the ensuing three weeks. On her beginning ambulation, on March 6, signs and symptoms of left iliofemoral thrombophlebitis were noted, for which systemic heparinization was begun (. . . heparin sodium in divided subcutaneous doses, totaling 150–300 mg per day. . . .). On March 16. . . , after 10 days of anticoagulation therapy, sudden signs of right common femoral arterial occlusion led to the diagnosis of common femoral arterial embolism. Successful femoral embolectomy was carried out. She was kept on adequate heparinization and made a satisfactory initial recovery until March 19, . . . when signs of sudden occlusion of the distal aorta appeared.

> . . . [P]rompt transperitoneal distal aortic and bilateral iliac embolectomies were performed. In the ensuing 24 hours, because unsatisfactory distal circulation persisted, the patient underwent left femoral exploration, with negative findings, and right popliteal exploration, revealing an embolus. She subsequently pursued a favorable course,...never showing more serious ischemic changes than a small area of superficial gangrene of the right great toe and several small areas of skin infarction of the right leg (Weismann and Tobin, 1958).

The report included a photograph of the emboli removed from the distal aorta and both iliac arteries, with the authors noting their ''unusual length and cylindrical shape, suggesting origin in [the] proximal aorta,'' as well as a corresponding photomicrograph of the embolus. The thromboemboli were described by the authors as ''pale, soft, salmon-colored clots'' that ''histologically . . . were comprised mostly of fibrin, platelets and leukocytes; red cells were rare.'' This appearance was distinguishable from the typical appearance of thrombi originating in the heart (i.e., mulberry-colored thrombi tending to contain cellular elements of the blood in approximately normal proportions), leading the authors to propose that ''the source for the emboli . . . to be aortic mural platelet-fibrin thrombi.''

A summary of the ten reported patients noted that the onset of arterial embolism began between 7 and 15 days, inclusive, of commencing heparin treatment (mean, day 10). Multiple thromboemboli occurred in nine patients; six of the patients died as a direct result of these complications; two survived with extensive amputations, and two were discharged with their extremities intact. The temporal time frame was consistent with the later realization by others that this syndrome represented an immune-mediated reaction initiated by the heparin.

The authors noted that further embolization stopped when the heparin was discontinued, leading to their recommendation that ''heparin should be promptly reduced in dosage, and, if possible, discontinued if the presence of fibrin–platelet thrombi adherent to the intima of the aorta is suspected.'' Aggressive surgical management of emboli was also recommended, as some limbs were salvageable in this way. The authors summarized well the clinical dilemma: ''In each instance there was a feeling of futility in the management of the problem, due to anticipation of further emboli from the same or similar sources. Heparin was badly needed to retard distal thrombosis; yet the agent was probably seriously altering the integrity and attachment of the thrombotic source'' (Weismann and Tobin, 1958).

B. Roberts and Colleagues

The communication of Weismann and Tobin was met with considerable skepticism. When a show of hands was asked to indicate those surgeons who had also observed similar events, none were raised (Weismann, personal communication, July 1998). However, a few years later, Brooke Roberts and colleagues from the

University of Pennsylvania in Philadelphia described a series of patients who were remarkably similar to those reported by Weismann and Tobin (Roberts et al., 1964; Barker et al., 1966; Kaupp and Roberts, 1972). The key features were summarized as follows:

> To witness a series of apparently paradoxical events is disconcerting as well as challenging. When such paradoxes involve totally unexpected results following the use of a major therapeutic agent, it is at first difficult to know whether the relationship is causal or merely coincidental. When, however, the same series of events has been seen repeatedly it is difficult to escape the conclusion that there is some causal relationship, even though the mechanism by which it is accomplished may be unknown. . . . During the last 9 years at the Hospital of the University of Pennsylvania we have seen a group of 11 patients who suffered unexplained arterial embolization for the first time while being treated with heparin for some condition that could not of itself reasonably be expected to cause arterial emboli. . . . All patients had been receiving heparin for 10 days or more when the initial embolus occurred. . . . All emboli removed were of a light color, seemingly made up primarily of fibrin and platelets, and microscopically appeared to be relatively free of red cells. . . . All patients in this group had multiple emboli. . . . Of the 4 deaths, 3 were attributed to cerebral vascular accidents presumably embolic in origin and 1 was thought to have resulted from a perforation of the small bowel 2 weeks after the removal of a mesenteric embolus (Roberts et al., 1964).

Roberts' group also viewed the likely pathogenesis as that of embolization of platelet–fibrin-rich material originating within the aorta, rather than the heart. Furthermore, they believed that the thrombi were initially formed on aortic ulcerations that acted as a nidus for thrombus formation. This pathogenesis was suggested by the observation that such adherent thrombi could be removed from the proximal aorta in a few of the patients (Roberts et al., 1964; Kaupp and Roberts, 1972).

C. An Immune Basis for Heparin-Induced Thrombosis?

The delay between initiation of heparin therapy and onset of embolization caused Roberts and colleagues (1964) to speculate that the etiology could represent an "antiheparin factor," resulting perhaps from "an antigen–antibody mechanism." Furthermore, the observation that the first 21 patients reported with this syndrome from both Hanover and Philadelphia had received heparin exclusively by subcutaneous or intramuscular, rather than intravenous, injection also was offered by Roberts' group as support for immune sensitization. Apparent heparin-induced thrombosis did not seem rare to these investigators: at least 13 of 110 (12%) patients with peripheral arterial emboli managed by the Philadelphia group over a decade were believed to have been *caused* by preceding heparin treatment (Barker et al., 1966).

III. HEPARIN-INDUCED THROMBOCYTOPENIA AND PARADOXICAL THROMBOSIS

A. Heparin-Induced Thrombocytopenia

Routine platelet count measurements were not a feature of hospital laboratory practice until the 1970s, and neither the Dartmouth nor Philadelphia surgeons reported thrombocytopenia in their patients with heparin-induced arterial thrombosis. Ironically, the first report of severe heparin-induced thrombocytopenia involved a patient who did not develop paradoxical thrombosis. Natelson and coworkers (1969) reported on a 78-year-old man with prostate carcinoma and pulmonary embolism, who on day 10 of treatment with therapeutic-dose heparin developed severe thrombocytopenia. Three days after discontinuing the heparin therapy, the patient's fibrinogen fell to 1 g/L, attributed to carcinoma-associated disseminated intravascular coagulation (DIC). Heparin treatment was restarted and, although fibrinogen levels normalized, the platelet count fell to 5×10^9/L, rising to 115×10^9/L 6 days after stopping heparin administration. Simultaneously, however, the fibrinogen value fell to less than 0.5 g/L. When heparin was given for the third time, the platelet count fell over 2 days to 10×10^9/L, although the fibrinogen values again normalized. In vitro studies showed that heparin added to the patient's citrated platelet-rich plasma produced platelet count reductions. This early report of severe heparin-induced thrombocytopenia is interesting, as it illustrates the dichotomy of heparin reproducibly producing severe thrombocytopenia while at the same time maintaining anticoagulant activity (correction of DIC). However, it remained for later workers to link thrombocytopenia and thrombosis to heparin therapy.

B. Rhodes, Dixon, and Silver: "Heparin Induced Thrombocytopenia with Thrombotic and Hemorrhagic Manifestations"

Laboratory evidence implicating an immune basis for heparin-induced thrombocytopenia was first provided by studies performed by a vascular surgeon (Donald Silver; Fig. 2), in collaboration with two residents (Glen R. Rhodes and R. H. Dixon). The first two patients described by Silver's group (Rhodes et al., 1973) developed severe thrombocytopenia (platelet count nadirs, 8 and 10×10^9/L), myocardial infarction, petechiae, and heparin resistance, with complete platelet count recovery on discontinuing heparin treatment. Both patients developed rapid

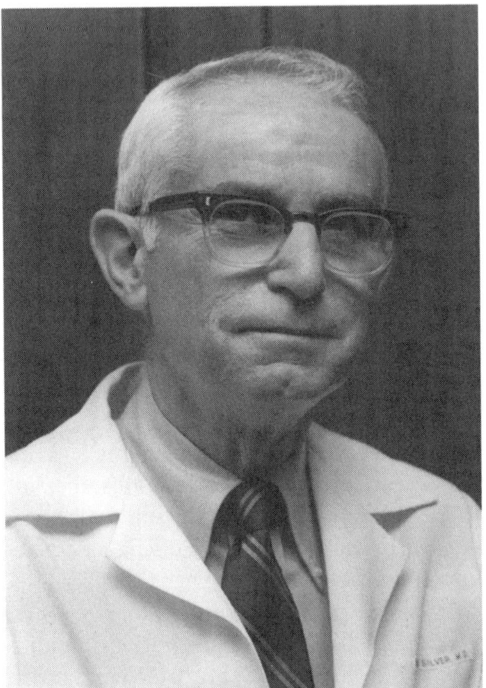

Figure 2 Photograph of Dr. Donald Silver, taken circa 1975.

recurrence of thrombocytopenia when heparin rechallenges were given within 1 week of platelet count recovery.

The immune basis of this syndrome was suggested by several laboratory observations. First, increased platelet consumption was suggested by increased numbers of marrow megakaryocytes, as well as immediate recurrence of thrombocytopenia on reexposure to heparin. Second, a circulating platelet-activating substance was found in both patients' blood: patient, but not control, serum resulted in aggregation of normal donor platelets in the presence of heparin. Third, the possible identity of the aggregating agent as an immunoglobulin G (IgG) was shown by fractionation of one patient's serum to show the presence of heparin-dependent, complement-fixing activities within the IgG fraction.

A second report from this group (Rhodes et al., 1977) represented the landmark study in establishing HIT as a distinct syndrome. Eight patients were reported with thrombocytopenia that occurred during intravenous therapeutic-dose or subcutaneous prophylactic-dose heparin. The mean platelet count nadir was 25 (range, $5–54 \times 10^9/L$). The predominance of thrombotic, rather than hemorrhagic, complications was demonstrated: seven patients had new or recurrent thromboembolic events, and the remaining patient had a stroke leading to evacuation of a temporal lobe hematoma. Complement-fixing, heparin-dependent antibodies were identified in five of the patients. The authors also cited the previous work by Weismann and Tobin (1958) and Roberts and colleagues (1964) as likely representing the identical syndrome. Thus, for the first time, the concept of an immune-mediated hypercoagulable state, with a predisposition to arterial thromboembolism that occurred in association with thrombocytopenia, was proposed.

C. Platelet-Activating Antibodies in the Pathogenesis of HIT

Although some limited studies of heparin-dependent platelet aggregation by patient serum were performed in the classic study by Rhodes and colleagues (1973), the next few years saw increasing emphasis on this characteristic feature of HIT antibodies. In 1975, National Institutes of Health investigators Fratantoni et al. described a patient who developed severe thrombocytopenia (4×10^9/L) and pulmonary embolism while receiving therapeutic-dose UFH to treat deep venous thrombosis. Recurrent thrombocytopenia resulted following heparin rechallenge. The patient's serum produced both aggregation and serotonin release from normal platelets in the presence of heparin. The platelet-activating factor was presumed, but not proved, to be caused by an antibody.

During the next 5 years, at least eight groups of investigators reported similar patients, confirming the presence of heparin-dependent, platelet-activating antibodies (Babcock et al., 1976; Green et al., 1978; Nelson et al., 1978; Trowbridge et al., 1978; Wahl et al., 1978; Cimo et al., 1979; Hussey et al., 1979; Cines et al., 1980). Babcock and colleagues (1976) described five patients who developed thrombocytopenia (mean platelet count nadir, 28×10^9/L) during heparin treatment; heparin-dependent antibodies were detected that produced platelet factor 3 activity (i.e., patient globulin fractions incubated with heparin, platelet-rich plasma, and celite-activated contact product shortened the clotting time following recalcification). Three patients developed thrombotic complications, and none developed hemorrhage. The five patients were observed within a 6-week time span, leading the authors to suggest that "this syndrome may occur more often than has previously been suspected."

A consistent theme was evident from these various reports. Patients developed arterial or venous thrombotic complications, in association with thrombocytopenia that generally began after 5 or more days of heparin treatment. A platelet-activating antibody that aggregated platelets suspended in citrated plasma was usually detected. The platelet count nadirs seen in some of the larger series (e.g., 33 and 48×10^9/L, respectively) observed by Cimo et al. (1979) and Hussey et al. (1979), were higher than in previous reports, indicating that as recognition of the syndrome grew, less severely thrombocytopenic patients were recognized.

D. The "White Clot Syndrome"

Jonathan Towne, a vascular surgeon in Milwaukee, reported with his colleagues (1979) that the pale thrombi characteristic of this syndrome consisted of fibrin–platelet aggregates (electron microscropy). These workers coined the term "white clot syndrome" to describe the characteristic appearance of these arterial thromboemboli. Ironically, their report is also the first to note the occurrence of phlegmasia cerulea dolens that progressed to venous limb gangrene in two of their patients (i.e., a syndrome of venous thrombosis without white arterial thrombi). Nonetheless, the designation of white clot syndrome has become virtually synonymous with HIT, both in North America and Europe (Benhamou et al., 1985; Stanton et al., 1988), despite the lack of specificity of these thrombi for HIT (see Chap. 12).

IV. NONIMMUNE HEPARIN-ASSOCIATED THROMBOCYTOPENIA

A. Nonimmune Mechanisms in Heparin-Associated Thrombocytopenia

Klein and Bell (1974) reported on two patients who developed severe thrombocytopenia, thrombotic complications, and DIC, with hypofibrinogenemia and microangiopathic red cell abnormalities (i.e., these patients likely had severe HIT). This experience prompted Bell to perform the first prospective study investigating the frequency of thrombocytopenia complicating therapeutic-dose unfractionated heparin (UFH) (Bell et al., 1976). Sixteen of 52 patients (31%) developed a platelet count fall to less than 100×10^9/L, and some of these patients developed hypofibrinogenemia and elevated fibrin(ogen) degradation products. The authors speculated that a "thromboplastic contaminant" extracted along with heparin from beef lung could explain the thrombocytopenia. A subsequent randomized controlled trial by Bell and Royall (1980) found the frequency of thrombocytopenia to be higher in patients who received bovine heparin (26%) compared with heparin of porcine intestinal origin (8%).

These investigators found no platelet-activating antibodies in plasma from the patients who developed thrombocytopenia (Alving et al., 1977), leading Bell (1988) to challenge the view that an immune pathogenesis explained HIT. However, the Johns Hopkins group did not report the occurrence of thrombotic complications in any of the 37 patients who developed thrombocytopenia in their prospective studies. Moreover, the apparent early onset of thrombocytopenia in many of their patients suggests that most of their patients likely did not have immune-mediated HIT.

B. Nonimmune (Type I) Versus Immune (Type II) Heparin-Induced Thrombocytopenia

A confusing situation arose. The terms ''heparin-induced thrombocytopenia'' or ''heparin-associated thrombocytopenia'' were often applied to any patient who developed thrombocytopenia during heparin therapy, whether presumed or proved to be caused by heparin-dependent antibodies, or otherwise. Investigators in Australia, led by Dr. Beng Chong (1981), also observed patients with thrombocytopenia in whom heparin-dependent, platelet-activating IgG antibodies could be identified. In a subsequent report that appeared in *Lancet*, two distinct syndromes of ''heparin-induced thrombocytopenia'' were described by Chong and colleagues (1982). The first, called ''group 1,'' developed severe, delayed-onset thrombocytopenia with thrombotic complications in association with IgG antibodies that caused platelet activation. In contrast, ''group 2'' patients had mild asymptomatic thrombocytopenia of early onset.

In 1989, at a Platelet Immunobiology Workshop in Milwaukee, it was suggested to Chong that terminology describing these two types of HIT be formalized. Accordingly, Chong recommended the terms in a review article that appeared in *Blut* (Chong and Berndt, 1989), although (in reverse of the *Lancet* article nomenclature) the early, nonimmune disorder was named ''HIT type I'' and the later-onset, immune disorder referred to as ''HIT type II.'' These terms subsequently became popular.

V. LABORATORY TESTING TO CHARACTERIZE THE HIT SYNDROME

A. A Sensitive and Specific Platelet Activation Assay for HIT

Many clinical laboratories began to use platelet aggregation assays (Fratantoni et al., 1975; Babcock et al., 1976) to diagnose HIT. Problems with this type of assay, however, included low sensitivity (Kelton et al., 1984) as well as technical limitations in simultaneous evaluation of multiple patient and control samples. In 1983–1984, while working as a research fellow in the McMaster University laboratory of John Kelton, Dave Sheridan overcame problems of low test sensitivity by showing that washed platelets, resuspended in a buffer containing physiological concentrations of divalent cations, were very sensitive to platelet activation by HIT sera (Sheridan et al., 1986). The assay, known as the ''platelet serotonin release assay (SRA),'' was adapted from a method of platelet washing developed at McMaster University by the laboratory of Dr. Fraser Mustard. In particular, the emphasis on using physiological calcium concentrations was based on observations that "artifacts" of agonist-induced platelet activation were caused by use of citrate anticoagulation resulting in low plasma calcium concentrations. One example of an artifact induced by citrate is that of two-phase aggregation triggered by ADP. At physiological calcium concentrations, only weak single-phase aggregation without thromboxane generation is triggered by ADP (Kinlough-Rathbone et al., 1983). Fortuitously, the washed platelet technique previously developed at McMaster University by Mustard and colleagues that Sheridan evaluated for its HIT serum-sparing properties rendered platelets far more sensitive to the platelet-activating properties of HIT antibodies than assays based on citrated platelet-rich plasma. Modified washed platelet assays have subsequently been developed by other investigators (see Chap. 11).

Sheridan and colleagues also made the observation that heparin concentrations strongly influenced platelet activation by HIT sera: therapeutic (0.05–1 U/mL), but not high (10–100 U/mL), heparin concentrations resulted in platelet activation, i.e., the characteristic "two-point" serotonin release activation profile of HIT. Later, Greinacher and colleagues (1994) showed that high heparin concentrations in solution release platelet factor 4 (PF4) from PF4–heparin complexes bound covalently to a solid phase, with a corresponding decrease in binding of HIT antibodies to the surface. Thus, the inhibition of platelet activation by high heparin concentrations probably results from a similar disruption of the multimolecular antigen complex on the platelet surface.

The high sensitivity of washed platelets to activation by HIT antibodies led to new insights into the pathogenesis of platelet activation. For example, two years after describing their washed platelet assay for HIT, Kelton and co-workers (1988) reported that the platelet activation process was critically dependent on the platelet Fc receptor. This represented a fundamental new pathobiological mechanism in a drug-induced thrombocytopenic disorder.

B. Prospective Studies of Serologically Defined HIT

Although several prospective studies of the frequency of HIT were performed (see Chap. 4), until the 1990s, none had systematically evaluated serum or plasma from study participants for HIT antibodies. Often, the distinction between "early" and "late" thrombocytopenia was blurred. Thus, the relative frequency and clinical importance of immune versus nonimmune HIT were unclear. This is illustrated by a prospective study reported by Powers and colleagues (1979) that found HIT to be "uncommon" during treatment with porcine mucosal heparin, as only 4 of 120 (3%) patients developed thrombocytopenia, in contrast with the 26–31% frequency of thrombocytopenia reported for bovine lung heparin. However, 2 of these 120 patients may have died as a result of HIT-associated thrombosis (Warkentin and Kelton, 1990), underscoring the need for a specific laboratory marker for this immune-mediated syndrome.

In a prospective study of HIT that performed systematic testing for HIT antibodies (Warkentin et al., 1995), the author showed a dramatic clinical effect for HIT. Of 665 patients participating in a clinical trial of UFH versus low molecular weight heparin (LMWH) after orthopedic surgery, 9 patients developed ''late'' thrombocytopenia serologically confirmed to represent HIT. These patients had a thrombotic event rate far greater than controls. Moreover, the spectrum of thrombosis in HIT patients included venous thromboembolism, rather than only the classic problem of arterial thrombosis. This study also showed that early postoperative thrombocytopenia occurred frequently, but was not explained by HIT antibodies (see Chap. 4).

VI. THE TARGET ANTIGEN OF HIT: PLATELET FACTOR 4–HEPARIN

In 1992, Jean Amiral, working in the laboratory of Dominique Meyer, reported that the antigen recognized by HIT antibodies was a complex between heparin and platelet factor 4, an endogenous platelet α-granule protein (Amiral et al., 1992). This important discovery led to an explosion of basic studies in numerous laboratories that led to further characterization of the basic pathogenesis of HIT (see Chaps. 6–8). Amiral's discovery also led to the development of new assays for HIT antibodies based on enzyme immunoassay techniques (see Chap. 11).

VII. TREATMENT OF THROMBOSIS COMPLICATING HIT

The treatment of HIT is discussed in Chapters 13–15. Here we will discuss only a few vignettes relating to the initial use of selected treatments for HIT.

A. Danaparoid Sodium

In 1982, a 48-year-old vacationing American developed deep venous thrombosis and pulmonary embolism following a transatlantic flight to Germany. Heparin treatment was complicated by thrombocytopenia and progression of venous thrombosis. Professor Job Harenberg of Heidelberg University, who had performed phase I evaluations of the experimental glycosaminoglycan anticoagulant danaparoid, requested this agent from the manufacturer (NV Organon, The Netherlands). The platelet count recovered and the venous thrombosis resolved (Harenberg et al., 1983, 1997). Over the next 6 years, this patient developed recurrent thromboembolic events, each time successfully treated with danaparoid. This favorable experience led to a named-patient, compassionate-release program ending in March 1997, during which time somewhat over 750 patients were treated with this agent. Additionally, Chong performed the first randomized, controlled clinical trial evaluating danaparoid (see Chap. 14).

B. Recombinant Hirudin

The medicinal leech, *Hirudo medicinalis*, has been used for medical purposes for many centuries. Given the observation that the medicinal leech can prevent clotting of blood it has ingested, crude preparations derived from this animal were given experimentally at the beginning of this century. However, because this treatment's daily cost (75 Reichsmark) in 1908 was equivalent to the monthly salary of a factory worker, it was judged to be infeasible. After World War I, Haas, at Justus-Liebig University in Giessen, began his experiments using crude extracts of leech heads for hemodialysis. The major complication in these animal experiments was severe bleeding. The first human hemodialysis patients were treated by him with hirudin during dialysis when a more purified, but still crude protein extract of leech heads became available (Haas, 1925).

In 1956, Dr. F. Markwardt began his work to extract the active component of the leech at the Ernst-Moritz-Arndt University, in Greifswald. Still today, elderly peasants in the small villages around Greifswald tell stories of how they earned their pocket money by collecting leeches for the researchers at the nearby medical school.

The production of large amounts of hirudin by recombinant technology allowed assessment of this direct thrombin inhibitor in clinical trials. Dr. Andreas Greinacher, at that time working at the Justus-Liebig University in Giessen, first used a recombinant hirudin (lepirudin) to anticoagulate a patient who developed acute HIT following heart transplantation. After Greinacher's move to Greifswald, he further assessed the use of hirudin in patients with HIT in two clinical studies that led to the first approval of a drug for parenteral anticoagulation of patients with HIT in both the European Community (March 1997) and in the United States (March 1998) (Greinacher et al., 1999).

C. Warfarin-Induced Venous Limb Gangrene

A theme of this book is the central importance of increased thrombin generation in the pathogenesis of thrombosis complicating HIT. The recognition that warfarin therapy can be deleterious in some patients with HIT illustrates the importance of uncontrolled thrombin generation in HIT.

In December 1992, in Hamilton, Canada, while receiving ancrod and warfarin treatment for deep vein thrombosis complicating HIT, a 35-year-old woman developed progressive venous ischemia, culminating in venous limb gangrene.

This occurred despite a supratherapeutic international normalized ratio (INR). The following day, Kelton observed an area of skin necrosis on the abdomen of this patient, suggesting the diagnosis of warfarin-induced skin necrosis. The author questioned whether the warfarin had also contributed to the pathogenesis of the venous limb gangrene. This hypothesis was directly tested just 2 months later when a second young woman developed severe phlegmasia cerulea dolens of an upper limb during treatment of deep vein thrombosis complicating HIT with ancrod and warfarin. Treatment with vitamin K and plasma given by pheresis reversed the phlegmasia. Further laboratory studies supported this hypothesis of a disturbance in procoagulant–anticoagulant balance during treatment of HIT with warfarin (Warkentin et al., 1997; see Chaps. 3, 12 and 13).

Increasingly, HIT became viewed as a syndrome characterized by multiple prothrombotic events, including not only platelet and endothelial cell activation, but also profound activation of coagulation pathways. This conceptual framework provides a rationale for antithrombotic therapy that reduces thrombin generation in patients with HIT (Warkentin et al., 1998).

REFERENCES

Alving BM, Shulman NR, Bell WR, Evatt BL, Tack KM. In vitro studies of heparin-associated thrombocytopenia. Thromb Res 11:827–834, 1977.

Amiral J, Bridey F, Dreyfus M, Vissac AM, Fressinaud E, Wolf M, Meyer D. Platelet factor 4 complexed to heparin is the target for antibodies generated in heparin-induced thrombocytopenia [letter]. Thromb Haemost 68:95–96, 1992.

Babcock RB, Dumper CW, Scharfman WB. Heparin-induced thrombocytopenia. N Engl J Med 295:237–241, 1976.

Barker CF, Rosato FE, Roberts B. Peripheral arterial embolism. Surg Gynecol Obstet 123: 22–26, 1966.

Bell WR. Heparin-associated thrombocytopenia and thrombosis. J Lab Clin Med 111: 600–605, 1988.

Bell WR, Royall RM. Heparin-associated thrombocytopenia: a comparison of three heparin preparations. N Engl J Med 303:902–907, 1980.

Bell WR, Tomasulo PA, Alving BM, Duffy TP. Thrombocytopenia occurring during the administration of heparin. A prospective study in 52 patients. Ann Intern Med 85: 155–160, 1976.

Benhamou AC, Gruel Y, Barsotti J, Castellani L, Marchand M, Guerois C, Leclerc MH, Delahousse B, Griguer P, Leroy J. The white clot syndrome or heparin associated thrombocytopenia and thrombosis (WCS or HATT). Int Angiol 4:303–310, 1985.

Best CH. Preparation of heparin, and its use in the first clinical cases. Circulation 19:79–86, 1959.

Chong BH, Berndt MC. Heparin-induced thrombocytopenia. Blut 58:53–57, 1989.

Chong BH, Grace CS, Rozenberg MC. Heparin-induced thrombocytopenia: effect of heparin platelet antibody on platelets. Br J Haematol 49:531–540, 1981.

Chong BH, Pitney WR, Castaldi PA. Heparin-induced thrombocytopenia: association of thrombotic complications with heparin-dependent IgG antibody that induces thromboxane synthesis and platelet aggregation. Lancet 2:1246–1249, 1982.

Cimo PL, Moake JL, Weinger RS, Ben-Menachem Y, Khalil KG. Heparin-induced thrombocytopenia: association with a platelet aggregating factor and arterial thromboses. Am J Hematol 6:125–133, 1979.

Cines DB, Kaywin P, Bina M, Tomaski A, Schreiber AD. Heparin-associated thrombocytopenia. N Engl J Med 303:788–795, 1980.

Crafoord C. Preliminary report on post-operative treatment with heparin as a preventive of thrombosis. Acta Chir Scand 79:407–426, 1937.

Fratantoni JC, Pollet R, Gralnick HR. Heparin-induced thrombocytopenia: confirmation of diagnosis with in vitro methods. Blood 45:395–401, 1975.

Green D, Harris K, Reynolds N, Roberts M, Patterson R. Heparin immune thrombocytopenia: evidence for a heparin–platelet complex as the antigenic determinant. J Lab Clin Med 91:167–175, 1978.

Greinacher A, Pötzsch B, Amiral J, Dummel V, Eichner A, Mueller-Eckhardt C. Heparin-associated thrombocytopenia: isolation of the antibody and characterization of a multimolecular PF4-heparin complex as the major antigen. Thromb Haemost 71: 247–251, 1994.

Greinacher A, Völpel H, Janssens U, Hach-Wunderle V, Kemkes-Matthes B, Eichler P, Mueller-Velten HG, Pötzsch B, for the HIT Investigators Group. Recombinant hirudin (lepirudin) provides safe and effective anticoagulation in patients with heparin-induced thrombocytopenia. Circulation 99:73–80, 1999.

Haas G. Versuche der Blutauswaschung am Lebenden mit Hilfe der Dialyse. Klin Wochenschr 4:13–14, 1925.

Harenberg J, Zimmermann R, Schwarz F, Kubler W. Treatment of heparin-induced thrombocytopenia with thrombosis by new heparinoid [letter]. Lancet 1:986–987, 1983.

Harenberg J, Huhle G, Piazolo L, Wang LU, Heene DL. Anticoagulation in patients with heparin-induced thrombocytopenia type II. Semin Thromb Hemost 23:189–196, 1997.

Howell WH, Holt E. Two new factors in blood coagulation—heparin and pro-antithrombin. Am J Physiol 47:328–341, 1918.

Hussey CV, Bernhard VM, McLean MR, Fobian JE. Heparin induced platelet aggregation: in vitro confirmation of thrombotic complications associated with heparin therapy. Ann Clin Lab Sci 9:487–493, 1979.

Kaupp HA, Roberts B. Arterial embolization during subcutaneous heparin therapy. Case report. J Cardiovasc Surg 13:210–212, 1972.

Kelton JG, Sheridan D, Brain H, Powers PJ, Turpie AG, Carter CJ. Clinical usefulness of testing for a heparin-dependent platelet-aggregating factor in patients with suspected heparin-associated thrombocytopenia J Lab Clin Med 103:606–612, 1984.

Kelton JG, Sheridan D, Santos A, Smith J, Steeves K, Smith C, Brown C, Murphy WG. Heparin-induced thrombocytopenia: laboratory studies. Blood 72:925–930, 1988.

Kinlough-Rathbone RL, Packham MA, Mustard JF. Platelet aggregation. In: Harker LA, Zimmerman TS, eds. Methods in Hematology. Measurements of Platelet Function. Edinburgh: Churchill Livingstone, 1983, pp. 64–91.

Klein HG, Bell WR. Disseminated intravascular coagulation during heparin therapy. Ann Intern Med 80:477–481, 1974.

Mason EC. Blood coagulation. The production and prevention of experimental thrombosis and pulmonary embolism. Surg Gynecol Obstet 39:421–428, 1924.

McLean J. The thromboplastic action of cephalin. Am J Physiol 41:250–257, 1916.

Natelson EA, Lynch EC, Alfrey CP Jr, Gross JB. Heparin-induced thrombocytopenia. An unexpected response to treatment of consumption coagulopathy. Ann Intern Med 71:1121–1125, 1969.

Nelson JC, Lerner RG, Goldstein R, Cagin NA. Heparin-induced thrombocytopenia. Arch Intern Med 138:548–552, 1978.

Powers PJ, Cuthbert D, Hirsh J. Thrombocytopenia found uncommonly during heparin therapy JAMA 241:2396–2397, 1979.

Rhodes GR, Dixon RH, Silver D. Heparin induced thrombocytopenia with thrombotic and hemorrhagic manifestations. Surg Gynecol Obstet 136:409–416, 1973.

Rhodes GR, Dixon RH, Silver D. Heparin induced thrombocytopenia: eight cases with thrombotic–hemorrhagic complications. Ann Surg 186:752–758, 1977.

Roberts B, Rosato FE, Rosato EF. Heparin—a cause of arterial emboli? Surgery 55:803–808, 1964.

Sheridan D, Carter C, Kelton JG. A diagnostic test for heparin-induced thrombocytopenia. Blood 67:27–30, 1986.

Shionoya T. Studies on experimental extracorporeal thrombosis. III. Effects of certain anticoagulants (heparin and hirudin) on extracorporeal thrombosis and on the mechanism of thrombus formation. J Exp Med 46:19–26, 1927.

Stanton PE Jr, Evans JR, Lefemine AA, Vo RN, Rannick GA, Morgan CV Jr, Hinton JP, Read M. White clot syndrome. South Med J 81:616–620, 1988.

Towne JB, Bernhard VM, Hussey C, Garancis JC. White clot syndrome. Peripheral vascular complications of heparin therapy. Arch Surg 114:372–377, 1979.

Trowbridge AA, Caraveo J, Green JB III, Amaral B, Stone MJ. Heparin-related immune thrombocytopenia. Studies of antibody–heparin specificity. Am J Med 65:277–283, 1978.

Wahl TO, Lipschitz DA, Stechschulte DJ. Thrombocytopenia associated with antiheparin antibody. JAMA 240:2560–2562, 1978.

Warkentin TE, Kelton JG. Heparin and platelets. Hematol Oncol Clin North Am 4:243–264, 1990.

Warkentin TE, Levine MN, Hirsh J, Horsewood P, Roberts RS, Gent M, Kelton JG. Heparin-induced thrombocytopenia in patients treated with low-molecular-weight heparin or unfractionated heparin. N Engl J Med 332:1330–1335, 1995.

Warkentin TE, Elavathil LJ, Hayward CPM, Johnston MA, Russett JI, Kelton JG. The pathogenesis of venous limb gangrene associated with heparin-induced thrombocytopenia. Ann Intern Med 127:804–812, 1997.

Warkentin TE, Chong BH, Greinacher A. Heparin-induced thrombocytopenia: towards consensus. Thromb Haemost 79:1–7, 1998.

Weismann RE, Tobin RW. Arterial embolism occurring during systemic heparin therapy. Arch Surg 76:219–227, 1958.

2
Differential Diagnosis of Acute Thrombocytopenia

Volker Kiefel
Institute of Transfusion Medicine, University of Rostock, Rostock, Germany

I. INTRODUCTION

Platelet count is affected by the rate of platelet production, the platelet life span, and the distribution of platelets among different compartments (Wintrobe et al., 1981). These three aspects of platelet kinetics have been extensively studied with platelets radiolabeled with ^{51}Cr (Aster and Jandl, 1964) or ^{111}In (Heaton et al., 1979).

Platelet production is equivalent to platelet turnover in a ''steady state'' and can be estimated by determining platelet mean life span and count: approximately 44 $\times$ 10^9/L per day of platelets are produced by normal persons (Branehög et al., 1974). Platelet turnover is decreased in certain marrow disorders (e.g., aplastic anemia and hereditary thrombocytopenia) and often as a result of cytotoxic drugs used for the therapy of malignant disease. Platelet distribution is mainly influenced by spleen size. Normally, approximately 30% of platelets are sequestered in the spleen. In patients with splenomegaly, this fraction can increase to 90%, and mild-to-moderate thrombocytopenia can result. Conversely, in splenectomized subjects, more than 90% of the total platelet mass is circulating.

This chapter will focus on the differential diagnosis of thrombocytopenic states that are characterized by a shortened platelet survival that is mediated by immune mechanisms. Pathological conditions of enhanced platelet destruction caused by nonimmune mechanisms will also be briefly discussed. Autoantibodies responsible for autoimmune thrombocytopenic purpura (AITP), acquired platelet

Table 1 Antigens on Platelet Glycoproteins, Determined Under Reducing Conditions

Glycoproteins	Number of subunits	Molecular weight		Antigenic determinants for[a]
GP IIb/IIIa, CD41/CD61	3	IIb_{α}	125,000	allo, auto, drug
		II_{β}	22,000	
		IIIa	105,000	
GP Ib/IX/V, CD 42	4	Ib_{α}	135,000	allo, auto, drug
		Ib_{β}	22,000	
		IX	17,000	
		V	85,000	
GP Ia/IIa, VLA-2, CD 49b/CD29	2	Ia	165,500	allo, auto
		IIa	150,000	
GP IV, GP IIIb, CD36	1		88,000	iso, auto
CD109	1		175,000	allo
HLA Class I	2	heavy chain	45,000	allo
		β_2M	12,000	

[a] allo, alloantibody; auto, autoantibody; drug, drug-dependent antibody; VLA, very late activation antigen; β_2M, β_2-microglobulin.

dysfunction, cyclic thrombocytopenia, and some forms of drug-induced immune thrombocytopenia (e.g., gold-induced thrombocytopenia), react with monomorphic epitopes on platelet glycoproteins present on platelets of all healthy individuals. Alloantibodies recognize polymorphic, genetically determined epitopes on platelet glycoproteins. They are a specific finding in sera of patients with post-transfusion purpura. Other alloimmune thrombocytopenic disorders will not be discussed here. Drug-dependent antibodies can mediate platelet destruction by recognizing monomorphic determinants on platelet glycoproteins in the presence of the causative drug. Table 1 gives an overview of the platelet glycoproteins known to carry antigenic determinants.

II. AUTOIMMUNE THROMBOCYTOPENIC PURPURA

A. Pathogenesis

Thrombocytopenia in AITP results from rapid clearance of platelets sensitized with autoantibodies, usually of the IgG class, reacting with glycoproteins on the platelet surface (reviewed in Kiefel et al., 1992). Van Leeuwen and co-workers (1982a) were the first to identify the glycoprotein (GP) IIb/IIIa complex as the major target antigen recognized by platelet autoantibodies in AITP, a finding confirmed by others. Epitopes of some antibodies have been assigned to GP IIIa

(Beardsley et al., 1984) or GP IIb (Tomiyama et al., 1987). The other major target antigen is the platelet GP Ib/IX complex (Woods et al., 1984; Kiefel et al., 1991). Other ''rare'' autoantibodies have been shown to react with GP Ia/IIa (Castaldi et al., 1989), GP V (Mayer and Beardsley, 1996), GMP-140 (CD62), and the thrombopoietin receptor (Malloy et al., 1995).

B. Clinical Manifestations

In its various manifestations AITP is a relatively common disorder. Different forms are usually distinguished by clinical criteria.

Acute Postinfectious Autoimmune Thrombocytopenia

Acute AITP usually affects children younger than 10 years of age, boys and girls equally. The thrombocytopenia typically begins suddenly 10 days to 3 weeks after an acute viral infection (Waters, 1992). The incidence of AITP in childhood is estimated at 1:25,000 children per year. Bleeding symptoms may be severe in patients with platelet counts of fewer than 10×10^9/L. However, most patients recover within 3 months, even if they have not been treated with corticosteroids or intravenous IgG (ivIgG). By convention, AITP is referred to as ''chronic'' if thrombocytopenia persists for more than 6 months. However, about 90% of children with AITP develop the acute self-limited form.

Chronic AITP

Chronic AITP is the most common form of immune thrombocytopenia in adults, with women more frequently affected (3:1). It may occur as ''idiopathic'' immune thrombocytopenia or as ''secondary AITP'': that is, observed together with other immunological diseases, such as systemic lupus erythematosus (Waters, 1992), rheumatoid arthritis (Hegde et al., 1983), Crohn's disease (Kosmo et al., 1986), primary biliary cirrhosis (Panzer et al., 1990); malignant diseases, such as lymphoproliferative disorders (Hegde et al., 1983) and solid tumors (Mueller-Eckhardt et al., 1983a); infectious diseases including viral hepatitis (Pawlotsky et al., 1995; Ibarra et al., 1986), human immunodeficiency virus (HIV) infection (Van der Lelie et al., 1987; Walsh et al., 1985); after bone marrow transplantation (Benda et al., 1989); and in diseases of unknown origin, such as sarcoidosis (Henke et al., 1986). AITP with concomitant warm-type autoimmune hemolytic anemia is known as Evans's syndrome (Waters, 1992).

Onset of hemorrhagic diathesis is often insidious in chronic AITP. Most commonly, patients present with hemorrhagic manifestations of the skin, and in more severe forms, mucosal bleeding (''wet purpura'') with bloody blisters in the mouth, oozing from gums, epistaxis, melena, and menorrhagia (Crosby, 1975). Concerns about life-threatening intracranial hemorrhage are an important reason for therapy in AITP. The clinical course in AITP is difficult to predict, and it is estimated that in 10% of patients in childhood with acute AITP it will become chronic. The likelihood of chronic thrombocytopenia is much higher in adults. Many patients experience remissions and relapses that occur spontaneously or following infections. Chronic AITP may be an early manifestation of systemic lupus erythematosus.

C. Diagnosis

Clinical diagnosis of idiopathic AITP is based on its typical clinical picture and the exclusion of other causes for thrombocytopenia: isolated thrombocytopenia without evidence of impaired thrombocytopoiesis (normal numbers of megakaryocytes in the bone marrow). Moreover, spleen size is normal and no other conditions known to enhance platelet clearance are found, such as disseminated intravascular coagulation (DIC), thrombotic thrombocytopenia purpura (TTP), or large hemangiomas characteristic of the Kasabach-Meritt syndrome. Familial thrombocytopenia implies a nonimmune pathogenesis (Greinacher and Mueller-Eckhardt, 1994), for most patients with hereditary thrombocytopenia do not have enhanced platelet destruction (Najean and Lecompte, 1990).

It may be difficult to diagnose AITP on clinical grounds in patients with malignancy, because immune thrombocytopenia may coexist with splenomegaly or neoplastic marrow infiltration. Moreover, not all "platelet antibody tests" are diagnostically helpful (George et al., 1996). In particular, "platelet-associated immunoglobulin G" (PAIgG) assays developed as "platelet Coombs tests" focused on technical considerations, rather than on clinical usefulness (Dixon et al., 1975; Mueller-Eckhardt et al., 1978; Hegde et al., 1985; Follea et al., 1982; Morse et al., 1981; Kunicki et al., 1982; Leporrier et al., 1979; McMillan et al., 1979; Court and LoBuglio, 1986; Kiefel et al., 1987a). However, it appears that platelet-bound IgG in these assays bears little or no direct relation to immune-mediated platelet destruction (Mueller-Eckhardt et al., 1982; Kiefel et al., 1986). Rather, PAIgG reflects IgG stored in the platelet α-granules (George, 1990). However, with the advent of platelet glycoprotein-specific assays (McMillan et al., 1987; Kiefel et al., 1987b; Kiefel, 1992), it is evident that IgG bound to GPs IIb/IIIa or Ib/IX is specific for AITP.

D. Therapeutic Considerations

Therapy should be based on the degree of hemorrhagic diathesis observed. Thus, patients with "wet purpura" are generally treated more aggressively because they are considered to be at greatest risk for bleeding. In children with severe acute AITP, it is important to reduce physical activity. Drugs that inhibit platelet function, such as acetylsalicylic acid, should be avoided. If therapy is necessary, prednisone at an initial dose of 1 mg/kg body weight should be given for a limited period. The ivIgG preparations are very effective in childhood AITP (Imbach et al., 1981, 1985), with doses of 2 g/kg body weight (0.4 g/kg daily for 5 days or 1 g/kg for 2 days) usually effective for a limited time in adult patients. Alternatively, blockade of immune phagocytosis with sensitized autologous red blood cells has been proposed (Salama et al., 1983; Becker et al., 1986): IgG anti-D (Rh_O) may be given intravenously to rhesus (D)-positive patients with AITP. Two doses of approximately 20 μg/kg body weight result in an increase in platelets in most patients. Although the therapeutic effect of anti-D appears less rapid than with high-dose ivIgG, it is often more sustained. Immunosuppressive therapy with azathioprine (Quiquandon et al., 1990) alone or together with corticosteroids may be attempted in patients refractory to other forms of treatment. Refractory patients with dangerous bleeding complications have been successfully treated with cyclophosphamide (Reiner et al., 1995). One of the most effective therapeutic measures in AITP is splenectomy. It should not be performed in children younger than 6 years of age and not in the first 6 months of initially diagnosed acute AITP. It results in partial or complete remissions in 50–80% of patients (Shulman and Jordan, 1987). Possibly, patients with predominantly splenic sequestration of platelets have a higher chance of remission after splenectomy (Najean et al., 1997). A good response to ivIgG may indicate a higher remission rate after splenectomy (Law et al., 1997). Therapy of AITP has been reviewed (Berchtold and McMillan, 1989; George et al., 1996; Waters, 1992; Eden and Lilleyman, 1992).

E. Other Manifestations of Autoimmunity Against Platelets

Acquired Antibody-Mediated Platelet Dysfunction

In ''typical'' AITP, platelet autoantibodies induce thrombocytopenia with relatively moderate bleeding tendency that often is less pronounced than that observed with similar platelet counts caused by impaired thrombocytopoiesis (Waters, 1992). Therefore, it has been concluded that platelet autoantibodies normally do not, or only slightly, affect platelet function. In 1986, the first case of a patient with normal platelet counts, but an IgG1 autoantibody-induced platelet dysfunction resembling Glanzmann's thrombasthenia, was described (Niessner et al., 1986). Interestingly, patients with antibody-mediated platelet dysfunction may develop immune thrombocytopenia (Kubota et al., 1989) and vice versa (Meyer et al., 1991).

Cyclic Thrombocytopenia

Cyclic thrombocytopenia, which predominantly occurs in women, is characterized by rhythmic fluctuations of platelet counts. These fluctuations are in phase with the menstrual cycle, lowest platelets counts being observed during menses. Normal to high platelet counts are observed at midcycle (Tomer et al., 1989). In many patients with this condition, thrombocytopenia is the result of accelerated platelet clearance, as determined with ^{111}In-labeled platelets. In two of the three patients described by Tomer, autoantibodies with GP Ib/IX specificity were identified during both the thrombocytopenic period and during the period with normal platelet counts. These authors correlated platelets counts with changing densities of the Fcγ-receptor on the patients' autologous monocytes. In one patient studied by Menitove, IgG anti-GP IIb/IIIa was found (Menitove et al., 1989). In another case, an IgM anti-GP IIb/IIIa has been reported (Kosugi et al., 1994). Data from another group suggest that the pathophysiology underlying the clinical picture of cyclic thrombocytopenia may be heterogeneous: an autoimmune form with cyclic changes in platelet destruction and a distinct condition with cyclic changes in thrombocytopoiesis (Nagasawa et al., 1995).

Onyalai

An exceptionally severe variant of AITP, onyalai, is observed in some black populations in southern Africa. Whites living in the same regions do not appear to suffer from this disease. In a series of 103 patients (Hesseling, 1987), all patients presented with hemorrhagic bullae of the mucous membranes of the oropharynx. Six died, four of cerebral hemorrhage and two of hemorrhagic shock. Clinical diagnosis is based on the critera of AITP and, in addition, to the presence of hemorrhagic bullae (Hesseling, 1992). Antibodies against GP IIb/IIIa—often of the IgM class—have been implicated. The bone marrow contains normal counts of megakaryocytes, but patients may be anemic at presentation owing to blood loss. Therapeutic options are discussed elsewhere (Hesseling, 1992).

III. POSTTRANSFUSION PURPURA

A. Pathogenesis

Posttransfusion purpura (PTP) is a rare, but severe, transfusion reaction. Typically, 6–8 days after transfusion of whole blood, packed red blood cells, or platelet concentrates, patients experience an abrupt platelet count drop. The patient's serum almost invariably contains a high-titered platelet-specific alloantibody, typically reacting with a determinant on the platelet GP IIb/IIIa complex. In most cases, it reacts with HPA-1a, but other specificities have been observed (Table 2). The duration of this immune-mediated thrombocytopenia is normally limited to 5–60 days. Although the patient's autologous platelets do not carry the corresponding alloantigen, nevertheless, they undergo enhanced destruction. The alloimmune response is anamnestic, for nearly all patients with PTP have a docu-

Table 2 Platelet Specific Alloantigens Implied in Cases of PTP

Alloantigen	Original designation	Percent positive	Localization	Refs.
HPA-1a	Pl^{A1}, Zw^{a}	97.5	GP IIIa	Shulman et al., 1961
HPA-1b	Pl^{A2}, Zw^{b}	30.8	GP IIIa	Taaning et al., 1985; Chapman et al., 1987
HPA-2b	Ko^{a}	11.8	GP Ibα	Lucas et al., 1998
HPA-3a	Bak^{a}, Lek^{a}	86.1	GP IIb	Boizard and Wautier, 1984; Keimowitz et al., 1986
HPA-3b	Bak^{b}	62.9	GP IIb	Kickler et al., 1988; Kiefel et al., 1989
HPA-4b	Yuk^{b}, Pen^{a}	>99.8[a] >99.7[b]	GP IIIa	Simon et al., 1988
HPA-5b	Br^{a}, Zav^{a}	20.6	GP Ia	Christie et al., 1991

[a] Alloantigen frequency observed in Germany.
[b] Alloantigen frequency observed in Japan.

mented prior exposure to the platelet alloantigen during previous pregnancy or transfusion.

Although PTP was first described in 1961, its pathogenesis remains debated even today. It has been suggested that circulating HPA-1a antigen from the platelets of the immunizing blood product persists, and thus antigen–antibody complexes are adsorbed onto the autologous platelets (Shulman et al., 1961). Others have proposed that during the secondary, anamnestic immunization precipitating PTP, a second autorective antibody arises, causing the patient's severe thrombocytopenia. It is our experience that alloantibodies observed in the early anamnestic response in PTP are always high-titered. Moreover, they can be eluted from the autologous (alloantigen-negative) platelets in most cases studied (Kroll et al., 1993). Therefore, it can also be hypothesized that this pseudospecific alloantibody for a limited time cross-reacts with a structurally related epitope on the patient's autologous platelets.

B. Clinical Picture

The clinical course of PTP has been summarized by the Europen PTP study group (Mueller-Eckhardt et al., 1991). Women were predominantly affected (99 out of 104). Mean age was 58.4 years. In 28 of 51 patients, marked febrile transfusion reactions were observed following the transfusion that precipitated PTP. The interval between transfusion and onset of severe thrombocytopenia was generally 6–10 days. In 68 out of 84 patients, the initial platelet count was fewer than 10 ×

10^9/L. Bleeding persisted for 3–37 days (mean, 10.2 days). Most patients required treatment. Fatal bleeding is not rare, occurring in 7 of 75 patients (Shulman and Jordan, 1987) and in 2 of 38 patients (Kroll et al., 1993) in two studies.

C. Diagnosis

The diagnosis of PTP should be considered in all patients with a sudden drop in platelet count to fewer than 10×10^9/L. Thus, PTP and HIT may occur in similar clinical situations, (i.e., about 1 week after surgery). In PTP, however, thrombocytopenia is more pronounced and associated with bleeding, in contrast with the absence of petechiae and presence of thromboembolic complications characteristic of HIT (see Chap. 3).

Moreover, PTP only occurs following recent transfusion. PTP has occurred in association with delayed hemolytic transfusion reaction (Chapman et al., 1987; Maslanka and Zupanska, 1993). In a single case, PTP was observed concurrently with drug-dependent immune hemolytic anemia (Mueller-Eckhardt et al., 1987). Diagnosis is confirmed by detection of a platelet-specific alloantibody against an epitope on platelet GP IIb/IIIa, usually anti-HPA-1a. Platelets of the patient are always negative for the corresponding antigen. Eluates prepared from patients' autologous platelets usually contain anti-HPA-1a (Kroll et al., 1993).

D. Therapeutic Considerations

The efficacy of corticosteroids is uncertain. In contrast, high-dose ivIgG (Mueller-Eckhardt et al., 1983b) is clearly effective in most (Mueller-Eckhardt and Kiefel, 1988; Chong et al., 1986; Berney et al., 1985) but not all cases (Kroll et al., 1993). Thus, ivIgG is the treatment of choice for PTP. Platelet transfusions are ineffective, even if platelets from HPA-1a–negative donors are given (Gerstner et al., 1979). As the bleeding tendency is often pronounced, immediate therapy following clinical diagnosis is mandatory.

IV. PASSIVE IMMUNE THROMBOCYTOPENIA

Acute thrombocytopenia in humans resulting from experimental transfer of platelet autoantibodies has been observed in studies on the pathogenesis of AITP (Harrington et al., 1951). However, inadvertent transfer of platelet autoantibodies has not been recognized as a problem in clinical transfusion practice. In contrast, platelet alloantibodies with HPA-1a (Moilan et al., 1985; Ballem et al., 1987; Scott et al., 1988; Brunner-Bollinger et al., 1997) and HPA-5b (Warkentin et al., 1992) specificities can cause abrupt-onset immune thrombocytopenia. In three cases, the antibody was transfused with plasma, in one case by whole blood, and once by a red blood cell concentrate. The condition may be accompanied by a febrile transfusion reaction. It is important to investigate these cases to identify and exclude donors with "harmful" platelet alloantibodies.

V. DRUG-INDUCED IMMUNE THROMBOCYTOPENIA

A. Pathogenesis

Drugs can induce various immune-mediated cytopenias, such as immune hemolytic anemia, neutropenia, and drug-induced immune thrombocytopenia (DIT) (Salama and Mueller-Eckhardt, 1992). Different mechanisms are involved in causing DIT, with drug-dependent antibodies being most extensively investigated. Drug-dependent antibodies typically react with monomorphic epitopes on virtually the same platelet glycoproteins recognized by platelet-specific autoantibodies: GP Ib/IX (van Leeuwen et al., 1982b; Kunicki et al., 1978; Berndt et al., 1985), GP V (Stricker and Shuman, 1986) or GP IIb/IIIa (Christie et al., 1987, 1993; Pfueller et al., 1990; Visentin et al., 1991). They bind to only the platelet target antigen in the presence of the causative drug: thus, if the drug is removed from the buffer during in vitro studies, the antibody detaches (see Fig. 2). The antibody specifically recognizes the antigen on platelet glycoprotein by the Fab fragment (Christie et al., 1985). The precise role of the drug in antigen–antibody binding is unclear. Experimental studies suggest that in some individuals, the drug induces conformational change either in the antibody or in the platelet glycoprotein to induce complementarity required for antibody binding (Shulman and Jordan, 1987).

The drugs most commonly implicated in DIT are quinidine and quinine. Many substances have been suspected to induce this condition, but only a few have been documented by appropriate laboratory analysis (Aster and George, 1990). Table 3 lists drugs implicated in the author's laboratory. Sometimes a metabolite, rather than the drug itself, mediates drug-dependent antibody binding to the platelet surface (Eisner and Shahidi, 1972; Eisner and Kasper, 1972; Kiefel et al., 1987c; Meyer et al., 1993). Similar observations have been made for drug induced immune hemolysis (Salama and Mueller-Eckhardt, 1985).

B. Clinical Picture and Therapy

Thrombocytopenia begins at least 7 days after the first exposure to the drug (Shulman and Jordan, 1987). Drug-dependent antibodies can persist; thus, reexposure to the drug can cause a sudden drop in platelet count, and is not recommended as a diagnostic maneuver. DIT often causes severe thrombocytopenia and bleeding.

The most important measure is to discontinue the offending drug. This is normally followed by a rise of platelet count. If bleeding symptoms are life-

Table 3 Drugs Inducing DIT

Drug	*n*	Comments
Quinidine	18	
Quinine	3	
Quinidine + quinine	5	
Trimethoprim–sulfamethoxazole	6	1 metabolite—specific ddAb (sulfamethoxazole)
Rifampicin (rifampin)	4	
Nomifensine	2	
Paracetamol (acetaminophen)	1	1 metabolite—specific ddAb
Carbamazepine	4	
Diclofenac	5	
Ibuprofen	3	1 metabolite—specific ddAb
Ranitidine	1	
Vancomycin	1	

Source: Institute for Clinical Immunology and Transfusion Medicine, University of Giessen.

threatening, transfusion of large doses of platelets, together with ivIgG should be considered.

C. Other Forms of Drug-Induced Immune Thrombocytopenia

Some drugs cause autoimmune cytopenias by inducing autoantibodies indistinguishable from those encountered in ''idiopathic'' autoimmune cytopenia. A well-known example is α-methyldopa, which in 10–36% of patients induces formation of red blood cell autoantibodies (Petz and Garratty, 1980). However, only 1% of patients develop clinical hemolysis. Similarly, autoimmune thrombocytopenia has been observed during the course of gold therapy (von dem Borne et al., 1986). The antibodies found in these patients do not require the presence of the drug for binding to platelets in vitro (i.e., they resemble autoantibodies).

Abciximab (ReoPro), a monoclonal antibody Fab moiety reacting with GP IIb/IIIa that has therapeutic platelet inhibitory effects, causes severe immune thrombocytopenia in about 2% of patients treated. In contrast to other forms of DIT, thrombocytopenia appears rapidly, within hours following even first exposure to the drug. Platelet transfusions (Kereiakes et al., 1996) appear to be effective more than ivIgG and corticosteroids.

VI. CONSUMPTIVE THROMBOHEMORRHAGIC DISORDERS

A. Pathogenesis

A heterogeneous group of events, including sepsis, malignancies, trauma, obstetric complications, snake venoms, and hemolytic transfusion reactions, can be complicated by a systemic syndrome characterized by dysregulated thrombin formation, leading to activation and consumption of coagulation factors, and resulting in the formation of intravascular fibrin thrombi. Secondary plasmin generation helps lyse the fibrin formed. Additionally, the vessel wall and platelets are usually involved in this pathological process of "disseminated intravascular coagulation" (DIC). Indeed, thrombocytopenia is a common clinical manifestation of DIC (Mammen, 1998). Both bleeding and widespread thrombotic microvascular occlusion, leading to organ failure, can result from DIC.

B. Clinical Disorders

Septicemia

Disseminated intravascular coagulation can complicate infections, especially with gram-negative bacteria (Marder et al., 1994; Mammen, 1998). It has been suggested that thrombocytopenia in septic patients is the consequence of immune-mediated platelet damage, based on the observation of elevated PAIgG levels (Kelton et al., 1979). However, this does not prove an autoimmune basis for the thrombocytopenia (Shulman and Reis, 1994), for PAIgG is elevated in thrombocytopenia of nonimmune origin.

The pathogenesis of DIC in sepsis is multifactorial, and includes direct endothelial damage and platelet activation by endotoxins, resulting in exposure of procoagulant material. In addition, the cytokines interleukin-1 and tumor necrosis factor increase tissue factor activity, thereby shifting the balance toward a prothrombotic tendency (Mammen, 1998). Plasminogen activator inhibitor-1 (PAI-1) blocks plasmin generation during the course of sepsis, thereby contributing to fibrin deposition in the microcirculation (Müller-Berghaus, 1987).

Malignant Disease

About 9–15% of patients with cancer have DIC at some point during their disease (Pasquini et al., 1995). Overt bleeding is uncommon; rather, recurrent thromboembolism is characteristic, an entity known as Trousseau's syndrome. An exception: acute promyelocytic leukemia is often accompanied by a severe DIC and bleeding, often induced or worsened by chemotherapy (Marder et al., 1994).

Other Conditions

Diseminated intravascular coagulation occurs in obstetric situations characterized by release of thrombogenic material [e.g., the retained dead fetus syndrome (Baglin, 1996; Marder et al., 1994), amniotic fluid embolism, or placental separation]. Bites of certain snakes may cause hypofibrinogenemia induced by enzymes that clot fibrinogen or directly activate platelets. Severe hemolytic transfusion reactions can cause DIC, especially in association with red cell antibodies, causing intravascular complement-mediated hemolysis (e.g., ABO-incompatible transfusion). DIC seems to be aggravated by complement-mediated damage of endothelial cells. Whether red cell lysis alone (not mediated by complement) is able to induce DIC in humans remains unclear (Mollison et al., 1993; Baglin, 1996). Other conditions associated with DIC are trauma and localized processes in which activation of coagulation occurs within giant hemangiomas (Kasabach-Merrit syndrome) or aortic aneurysms.

C. Diagnosis

''Global'' coagulation tests, such as prothrombin and activated partial thromboplastin times, are usually prolonged; fibrinogen concentrations are often reduced. However, these parameters can be normal in DIC. Fibrin degradation products mirror the action of plasmin on fibrin clots, and therefore are elevated in most patients with DIC. The D-dimer test readily assesses cross-linked fibrin degradation. Elevated prothrombin fragment F1 + 2 levels reflect thrombin activation as one of the central mechanisms underlying DIC. Examination of a blood smear sometimes will show red cell fragmentation in DIC. On the other hand, a high percentage of red cell fragmentation suggests a microangiopathic hemolytic disorder (discussed subsequently). Laboratory diagnosis (Marder et al., 1994) and therapy (Baglin, 1996; Marder et al., 1994; Humphries, 1994) of DIC are reviewed elsewhere.

VII. THROMBOTIC THROMBOCYTOPENIC PURPURA AND THE HEMOLYTIC–UREMIC SYNDROME

Thrombotic thrombocytopenic purpura (TTP) is a severe disease characterized by intravascular platelet aggregation, nonimmune hemolytic anemia, neurological symptoms and signs, and renal failure. Red cell fragmentation, hemolysis with a negative direct antiglobulin test, and platelet-rich thrombi occluding small blood vessels are characteristic.

Different hypotheses have been proposed to explain the peculiar phenomenon of platelet deposition within the precapillary arterioles (Moake and Eisenstaedt, 1994). Serum of patients with TTP and the hemolytic–uremic syndrome (HUS) contains unusually large von Willebrand factor (vWF) forms (Moake et al., 1982) that may mediate platelet aggregation. Recent findings suggest deficiency of a vWF-cleaving protease (''depolymerase'') in patients with chronic, relapsing TTP (Furlan et al., 1997). An IgG inhibitor of the vWF-cleaving protease (Furlan et al., 1998) may be responsible for acute, self-limited TTP. Various disorders can be associated with a TTP-like illness, including treatment with immunosuppressive drugs, metastatic cancer or its therapy (Gordon and Kwaan, 1997), and infections.

Vascular damage in HUS is usually confined to the kidneys, and neurological sequelae are less pronounced than in TTP (Moake and Eisenstaedt, 1994). HUS developing after bloody diarrhea is associated with strains of verocytotoxin-producing *Escherichia coli* serotype 0157 (Taylor and Monnens, 1998).

The cornerstone of therapy for TTP is transfusion of homologous plasma, usually given by plasmapheresis. Corticosteroids may be effective in conditions of immune-mediated inhibition of the vWF-cleaving protease. Clinical features and therapeutic options in TTP/HUS are reviewed in detail elsewhere (Remuzzi, 1987; Moake and Eisenstaedt, 1994; George and Aster, 1990).

VIII. TECHNIQUES FOR CHARACTERIZATION OF PLATELET ANTIBODIES

Laboratory testing for immune-mediated thrombocytopenia requires specific knowledge of the underlying clinical problem. For example, an accurate drug history is needed to evaluate DIT in vitro.

A. Analysis of Platelet Autoantibodies and Alloantibodies in Serum Samples

Often, only serum samples from a thrombocytopenic patient are available for study. Depending on the clinical problem, it may be useful to screen for platelet-reactive serum antibodies. A reliable, standardized immunoglobulin-binding assay for platelet antibodies is the platelet suspension immunofluorescence test (von dem Borne et al., 1978). A simplified alternative is more convenient for large-scale screening (Schneider and Schnaidt, 1981), but may be less sensitive. Usually a ''panel'' of platelets with different alloantigens is employed: platelet suspensions are incubated with the serum to be studied and immunoglobulin binding to platelets is determined by platelet immunofluorescence. Reactivity with all platelets from the panel is often observed with platelet autoantibodies, but may also occur with antibodies against ''high-frequency'' antigens (e.g., Yuk^a, Nak^a), or mixtures of alloantibodies, if the panel does not include antigen-negative platelet suspensions. The most compelling way to exclude that a broadly reactive antibody is an autoantibody is to test the serum against autologous platelets. With the rare exception of PTP, alloantibodies do not react with autologous platelets.

Whenever possible, the platelet glycoprotein target of the antibodies should be identified. This is important because many sera of patients who have previously been exposed to allogeneic blood cells via transfusion or pregnancy contain "contaminating" alloantibodies reacting with HLA class I antigens present in high density on platelets.

Laboratory diagnosis of AITP, PTP, DIT, and certain thrombocytopenic states in newborns is based on the characterization of platelet-specific antibodies. This may be accomplished with assays that include electrophoretic determination of molecular weight of glycoproteins, including immunoblot (Herman et al., 1986; Huisman, 1986) or (radio-) immunoprecipitation (Mulder et al., 1984; Santoso et al., 1989; Smith et al., 1993). These techniques are cumbersome and time-consuming. Therefore, assays that allow identification of target antigens with well-characterized monoclonal antibodies are now preferred. These include the monoclonal antibody immobilization of platelet antigens (MAIPA) assay (Kiefel

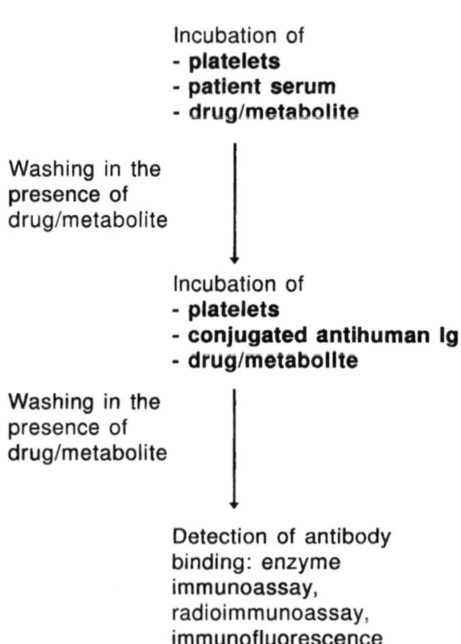

Figure 1 Summary of drug-dependent antibody detection in immunoglobulin-binding assays.

et al., 1987b; Kiefel, 1992) and the immunobead assay (McMillan et al., 1987). These monoclonal antibody-based immunoassays are suitable to detect, and discriminate among, antibodies against GP IIb/IIIa, GP Ia/IIa, GP Ib/IX, GP V, HLA class I antigen, and other structures of the platelet membrane.

Virtually all antibodies reacting with the HLA class I antigens, and most antibodies against GP Ia/IIa, are alloantibodies. In contrast, GP IIb/IIIa and GP Ib/IX/V carry determinants recognized by autoantibodies, drug-dependent antibodies, and alloantibodies (see Tables 1 and 2). The serological diagnosis of PTP is based on detection of platelet alloantibodies, mainly against GP IIb/IIIa.

B. Characterization of Platelet-Bound Antibodies

Determination of specific autoantibodies against GPs IIb/IIIa and Ib/IX on a patient's autologous platelets performed with "direct" glycoprotein-specific immunoassays (McMillan et al., 1987) is much more specific than quantitation of PAIgG. As an alternative, testing of eluates prepared at pH 2.8 from autologous patient platelets in an antibody-binding assay (platelet immunofluorescence) is also specific for AITP (Kiefel et al., 1996). Direct immunoprecipitation detected

Table 4 Interpretation of Immunoglobulin-Binding Assays for Detection of Drug-Dependent Antibodies

Platelets	Drug or metabolite	Serum	Reaction	Interpretation
+	+	Patient	+ [a]	Drug-dependent antibody
+	−	Patient	− [b]	
+	+	Normal donor serum	− [c]	
+	−	Normal donor serum	− [d]	
+	+	Patient	+	Autoantibody (alloantibody)
+	−	Patient	+	
+	+	Normal donor serum	−	
+	−	Normal donor serum	−	
+	+	Patient	+	(Nonspecific) adsorption of immunoglobulins to platelets induced by the drug
+	−	Patient	−	
+	+	Normal donor serum	+	
+	−	Normal donor serum	−	
+	+	Patient	−	Negative result
+	−	Patient	−	
+	+	Normal donor serum	−	
+	−	Normal donor serum	−	

[a] The experiment for ddAb detection, as depicted in Figure 2; [b–d] Control experiments.

anti-HPA-5b on the patient's platelets in a case of passive alloimmune thrombocytopenia (Warkentin et al., 1992).

C. Determination of Drug-Dependent Antibodies

Drug-dependent antibodies against platelets can be characterized using various techniques. If antiglobulin-binding assays are used, they should include the following steps (Fig. 1). Test platelets should be incubated in buffer containing the drug, and the serum sample to be tested is added. Platelets are washed with buffer containing the same concentration of the drug. Following incubation in buffer with the conjugated antihuman IgG (also containing the same drug concentration as the incubation mixture), platelets are again washed, and binding of IgG is detected by enzyme-linked immunosorbent assay (ELISA) or by radioimmunoassay. With each experiment, several controls should be included (Table 4). Figure 2 shows a typical experiment with two quinidine-dependent platelet antibodies: evidently the drug-dependent antibodies do not remain fixed to the platelet mem-

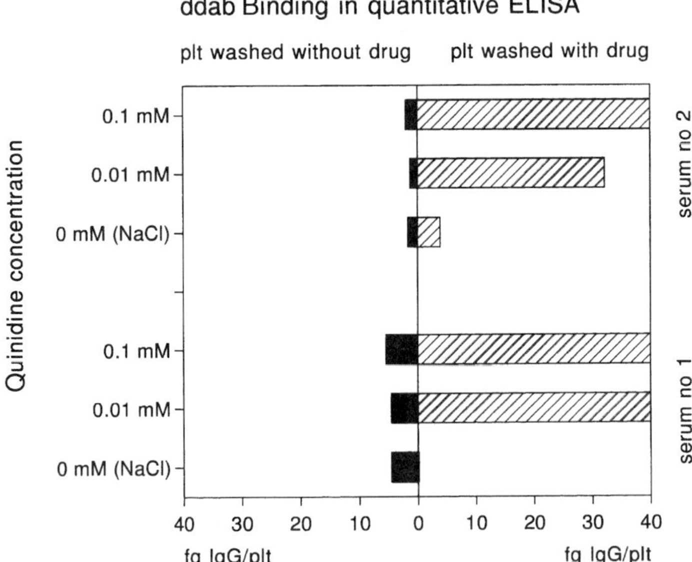

Figure 2 Quinidine-dependent antibodies binding to platelet in the presence (0.01 mM and 0.1 mM) and absence of the drug (0 mM drug, in normal saline). Antibody binding to platelets was detected only with quinidine added to the washing buffer at the same concentrations as the incubation mixture. ddab, drug-dependent antibodies; ELISA, enzyme-linked immunosorbent assay; IgG, immunoglobulin G; plt, platelets.

brane if the drug is not included in the washing buffer. As already discussed, drug-dependent antibodies can be caused by a drug metabolite, rather than by the drug itself. In this case, positive results are obtained only with metabolites. If metabolites are renally excreted, urine from a person ingesting the drug may be sufficient as a crude ''metabolite preparation'' (Kiefel et al., 1987c). This approach has also been explored for the detection of drug-dependent antibodies against red blood cells (Salama and Mueller-Eckhardt, 1985).

REFERENCES

Aster RH, George JN. Thrombocytopenia due to enhanced platelet destruction by immunologic mechanisms. In: Williams WJ, Beutler E, Erslev AJ, Lichtman MA, eds. Hematology. New York: McGraw-Hill, 1990, pp 1370–1398.

Aster RH, Jandl JH. Platelet sequestration in man. I. Methods. J Clin Invest 43:843–855, 1964.

Baglin T. Disseminated intravascular coagulation: diagnosis and treatment. Br Med J 312: 683–687, 1996.

Ballem PJ, Buskard NA, Decary F, Doubroff P. Post-transfusion purpura secondary to passive transfer of anti-Pl^{A1} by blood transfusion. Br J Haematol 66:113–114, 1987.

Beardsley DS, Spiegel JE, Jacobs MM, Handin RI, Lux SE. Platelet membrane glycoprotein IIIa contains target antigens that bind anti-platelet antibodies in immune thrombocytopenias. J Clin Invest 74:1701–1707, 1984.

Becker T, Küenzlen E, Salama A, Mertens R, Kiefel V, Weiß H, Lampert F, Gaedicke G, Mueller-Eckhardt C. Treatment of childhood idiopathic thrombocytopenic purpura with rhesus antibodies (anti-D). Eur J Pediatr 145:166–169, 1986.

Benda H, Panzer S, Kiefel V, Mannhalter C, Hinterberger W, Lechner K, Mueller-Eckhardt C. Identification of the target platelet glycoprotein in autoimmune thrombocytopenia occurring after allogeneic bone marrow transplantation. Blut 58: 151–153, 1989.

Berchtold P, McMillan R. Therapy of chronic idiopathic thrombocytopenic purpura in adults. Blood 74:2309–2317, 1989.

Berndt MC, Chong BH, Bull HA, Zola H, Castaldi PA. Molecular characterization of quinine/quinidine drug-dependent antibody platelet interaction using monoclonal antibodies. Blood 66:1292–1301, 1985.

Berney SI, Metcalfe P, Wathen NC, Waters AH. Post-transfusion purpura responding to high dose intravenous IgG: further observations on pathogenesis. Br J Haematol 61:627–632, 1985.

Boizard B, Wautier JL. Lek^{a}, a new platelet antigen absent in Glanzmann's thrombasthenia. Vox Sang 46:47–54, 1984.

Branehög I, Kutti J, Weinfeld A. Platelet survival and platelet production in idiopathic thrombocytopenic purpura (ITP). Br J Haematol 27:127–143, 1974.

Brunner-Bollinger S, Kiefel V, Horber FF, Nydegger UE, Berchtold P. Antibody studies in a patient with acute thrombocytopenia following infusion of plasma containing anti-Pl^{A1}. Am J Hematol 56:119–121, 1997.

Castaldi PA, Mehrabani PA, Fournier DJ, Berndt MC. Autoimmune thrombocytopenia associated with B-CLL and an IgG autoantibody directed against the human platelet GP Ia-IIa complex (VLA-2) [abstr]. Thromb Haemost 62:151, 1989.

Chapman JF, Murphy MF, Berney SI, Ord J, Metcalfe P, Amess JAL, Waters AH. Post-transfusion purpura associated with anti-Bak[a] and anti-Pl[A2] platelet antibodies and delayed hemolytic transfusion reaction. Vox Sang 52:313–317, 1987.

Chong BH, Cade J, Smith JA, Tatoulis J. An unusual case of post-transfusion purpura: good transient response to high-dose immunoglobulin. Vox Sang 51:182–184, 1986.

Christie DJ, Mullen PC, Aster RH. Fab-mediated binding of drug-dependent antibodies to platelets in quinidine- and quinine-induced thrombocytopenia. J Clin Invest 75: 310–314, 1985.

Christie DJ, Mullen PC, Aster RH. Quinine- and quinidine platelet antibodies can react with GP IIb/IIIa. Br J Haematol 67:213–219, 1987.

Christie DJ, Pulkrabek S, Putnam JL, Slatkoff ML, Pischel KD. Posttransfusion purpura due to an alloantibody reactive with glycoprotein Ia/IIa (anti-HPA-5b). Blood 77: 2785–2789, 1991.

Christie DJ, Sauro SC, Cavanaugh AL, Kaplan ME. Severe thrombocytopenia in an acquired immunodeficiency syndrome patient associated with pentamidine-dependent antibodies specific for glycoprotein IIb/IIIa. Blood 82:3075–3080, 1993.

Court WS, LoBuglio AF. Measurement of platelet surface-bound IgG by a monoclonal ^{125}I-anti-IgG assay. Vox Sang 50:154–159, 1986.

Crosby WH. Wet purpura, dry purpura. JAMA 232:744–745, 1975.

Dixon R, Rosse WF, Ebbert L. Quantitative determination of antibody in idiopathic thrombocytopenic purpura. Correlation of serum and platelet-bound antibody with clinical response. N Engl J Med 292:230–236, 1975.

Eden OB, Lilleyman JS. Guidelines for management of idiopathic thrombocytopenic purpura. Arch Dis Child 67:1056–1058, 1992.

Eisner EV, Kasper K. Immune thrombocytopenia due to a metabolite of *para*-aminosalicylic acid. Am J Med 53:790–796, 1972.

Eisner EV, Shahidi NT. Immune thrombocytopenia due to a drug metabolite. N Engl J Med 287:376–381, 1972.

Follea G, Mandrand B, Dechavanne M. Simultaneous enzymo-immunologic assays of platelet associated IgG, IgM, and C3. A useful tool in assessment of immune thrombocytopenias. Thromb Res 26:249–258, 1982.

Furlan M, Robles R, Solenthaler M, Wassmer M, Sandoz P, Lämmle B. Deficient activity of von Willebrand factor-cleaving protease in chronic relapsing thrombotic thrombocytopenic purpura. Blood 89:3097–3103, 1997.

Furlan M, Robles R, Solenthaler M, Lämmle B. Acquired deficiency of von Willebrand factor-cleaving protease in a patient with thrombotic thrombocytopenic purpura. Blood 91:2839–2846, 1998.

George JN. Platelet immunoglobulin G: its significance for the evaluation of thrombocytopenia and for understanding the origin of alpha-granule proteins. Blood 76:859–870, 1990.

George JN, Aster RH. Thrombocytopenia due to enhanced platelet destruction by nonimmunologic mechanisms. In: Williams WJ, Beutler E, Erslev AJ, Lichtman MA, eds. Hematology, 4th ed. New York: McGraw-Hill, 1990, pp 1351–1370.

George JN, Woolf SH, Raskob GE, Wasser JS, Aledort LM, Ballem PJ, Blanchette VS, Bussel JB, Cines DB, Kelton JG, Lichtin AE, McMillan R, Okerbloom JA, Regan DH, Warrier I. Idiopathic thrombocytopenic purpura: a practice guideline developed by explicit methods for the American Society of Hematology. Blood 88:3–40, 1996.

Gerstner JB, Smith MJ, Davis KD, Cimo PL, Aster RH. Posttransfusion purpura: therapeutic failure of Pl^{A1}-negative platelet transfusion. Am J Hematol 6:71–75, 1979.

Gordon LI, Kwaan HC. Cancer- and drug-associated thrombotic thrombocytopenic purpura and hemolytic uremic syndrome. Semin Hematol 34:140–147, 1997.

Greinacher A, Mueller-Eckhardt C. Hereditary types of thrombocytopenia, an important differential diagnosis in chronic thrombocytopenia, In: Sutor AH, Thomas KB, eds. Thrombocytopenia in Childhood. Stuttgart: Schattauer, 1994, pp 191–198.

Harrington WJ, Minnich V, Hollingsworth JW, Moore CV. Demonstration of a thrombocytopenic factor in the blood of patients with thrombocytopenic purpura. J Lab Clin Med 38:1–10, 1951.

Heaton WA, Davis HH, Welch MJ, Mathias CJ, Joist JH, Sherman LA, Siegel BA. Indium-111: a new radionuclide label for studying human platelet kinetics. Br J Haematol 42:613–622, 1979.

Hegde UM, Williams K, Devereux S, Bowes A, Powell D, Fisher D. Platelet associated IgG and immune thrombocytopenia in lymphoproliferative and autoimmune disorders. Clin Lab Haematol 5:9–15, 1983.

Hegde UM, Ball S, Zuiable A, Roter BLT. Platelet associated immunoglobulins (PAIgG and PAIgM) in autoimmune thrombocytopenia. Br J Haematol 59:221–226, 1985.

Henke M, Engler H, Engelhardt R, Löhr GW. Successful treatment of sarcoidosis-associated thrombocytopenia refractory to corticosteroids by a single course of human gammaglobulins. Klin Wochenschr 64:1209–1211, 1986.

Herman JH, Kickler TS, Ness PM. The resolution of platelet serologic problems using Western blotting. Tissue Antigens 28:257–268, 1986.

Hesseling PB. Onyalai in Namibia. Clinical manifestations, haematological findings, course and management of 103 patients in the Kavango territory. Trans R Soc Trop Med Hyg 81:193–196, 1987.

Hesseling PB. Onyalai. Baillieres Clin Haematol 5:457–473, 1992.

Huisman JG. Immunoblotting: an emerging technique in immunohematology. Vox Sang 50:129–136, 1986.

Humphries JE. Tranfusion therapy in acquired coagulopathies. Hematol Oncol Clin North Am 8:1181–1201, 1994.

Ibarra H, Zapata C, Inostroza J, Mezzano S, Riedemann S. Immune thrombocytopenic purpura associated with hepatitis A. Blut 52:371–375, 1986.

Imbach P, Barandun S, d'Apuzzo V, Baumgartner C, Hirt A, Morell A, Rossi E, Schöni M, Vest M, Wagner HP. High-dose intravenous gammaglobulin for idiopathic thrombocytopenic purpura in childhood. Lancet 1:1228–1231, 1981.

Imbach P, Berchtold W, Hirt A, Mueller-Eckhardt C, Rossi E, Wagner HP, Gaedicke G, Joller P, Müller B, Barandun S. Intravenous immunoglobulin versus oral corticosteroids in acute thrombocytopenic purpura in childhood. Lancet 2:464–468, 1985.

Keimowitz RM, Collins J, Davis K, Aster RH. Post-transfusion purpura associated with alloimmunization against the platelet-specific antigen, Bak[a]. Am J Hematol 21:79–88, 1986.

Kelton JG, Neame PB, Gauldie J, Hirsh J. Elevated platelet-associated IgG in the thrombocytopenia of septicemia. N Engl J Med 300:760–764, 1979.

Kereiakes DJ, Essell JH, Abbottsmith CW, Broderick TM, Runyon JP. Abciximab-associated profound thrombocytopenia: therapy with immunoglobulin and platelet transfusion. Am J Cardiol 78:1161–1163, 1996.

Kickler TS, Herman JH, Furihata K, Kunicki TJ, Aster RH. Identification of Bak[b], a new platelet-specific antigen associated with posttransfusion purpura. Blood 71:894–898, 1988.

Kiefel V. The MAIPA assay and its applications in immunohematology. Transfusion Med 2:181–188, 1992.

Kiefel V, Spaeth P, Mueller-Eckhardt C. Immune thrombocytopenic purpura: autoimmune or immune complex disease? Br J Haematol 64:57–68, 1986.

Kiefel V, Jäger S, Mueller-Eckhardt C. Competitive enzyme-linked immunoassay for the quantitation of platelet-associated immunoglobulins (IgG, IgM, IgA) and complement (C3c, C3d). Vox Sang 53:151–156, 1987a.

Kiefel V, Santoso S, Weisheit M, Mueller-Eckhardt C. Monoclonal antibody-specific immobilization of platelet antigens (MAIPA): a new tool for the identification of platelet reactive antibodies. Blood 70:1722–1726, 1987b.

Kiefel V, Santoso S, Schmidt S, Salama A, Mueller-Eckhardt C. Metabolite-specific (IgG) and drug-specific antibodies (IgG, IgM) in two cases of trimethoprim–sulfamethoxazole-induced immune thrombocytopenia. Transfusion 27:262–265, 1987c.

Kiefel V, Santoso S, Glöckner WM, Katzmann B, Mayr WR, Mueller-Eckhardt C. Posttransfusion purpura associated with an anti-Bak[b]. Vox Sang 56:93–97, 1989.

Kiefel V, Santoso S, Kaufmann E, Mueller-Eckhardt C. Autoantibodies against platelet glycoprotein Ib/IX: a frequent finding in autoimmune thrombocytopenic purpura. Br J Haematol 79:256–262, 1991.

Kiefel V, Santoso S, Mueller-Eckhardt C. Serological, biochemical and molecular aspects of platelet autoantigens. Semin Hematol 29:26–33, 1992.

Kiefel V, Freitag E, Kroll H, Santoso S, Mueller-Eckhardt C. Platelet autoantibodies (IgG, IgM, IgA) against glycoproteins IIb/IIIa and Ib/IX in patients with thrombocytopenia. Ann Haematol 72:280–285, 1996.

Kosmo MA, Bordin G, Tani P, McMillan R. Immune thrombocytopenia and Crohn's disease [letter]. Ann Intern Med 104:136, 1986.

Kosugi S, Tomiyama Y, Shiraga M, Kashiwagi H, Nakao H, Kanayama Y, Kurata Y, Matzuzawa Y. Cyclic thrombocytopenia associated with IgM anti-GPIIb-IIIa autoantibodies. Br J Haematol 88:809–815, 1994.

Kroll H, Kiefel V, Mueller-Eckhardt C. Posttransfusionelle Purpura: Klinische und immunologische Untersuchungen bei 38 Patientinnen. Infusionsthera Transfusionsmed 20:198–204, 1993.

Kubota T, Tanoue K, Murohashi I, Nara N, Yamamoto N, Yamazaki H, Aoki N. Autoantibody against platelet glycoprotein IIb/IIIa in a patient with non Hodgkin's lymphoma. Thromb Res 53:379–386, 1989.

Kunicki TJ, Johnson MM, Aster RH. Absence of the platelet receptor for drug-dependent antibodies in the Bernard-Soulier syndrome. J Clin Invest 62:716–719, 1978.

Kunicki TJ, Koenig MB, Kristopeit SM, Aster RH. Direct quantitation of platelet-associated IgG by electroimmunoassay. Blood 60:54–58, 1982.

Law C, Marcaccio M, Tam P, Heddle N, Kelton JG. High-dose intravenous immune globulin and the response to splenectomy in patients with idiopathic thrombocytopenic purpura. N Engl J Med 336:1494–1498, 1997.

Leporrier M, Dighiero G, Auzemery M, Binet JL. Detection and quantification of platelet-bound antibodies with immunoperoxidase. Br J Haematol 42:605–611, 1979.

Lucas GF, Pittman SJ, Davies S, Solanki T, Bruggemann K. Post-transfusion purpura (PTP) associated with anti-HPA-1a, anti-HPA-2b and anti-HPA-3a antibodies. Transfusion Med 7:295–299, 1998.

Malloy B, Noel P, Eaton D, Solberg L. Immune thrombocytopenia associated with an antibody to c-Mpl, the thrombopoietin (TPO) receptor [abstr.]. Blood 86(suppl 1): 279a, 1995.

Mammen EF. The haematological manifestations of sepsis. J Antimicrob Chemother 41(suppl A):17–24, 1998.

Marder VJ, Feinstein DI, Francis CW, Colman RW. Consumptive thrombohemorrhagic disorders. In: Colman RW, Hirsh J, Marder VJ, Salzman EW, eds. Hemostasis and Thrombosis. Basic Principles and Clinical Practice. 3rd ed. Philadelphia: JB Lippincott, 1994, pp 1023–1063.

Maslanka K, Zupanska B. Post-transfusion purpura and delayed haemolytic transfusion reaction. Transfusion Med 3:281–284, 1993.

Mayer JL, Beardsley DS. Varicella-associated thrombocytopenia: autoantibodies against platelet surface glycoprotein V. Pediatr Res 40:615–619, 1996.

McMillan R, Tani P, Mason D. A method that allows shipment of whole blood for the assay of platelet-associated IgG. Blood 54:1201–1202, 1979.

McMillan R, Tani P, Millard F, Berchtold P, Renshaw L, Woods VL. Platelet-associated and plasma anti-glycoprotein autoantibodies in chronic ITP. Blood 70:1040–1045, 1987.

Menitove JE, Pereira J, Hoffman R, Anderson T, Fried W, Aster RH. Cyclic thrombocytopenia of apparent autoimmune etiology. Blood 73:1561–1569, 1989.

Meyer M, Kirchmaier CM, Spangenberg P, Ströhl C, Breddin K. Acquired disorder of platelet function associated with autoantibodies against membrane glycoprotein IIb-IIIa complex—1. Glycoprotein analysis. Thromb Haemost 65:491–496, 1991.

Meyer T, Herrmann C, Wiegand V, Mathias B, Kiefel V, Mueller-Eckhardt C. Immune thrombocytopenia associated with hemorrhagic diathesis due to ibuprofen administration. Clin Invest 71:413–415, 1993.

Moake JL, Rudy CK, Troll JH, Weinstein MJ, Colannino NM, Azocar J, Seder RH, Hong SL, Deykin D. Unusually large plasma factor VIII:von Willebrand factor multimers in chronic thrombocytopenic purpura. N Engl J Med 307:1432–1435, 1982.

Moake JL, Eisenstaedt RS. Thrombotic thrombocytopenic purpura and the hemolytic uremic syndrome. In: Colman RW, Hirsh J, Marder VJ, Salzman EW, eds. Hemostasis and Thrombosis. Basic Principles and Clinical Practice. 3rd ed. Philadelphia: JB Lippincott, 1994, pp 1064–1075.

Moilan J, Scott E, Dalmasso A. Transfusion reaction with severe thrombocytopenia due to a passively acquired platelet specific antibody [abstr]. Transfusion 25:459, 1985.

Mollison PL, Engelfriet CP, Contreras M. Blood Transfusion in Clinical Medicine. 9th ed. Oxford: Blackwell Scientific, 1993.

Morse BS, Giuliani D, Nussbaum M. Quantitation of platelet-associated IgG by radial immunodiffusion. Blood 57:809–811, 1981.

Mueller-Eckhardt C, Mahn I, Schulz G, Mueller-Eckhardt G. Detection of platelet autoantibodies by a radioactive anti-immunoglobulin test. Vox Sang 35:357–365, 1978.

Mueller-Eckhardt C, Mueller-Eckhardt G, Kayser W, Voss RM, Wegner J, Küenzlen E. Platelet associated IgG, platelet survival, and platelet sequestration in thrombocytopenic states. Br J Haematol 52:49–58, 1982.

Mueller-Eckhardt C, Küenzlen E, Kiefel V, Vahrson H, Graubner M. Cyclophosphamide-induced immune thrombocytopenia in a patient with ovarian carcinoma successfully treated with intravenous gamma globulin. Blut 46:165–169, 1983a.

Mueller-Eckhardt C, Küenzlen E, Thilo-Körner D, Pralle H. High-dose intravenous immunoglobulin for post-transfusion purpura [letter]. N Engl J Med 308:287, 1983b.

Mueller-Eckhardt C, Allolio B, Salama A, Kiefel V, Deuss U. Nomifensine-dependent immune hemolytic anemia and posttransfusion purpura in the same patient. Transfusion 27:250–252, 1987.

Mueller-Eckhardt C, Kiefel V. High-dose IgG for post-transfusion purpura—revisited. Blut 57:163–167, 1988.

Mueller-Eckhardt C, Kroll H, Kiefel V, The members of the European PTP Study Group. Posttransfusion purpura. In: Kaplan-Gouet C, Schlegel N, Salmon C, McGregor J, eds. Platelet Immunology: Fundamental and Clinical Aspects. Paris: John Libbey Eurotext, 1991, pp 249–255.

Mulder A, van Leeuwen EF, Veenboer GJM, Tetteroo PAT, von dem Borne AEGK. Immunochemical characterization of platelet-specific alloantigens. Scand J Haematol 33:267–274, 1984.

Müller-Berghaus G. Septicemia and the vessel wall. In: Verstraete M, Vermylen J, Lijnen R, Arnout J, eds. Thrombosis and Haemostasis 1987. Leuven: Leuven University Press, 1987, pp 619–671.

Nagasawa T, Hasegawa Y, Kamoshita M, Ohtani K, Komeno T, Itoh T, Shinagawa A, Kojima H, Ninomiya H, Abe T. Megakaryopoiesis in patients with cyclic thrombocytopenia. Br J Haematol 91:185–190, 1995.

Najean Y, Lecompte T. Genetic thrombocytopenia with autosomal dominant transmission: a review of 54 cases. Br J Haematol 74:203–208, 1990.

Najean Y, Rain JD, Billotey C. The site of destruction of autologous ^{111}In-labeled platelets and the efficacy of splenectomy in children and adults with idiopathic thrombocytopenic purpura: a study of 578 patients with 268 splenectomies. Br J Haematol 97: 547–550, 1997.

Niessner H, Clemetson KJ, Panzer S, Mueller-Eckhardt C, Santoso S, Bettelheim P. Acquired thrombasthenia due to GP IIb/IIIa-specific autoantibodies. Blood 68:571–576, 1986.

Panzer S, Penner E, Nelson PJ, Prochatzka E, Benda H, Saurugger PN. Identification of the platelet glycoprotein Ib/IIIa complex as a target antigen in primary biliary cirrhosis-associated autoimmune thrombocytopenia. Evidence that platelet-reactive autoantibodies can also bind to the mitochondrial antigen M2. J Autoimmun 3:473–483, 1990.

Pasquini E, Gianni L, Aitini E, Nicolini M, Fattori PP, Cavazzini G, Desiderio F, Monti F, Forghieri ME, Ravaioli A. Acute disseminated intravascular coagulation syndrome in cancer patients. Oncology 52:505–508, 1995.

Pawlotsky JM, Bouvier M, Fromont P, Deforges L, Duval J, Dhumeaux D, Bierling P. Hepatitis C virus infection and autoimmune thrombocytopenic purpura. J Haematol 23:635–639, 1995.

Petz LD, Garratty G. Acquired Immune Hemolytic Anemias. New York: Churchill Livingstone, 1980.

Pfueller SL, Bilston RA, Jane S, Gibson J. Expression of the drug-dependent antigen for quinine-dependent antiplatelet antibodies on GP IIIa but not that on GP Ib, IIb or IX on human endothelial cells. Thromb Haemost 63:279–281, 1990.

Quiquandon I, Fenaux P, Caulier MT, Pagniez D, Huart JJ, Bauters F. Re-evaluation of the role of azathioprine in the treatment of adult chronic idiopathic thrombocytopenic purpura: a report of 53 cases. Br J Haematol 74:223–228, 1990.

Reiner A, Gernsheimer T, Slichter SJ. Pulse cyclophosphamide therapy for refractory autoimmune thrombocytopenic purpura. Blood 85:351–358, 1995.

Remuzzi G. Thrombotic thrombocytopenic purpura and allied disorders; In: Verstraete M, Vermylen J, Lijnen R, Arnout J, eds. Thrombosis and Haemostasis 1987. Leuven: Leuven University Press, 1987, pp 673–708.

Salama A, Mueller-Eckhardt C, Kiefel V. Effect of intravenous immunoglobulin in immune thrombocytopenia. Competitive inhibition of reticuloendothelial system function by sequestration of autologous red blood cells? Lancet 2:193–196, 1983.

Salama A, Mueller-Eckhardt C. The role of metabolite-specific antibodies in nomifensine-dependent immune hemolytic anemia. N Engl J Med 313:469–474, 1985.

Salama A, Mueller-Eckhardt C. Immune-mediated blood cell dyscrasias related to drugs. Semin Hematol 29:54–63, 1992.

Santoso S, Kiefel V, Mueller-Eckhardt C. Immunochemical characterization of the new platelet alloantigen system Br^a/Br^b. Br J Haematol 72:191–198, 1989.

Schneider W, Schnaidt M. The platelet adhesion immunofluorescence test: a modification of the platelet suspension immunofluorescence test. Blut 43:389–392, 1981.

Scott EP, Moilan-Bergeland J, Dalmasso AP. Posttransfusion thrombocytopenia associated with passive transfusion of a platelet-specific antibody. Transfusion 28:73–76, 1988.

Shulman NR, Aster RH, Leithner A, Hiller MC. Immunoreactions involving platelets. V. Post-transfusion purpura due to a complement-fixing antibody against a genetically controlled platelet antigen. A proposed mechanism for thrombocytopenia and its relevance in ''autoimmunity.'' J Clin Invest 40:1597–1620, 1961.

Shulman NR, Jordan JV. Platelet kinetics. In: Colman RW, Hirsh J, Marder VJ, Salzman

EW, eds. Hemostasis and Thrombosis. Basic Principles and Clinical Practice. Philadelphia: JB Lippincott, 1987, pp 431–451.

Shulman NR, Reis DM. Platelet immunology. In: Colman RW, Hirsh J, Marder VJ, Salzman EW, eds. Hemostasis and Thrombosis: Principles and Clinical Practice. 3rd ed. Philadelphia: JB Lippincott, 1994, pp 414–468.

Simon TL, Collins J, Kunicki TJ, Furihata K, Smith KJ, Aster RH. Posttransfusion purpura associated with alloantibody specific for the platelet antigen, Pen^a. Am J Hematol 29:38–40, 1988.

Smith JW, Hayward CPM, Warkentin TE, Horsewood P, Kelton JG. Investigation of human platelet alloantigens and glycoproteins using non-radioactive immunoprecipitation. J Immunol Methods 158:77–85, 1993.

Stricker RB, Shuman MA. Quinidine purpura: evidence that glycoprotein V is a target platelet antigen. Blood 67:1377–1381, 1986.

Taaning E, Morling N, Ovesen H, Svejgaard A. Post transfusion purpura and anti-Zw^b (-Pl^{A2}). Tissue Antigens 26:143–146, 1985.

Taylor CM, Monnens LAH. Advances in hemolytic uraemic syndrome. Arch Dis Child 78:190–193, 1998.

Tomer A, Schreiber AD, McMillan R, Cines DB, Burstein SA, Thiessen AR, Harker LA. Menstrual cyclic thrombocytopenia. Br J Haematol 71:519–524, 1989.

Tomiyama Y, Kurata Y, Mizutani H, Kanakura Y, Tsubakio T, Yonezawa T, Tarui S. Platelet glycoprotein IIb as a target antigen in two patients with chronic idiopathic thrombocytopenic purpura. Br J Haematol 66:535–538, 1987.

Van der Lelie J, Lange JMA, Vos JJE, van Dalen CM, Danner SA, von dem Borne AEGK. Autoimmunity against blood cells in human immunodeficiency virus (HIV) infection. Br J Haematol 67:109–114, 1987.

van Leeuwen EF, van der Ven JTM, Engelfriet CC, von dem Borne AEGK. Specificity of autoantibodies in autoimmune thrombocytopenia. Blood 59:23–26, 1982a.

van Leeuwen EF, Engelfriet CP, von dem Borne AEGK. Studies on quinine- and quinidine-dependent antibodies against platelets and their reaction with platelet in the Bernard-Soulier syndrome. Br J Haematol 51:551–560, 1982b.

Visentin GP, Newman PJ, Aster RH. Characteristics of quinine- and quinidine-induced antibodies specific for platelet glycoproteins IIb and IIIa. Blood 77:2668–2676, 1991.

von dem Borne AEGK, Verheugt FWA, Oosterhof F, von Riesz E, Brutel de la Riviere A, Engelfriet CP. A simple immunofluorescence test for the detection of platelet antibodies. Br J Haematol 39:195–207, 1978.

von dem Borne AEGK, Pegels JG, van der Stadt RJ, van der Plas-van Dalen CM, Helmerhorst FM. Thrombocytopenia associated with gold therapy: a drug-induced autoimmune disease. Br J Haematol 63:509–516, 1986.

Walsh C, Krigel R, Lennette E, Karpatkin S. Thrombocytopenia in homosexual patients. Prognosis, response to therapy, and prevalence of antibody to the retrovirus associated with the acquired immunodeficiency syndrome. Ann Intern Med 103:542–545, 1985.

Warkentin TE, Smith JW, Hayward CPM, Ali AM, Kelton JG. Thrombocytopenia caused by passive transfusion of anti-glycoprotein Ia/IIa alloantibody (anti-HPA-5b). Blood 79:2480–2484, 1992.

Waters AH. Autoimmune thrombocytopenia: clinical aspects. Semin Hematol 29:18–25, 1992.

Wintrobe MM, Lee GR, Boggs DR, Bithell TC, Foerster J, Athens JW, Lukens JN. Clinical Hematology. 8th ed. Philadelphia: Lea & Febiger, 1981, pp 1090–1127.

Woods VL, Kurata Y, Montgomery RR, Tani P, Mason D, Oh EH, McMillan R. Autoantibodies against platelet glycoprotein Ib in patients with chronic immune thrombocytopenic purpura. Blood 64:156–160, 1984.

3

Clinical Picture of Heparin-Induced Thrombocytopenia

Theodore E. Warkentin
McMaster University and Hamilton Health Sciences Coroporation, Hamilton, Ontario, Canada

I. INTRODUCTION

Heparin-induced thrombocytopenia (HIT) is a distinct clinicopathologic syndrome caused by platelet-activating antibodies that recognize complexes of platelet factor 4–heparin (PF4/H). Its strong association with venous and arterial thrombosis represents a striking paradox. However, thrombocytopenia itself is common in clinical medicine. Furthermore, heparin is usually given to patients who either have thrombosis, or who are judged to be at high risk for thrombosis. Thus, thrombocytopenia with or without thrombosis during heparin treatment does not necessarily indicate a diagnosis of HIT. Indeed, several disorders can closely resemble HIT (see Chap. 12).

On the other hand, HIT is associated with a wide spectrum of unusual thrombotic and other complications (Table 1). Unrecognized HIT may have been an important contributing factor in otherwise bizarre clinical events that have occurred in certain heparin-treated patients (Anderson et al., 1981; Solomon et al., 1988; Pfueller et al., 1990; Muntean et al., 1992). Laboratory documentation of HIT antibodies has been crucial in determining the clinical scope of the HIT syndrome. Accordingly, this chapter emphasizes clinical data obtained from large prospective and retrospective studies that have used diagnostic testing for HIT antibodies.

II. THROMBOCYTOPENIA

Thrombocytopenia, using the standard definition of a platelet count of less than 150×10^9/L, is the most common clinical effect of HIT, occurring in 85–90%

Table 1 Thrombotic and Other Sequelae of HIT

Venous thrombosis	Arterial thrombosis	Miscellaneous
Deep vein thrombosis, DVT (50%): new, progressive, recurrent; lower limb (often bilateral); upper limb (at site of venous catheter)	Aortic or iliofemoral thrombosis resulting in acute limb ischemia/infarction (5–10%) or spinal cord infarction (rare)	Heparin-induced skin lesions at heparin injection sites (10–20%): Erythematous plaques Skin necrosis
Warfarin-induced venous limb gangrene (~5–10% of DVT treated with warfarin)	Acute thrombotic stroke (3–5%)	Coumarin-induced skin necrosis complicating HIT involving "central" sites (breast, abdomen, thigh, leg, etc.) (rare)
Pulmonary embolism (25%): with or without right-sided cardiac intra-atrial or intraventricular thrombi	Myocardial infarction (3–5%)	Acute systemic reactions postintravenous heparin bolus (~25% of sensitized patients who receive an intravenous heparin bolus): Inflammatory: e.g., fever, chills, flushing Cardiorespiratory: e.g., tachycardia, hypertension, dyspnea; cardiopulmonary arrest (rare) Gastrointestinal: nausea, vomiting, diarrhea Neurological: transient global amnesia, headache
Cerebral dural sinus thrombosis (rare)	Cardiac intraventricular or intra-atrial thrombosis (in situ or via embolization of DVT (rare)	
Adrenal hemorrhagic infarction: bilateral (acute or chronic adrenal failure) or unilateral (rare)	Thrombosis involving miscellaneous arteries (rare): upper limb, renal, mesenteric, spinal, and other arteries (rare)	
	Embolization of thrombus from heart or proximal aorta can also contribute to microvascular ischemic syndromes	
Disseminated intravascular coagulation (DIC), with hypofibrinogenemia and acquired natural anticoagulant deficiency, causing multiple venous and arterial thromboses (rare)		

Estimated frequencies of the various complications of HIT are taken from reports with serological confirmation of the diagnosis (Warkentin et al., 1995a; Warkentin and Kelton, 1996; Warkentin et al., 1997). "Rare" indicates an estimated frequency $< 3\%$ of HIT patients.

of patients (Warkentin, 1998a). An even higher proportion develop "thrombocytopenia" if a definition appropriate for the clinical situation is used.

A. Timing

The characteristic delay of 5 or more days between initiation of heparin and onset of thrombocytopenia, was the major clue that led early investigators to recognize the immune pathogenesis of HIT (Roberts et al., 1964; Rhodes et al., 1973). King and Kelton (1984) noted that the onset of thrombocytopenia occurred between days 6 and 15 for more than 90% of patients in whom HIT occurred during their first exposure to heparin. In contrast, for patients who developed HIT during a repeat course of heparin, the onset of thrombocytopenia was often more rapid, occurring within 2 days. These data have been interpreted as indicating an ''anamnestic'' (Gr., *memory*) or ''secondary'' immune response in HIT, i.e., the immune system produces HIT antibodies more quickly on reencountering an antigen ''remembered'' within its memory cell repertoire. Recent data, however, suggest another explanation for these two temporal profiles of HIT, *typical* and *rapid* (discussed subsequently).

Typical Onset of HIT

A prospective study of serologically confirmed HIT showed that the platelet count typically begins to fall between days 5 and 10 (inclusive) of postoperative subcutaneous heparin prophylaxis (Warkentin et al., 1995a,b) (Fig. 1a–c). Note that the data refer to the day the platelet count begins to fall, and not the later day that an arbitrary threshold defining thrombocytopenia is crossed. This study also showed that most patients who developed thrombocytopenia beginning after day 5 had HIT, rather than another explanation for the thrombocytopenia. The data suggest the following clinical rule:

Rule 1

A thrombocytopenic patient whose platelet count fall began between days 5 and 10 of heparin treatment (inclusive) should be considered to have HIT unless proved otherwise (first day of heparin use is considered ''day 0'').

HIT-IgG antibodies generally are not detectable before day 5 of heparin treatment, but are readily detectable using sensitive assays when the platelet count first begins to fall due to HIT.

Diminishing Risk of HIT After Day 10

The risk of HIT decreases after the day 5–10 ''window'' passes (see Fig. 1c). In my experience, a platelet count fall after day 10 usually is caused by another pathological process, such as septicemia. A notable exception: sometimes an invasive procedure ''resets the clock''; that is, a platelet count fall that begins on day 12 of a course of heparin that consists of two 6-day treatments with heparin (before and after intervening surgery), likely is HIT. Perhaps, the surgery causes circumstances that favor seroconversion (e.g., release of PF4; see Chap. 6). Thode and colleagues (1997) reported on a patient who for 9 years uneventfully received unfractionated heparin (UFH) for hemodialysis; nevertheless, HIT complicating hemodialysis began shortly after the patient underwent parathyroidectomy.

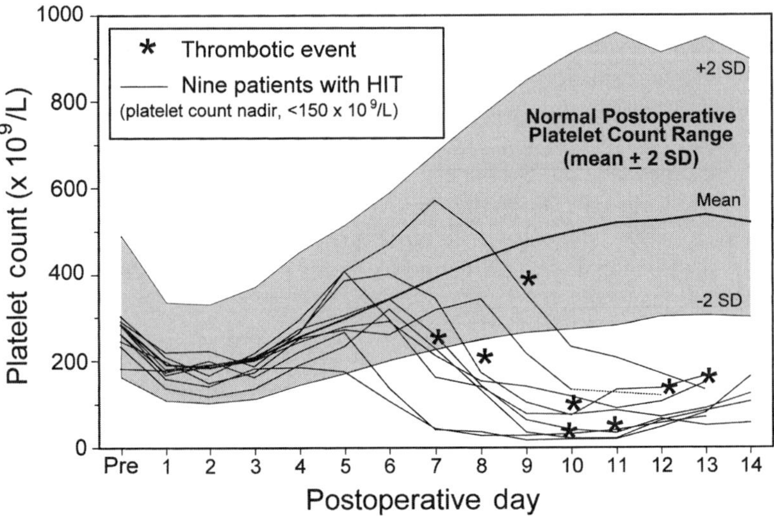

(a)

Figure 1 (a) Serial platelet counts of nine patients with HIT. The bold line and shaded area indicate the mean (± 2 SD) platelet count in the reference population (367 patients negative for HIT antibodies). The reference population indicates the occurrence of postoperative thrombocytopenia (days 1–3) followed by postoperative thrombocytosis (maximal values at days 11–14). Nine patients developed serologically confirmed HIT, with a platelet count fall to $< 150 \times 10^9$/L; eight of the nine patients developed HIT-associated thrombosis (indicated by asterisks). Three patients developed thrombosis while the platelet counts were falling relative to the postoperative peak, but before the platelet count fell to $< 150 \times 10^9$/L (38% fall to 355; 29% fall to 228; 61% fall to 172). (b) Cumulative frequency of thrombosis in patients with and patients without HIT. HIT is defined as a platelet count fall to $< 150 \times 10^9$/L. The data indicate that HIT is strongly associated with thrombosis. (c) Day of onset of HIT for 18 patients with definite or probable HIT observed in a clinical trial. HIT began between days 5–10, inclusive, in all 18 patients, and did not begin in any patients on day 11 or later. Length of heparin treatment and platelet count monitoring was variable; the remaining number of patients at risk for HIT for each day of follow-up is shown (n). *For one of the patients, the platelet count began to fall on day 5 after receiving UFH ''flushes'' through an intra-arterial catheter placed at the time of surgery. †The platelet count fell abruptly on day 12, together with symptoms and signs of an acute systemic reaction, following administration of a 5000 U intravenous UFH bolus (see Fig. 1a, Chap. 4). However, the first clinical manifestation of HIT was on day 9 (erythematous skin lesions at heparin injection sites), and HIT antibodies were first detected on day 5 by serotonin release assay. ‡The platelet count fell abruptly on day 10 after administration of a 5000 U intravenous UFH bolus, followed by therapeutic-dose UFH infusion. However, positive HIT antibodies were first detected by PF4/H-EIA on day 6 of treatment with subcutaneous UFH, 7500 U twice daily. (a, c, Warkentin et al., 1995a,b; b, Warkentin et al., 1995a.)

Cumulative incidence of thrombosis (%)
100
80
60
40
20
0
Heparin-induced thrombocytopenia (n=9)
No heparin-induced thrombocytopenia (n=656)
P<0.001
1 2 3 4 5 6 7 8 9 10 11 12 13 14
Postoperative day

(b)

Number of HIT patients
7 6 5 4 3 2 1 0
>50% Platelet count fall but nadir≥150 x 10⁹/L
>50% Platelet count fall and nadir <150 x 10⁹/L
n=665 654* 636 587 536 483† 443‡ 386 331 267
≤4 5 6 7 8 9 10 11 12 ≥13
Onset of HIT (days after starting heparin)

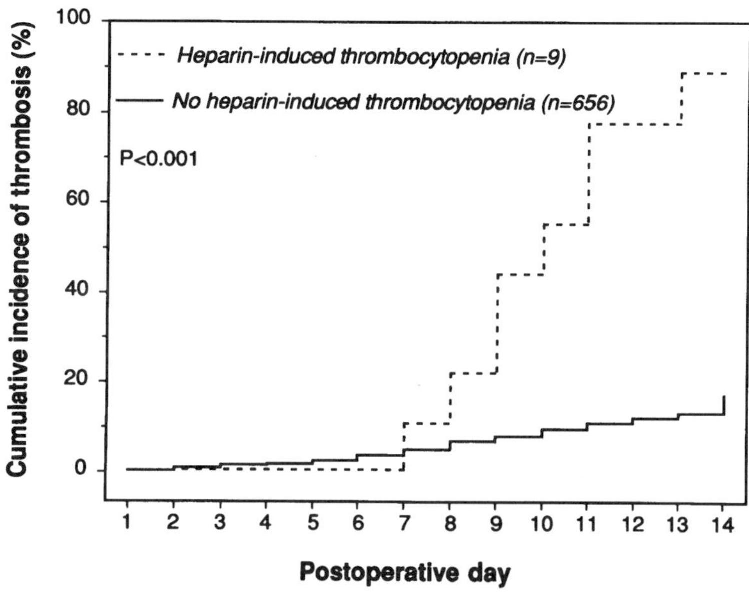

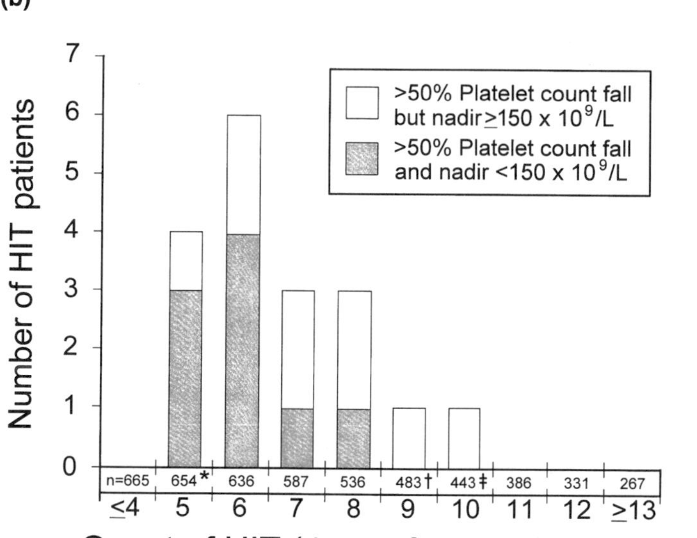

(c)

Rapid Onset of HIT

Sometimes, patients develop *rapid-onset HIT*. This is defined as an unexpected fall in the platelet count that begins soon after heparin is started. Indeed, it is generally evident on the first postheparin platelet count, whether obtained minutes, hours, or a day later. Patients who develop such a rapid fall in the platelet count, and who are confirmed serologically to have HIT antibodies, invariably have received heparin in the past (Warkentin and Kelton, 1998). A characteristic feature of this prior heparin exposure has been recently identified: it invariably includes a *recent* exposure to heparin, generally within the past 2–3 weeks, and almost invariably within the past 100 days (Fig. 2a,b).

This temporal profile of onset of HIT can be explained as follows: the rapid fall in platelet count represents abrupt onset of platelet activation caused by residual circulating HIT antibodies that resulted from the recent heparin treatment, rather than antibodies newly generated by the subsequent course of heparin.

This explanation is supported by other observations. First, for patients with typical onset of HIT, there was no difference in its median day of onset, irrespective of whether or not patients had previously been exposed to heparin. Second, patients did not generally develop thrombocytopenia that began between days 2 and 4. Had there truly been an anamnestic immune response more rapid than the usual 5- to 10-day period, one might have expected to identify such a group of patients. Third, patients reexposed to heparin following disappearance of HIT antibodies do not necessarily form HIT antibodies again; those who do, appear to form antibodies after day 5 (Gruel et al., 1990; Warkentin and Kelton, 1998).

Figure 2 (a) A 49-year-old patient exhibiting both typical- and rapid-onset HIT: The platelet count began to fall on day 6 of subcutaneous (sc) UFH injections given for antithrombotic prophylaxis following neurosurgery (typical HIT). An abrupt fall in platelet count occurred twice on day 18, each after a 5000-U intravenous (iv) UFH bolus (rapid HIT). Symptoms and signs of acute systemic reaction occurred 10 min after each bolus (dyspnea, tachypnea, hypertension, chest tightness, restlessness). Note that the patient's platelet count never fell below 150×10^9/L, even though her serum tested strongly positive for HIT antibodies by serotonin release assay. She developed proximal deep venous thrombosis (DVT) shortly after developing HIT. (b) HIT after stopping heparin: A 68-year-old woman who received UFH for heart surgery was noted to have a platelet count of 40×10^9/L on postoperative day 19, and a "rash" of her lower extremities. She presented on day 38 with symptomatic deep venous thrombosis (DVT) and developed rapid-onset recurrent thrombocytopenia after receiving intravenous (iv) unfractionated heparin (UFH). The patient was successfully treated with danaparoid sodium (D.S.) and warfarin. In retrospect, the thrombocytopenia first observed on postoperative day 19 almost certainly was caused by HIT.

TYPICAL HIT
RAPID HIT
Platelet count (x 10⁹/L)
Neurosurgery (perioperative hemodilution)
Day 6 of s.c. UFH prophylaxis
DVT symptoms
UFH i.v. bolus (twice) followed by acute dyspnea and hypertension
39% platelet count fall to 208 x 10⁹/L
Platelet count nadir 160 x 10⁹/L
UFH in art. line
UFH, 5000u q12h s.c.
Warfarin
Ancrod
Days after starting heparin

(a)

Platelet count (x 10⁹/L)
Coronary bypass surgery (intraoperative but no postoperative heparin)
Day 38: DVT
Abrupt platelet fall from 149 to 27 x 10⁹/L on i.v. therapeutic UFH
Warfarin
UFH
D.S.
Days after starting heparin

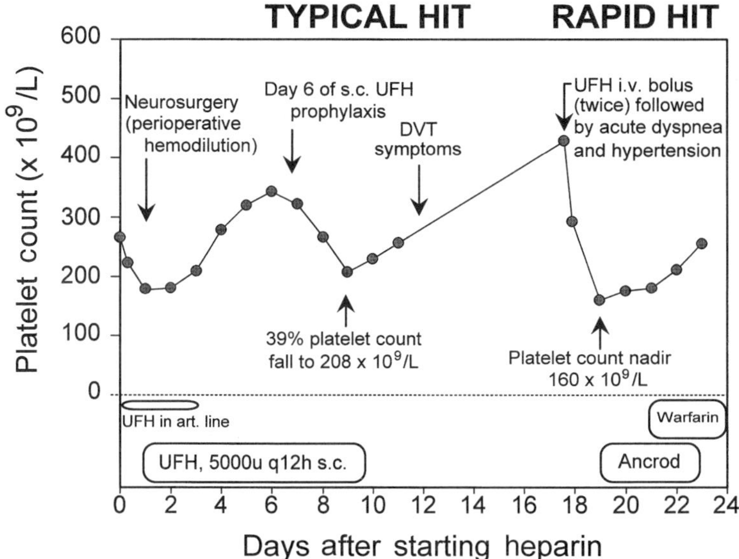

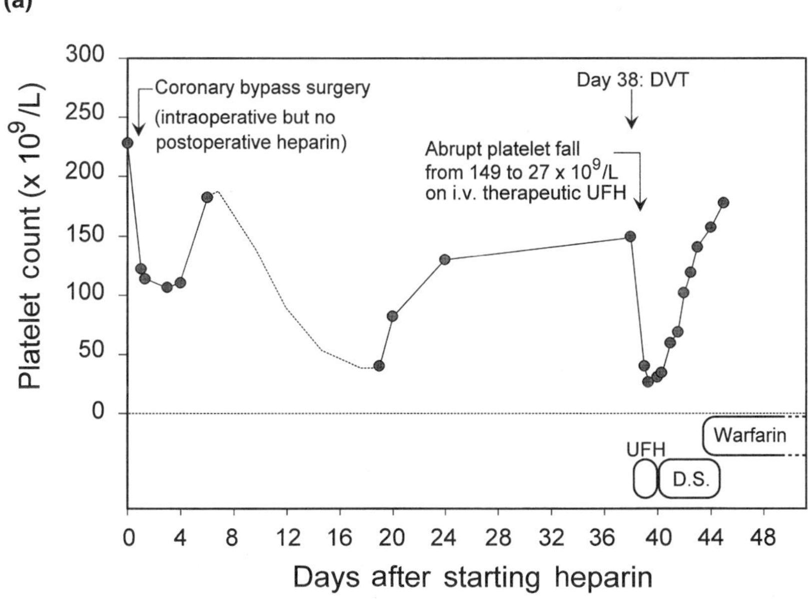

(b)

HIT Antibodies Are Transient

There is a plausible biological basis to explain why patients who develop rapid-onset HIT have received heparin in the recent, rather than in the remote, past: HIT antibodies are transient and become undetectable at a median of 50 days after first testing positive; in about 90% of patients, HIT antibodies are no longer detectable at 100 days (Warkentin and Kelton, 1998).

Rule 2

A rapid fall in the platelet count soon after starting heparin therapy is unlikely to represent HIT unless the patient has received heparin in the recent past, usually within the past 100 days.

To summarize, the rapid fall in platelet count appears to be caused by the repeat administration of heparin to a patient with residual circulating HIT antibodies, rather than resulting from a rapid regeneration of HIT antibodies.

A Hypothesis to Explain the Timing of HIT

There is a possible explanation for these unusual temporal features of HIT: because the HIT antigen is a "cryptic autoantigen" (or neoantigen) comprising two *autologous* substances (PF4 and heparin), it is possible that the typical IgG response in HIT, occurring as early as day 5 even in patients never previously exposed to heparin, could actually represent a secondary (anamnestic) immune response (i.e., the immune system has previously been exposed to this self-PF4/H antigen. This might explain why there is the same minimum time (5 days) to formation of detectable levels of HIT–IgG antibodies, irrespective of previous heparin use or even a history of HIT itself.

Implications for Repeat Use of Heparin in a Patient with a History of HIT

The (1) transient nature of the HIT antibody, the (2) apparent minimum of 5 days to regenerate clinically significant HIT antibodies even in a patient who once had HIT, and (3) the observation that HIT antibodies do not necessarily recur, despite heparin rechallenge in a patient with definite prior HIT, all suggest that it may be safe to readminister heparin to such patients. Fortunately, this potentially risky situation is not frequently necessary, as there are several alternative anticoagulants that can be substituted for heparin (see Chaps. 13–17).

However, UFH is the unparalleled drug of choice in certain therapeutic settings, particularly heart surgery when using cardiopulmonary bypass, or vascular surgery. Furthermore, there are important disadvantages of newer anticoagulants for these procedures (see Chap. 17). In my opinion, therefore, for patients with a remote history of HIT (>100 days) who require cardiac or vascular surgery, a rational approach is to prove serologically that HIT antibodies are no longer present, and then to give heparin for a brief time to permit the surgery (Olinger et al., 1984; Warkentin and Kelton, 1998). We have even used this approach successfully in a patient who required heparin for major vascular surgery 1 month following an episode of HIT, when the HIT antibodies had just become undetectable. After surgery, it seems prudent to avoid postoperative heparin completely, and to administer an alternative anticoagulant, such as danaparoid or lepirudin, as indicated. The actual risk of recurrent HIT beginning 5–10 days later, either following a transient intraoperative heparin exposure, or even during prolonged postoperative heparin use, is unknown, but may be low.

Sensitization by Incidental Heparin Exposure

Sensitizing exposures to heparin can be relatively obscure. For example, incidental use of intraoperative line ''flushes'' that were not even documented in the medical records has led to HIT antibody formation or acute onset of HIT, with tragic consequences (Brushwood, 1992; Ling and Warkentin, 1998). Greinacher and colleagues (1992) reported a patient who developed recurrent HIT when reexposed to heparin present in prothrombin complex concentrates. Physicians should suspect possible heparin exposure in a patient whose clinical course suggests HIT, especially if the patient was recently hospitalized or has undergone procedures in which heparin exposure may have occurred.

HIT After Stopping Heparin Administration

Rarely, HIT begins several days after discontinuing heparin therapy, or persists for several weeks despite stopping heparin administration (Castaman et al., 1992; see Fig. 2B). A dramatic case encountered by the author was a female outpatient who presented with transient global amnesia and a platelet count of 40×10^9/L 7 days after receiving two doses of UFH; this patient's serologically proved HIT persisted for several months. This unusual clinical course could result from high-titer HIT antibodies that activate platelets for several weeks, perhaps by heparin-independent activation (anti-PF4 reactivity), or because the HIT antibodies are reactive against PF4 bound to endothelial cell surface glycosaminoglycans.

B. Severity of Thrombocytopenia

Figure 3 shows the platelet count nadirs of 142 patients with laboratory-proved HIT in one medical community: the median platelet count nadir was approximately 60×10^9/L (Warkentin, 1998a). This contrasts with ''typical'' drug-induced immune thrombocytopenic purpura (DITP; e.g., caused by quinine/quinidine, sulfa antibiotics, or rifampin [see Chap. 2]), for which the median platelet count nadir is 15×10^9/L or less, and patients usually develop bleeding

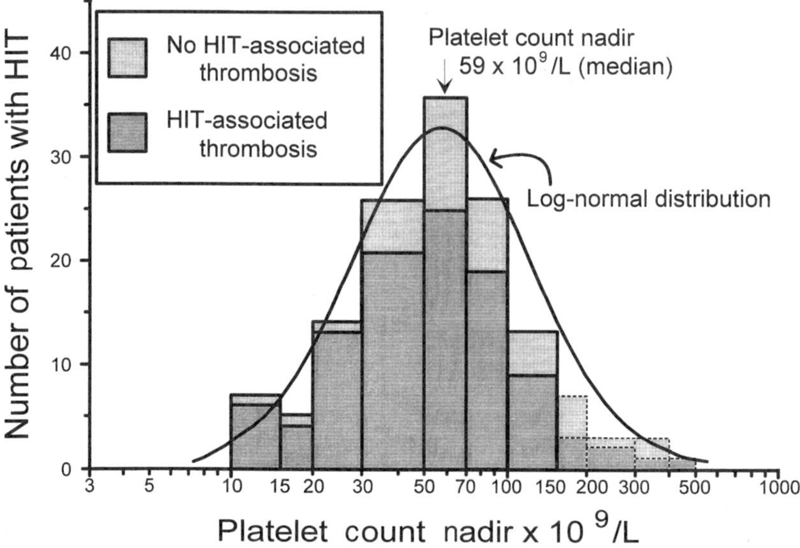

Figure 3 Platelet count nadirs in 142 patients with serologically confirmed HIT: The data are taken from a study of 127 patients with serologically confirmed HIT that used a definition of $< 150 \times 10^9$/L (Warkentin and Kelton, 1996), together with a group of 15 patients diagnosed with serologically confirmed HIT over the same time period whose platelet count nadir was $> 150 \times 10^9$/L. There is a lognormal distribution of the platelet count nadirs, with a median platelet count of 59×10^9/L. HIT is only occasionally complicated by very severe thrombocytopenia. HIT-associated thrombosis occurred in most patients irrespective of the severity of the platelet count nadir. (From Warkentin, 1998a).

(Pedersen-Bjergaard et al, 1997). The platelet count is 15×10^9/L or fewer in only about 5% of patients with HIT. But even in this minority of HIT patients with very severe thrombocytopenia, thrombosis, rather than bleeding, predominates.

Definition of Thrombocytopenia

Figure 3 illustrates that HIT is associated with thrombosis even when the platelet count nadir is more than 150×10^9/L. This suggests that the standard definition of thrombocytopenia ($< 150 \times 10^9$/L) may be inadequate for many patients with HIT. Particularly in postoperative patients, a major fall in the platelet count can occur without the nadir falling to less than 150×10^9/L (see Fig. 2A). Indeed, studies indicate a 50% or greater fall in the platelet count from the postoperative peak is strongly associated with HIT antibodies, even when the platelet count nadir remains higher than 150×10^9/L (Warkentin et al., 1995b; Ganzer et al., 1997). Moreover, this patient subgroup is at increased risk for thrombosis.

Rule 3

A platelet count fall of more than 50% from the postoperative peak between days 5 and 14 after surgery associated with heparin treatment can indicate HIT even if the platelet count remains higher than 150×10^9/L.

It is uncertain whether a greater than 50% platelet count fall definition is appropriate for medical patients. Regardless of the patient population, a clinician should have a high index of suspicion when unexpected large-percentage declines in the platelet count occur during heparin treatment, irrespective of whether an arbitrary threshold for ''thrombocytopenia'' is crossed.

Platelet Count Monitoring in Patients Receiving Heparin

In postoperative patients, the onset of HIT coincides with rising platelet counts (postoperative thrombocytosis); thus, the platelet count profile of HIT resembles an ''inverted V'' (/\; see Fig. 1A). The postoperative peak platelet count preceding HIT is often higher than the preoperative platelet count. Therefore, the postoperative peak platelet count is the appropriate baseline for calculating the magnitude of a subsequent platelet count fall (Table 2). It may be prudent to repeat the platelet count, test for HIT antibodies, and, possibly, to stop heparin and initiate alternative anticoagulant therapy pending the HIT test results, in a patient whose platelet count falls by more than 30% during the typical day 5- to 10-time period for HIT. However, there is no consensus on the frequency of, and management responses to, platelet count monitoring among the different patient populations who receive heparin (see Chap. 4).

HIT-Associated Thrombosis Without Thrombocytopenia

Anecdotal reports indicate that HIT-associated thrombosis can occur in the absence of thrombocytopenia, as conventionally defined (Phelan, 1983; Hach-Wunderle et al., 1994; Warkentin, 1996a, 1997). However, most of these patients do have an associated fall in the platelet count, although the nadir remains higher than 150×10^9/L. A study suggested that HIT antibody formation without thrombocytopenia is not associated with a thrombosis rate greater than control patients (Warkentin et al., 1995a,b). However, even a platelet fall of more than 50% that remained higher than 150×10^9/L was associated with an increased risk for thrombosis (Fig. 4). The importance of thrombocytopenia vis-a-vis HIT antibody formation alone is evidence that in vivo platelet activation contributes to the pathogenesis of HIT-associated thrombosis.

Platelet Count Recovery Following Discontinuation of Heparin

The median time to platelet count recovery to more than 150×10^9/L after stopping heparin administration is about 4 days, although several more days may be

Table 2 Determining the Day of Onset of Thrombocytopenia: A 35-Year-Old Woman Who Developed HIT After Heart Surgery

Day	Pre-operative	Day 0 (surgery)	Day 1	Day 2	Day 3	Day 4	Day 5	Day 6	Day 7	Day 8	Day 9	Day 10	Day 11
Heparin used		UFH during CPB	Line flushes	Nil	Nil	UFH 5000 b.i.d. sc	UFH 5000 b.i.d. sc	UFH 5000 b.i.d. sc	UFH 5000 b.i.d. sc	D.S.	D.S.	D.S.	D.S.
Platelet count	227	98	137	209	255	300	374	378	310	224 (PE[a])	166	171	161 (nadir)
Percent platelet count fall	Platelet fall during days 0–4 is unlikely to be HIT unless there was recent heparin use (past 100 days) and the magnitude of the platelet fall is greater than expected.						Rising platelet count	Peak platelet count	18% (378 → 310)	41% (378 → 224)	56% (378 → 166)	No further fall	57% (378 → 161)

[a] Pulmonary embolism (PE) occurred on postoperative day 8, in association with a platelet count fall of 41%, from 378 (postoperative peak) to 224×10^9/L. The platelet count began to fall on day 7. The case illustrates why it is wrong to use the preoperative platelet count value as the "baseline," as the fall in platelet count, from 227 (preoperative) to 224 (day 7) would be considered trivial, even though HIT-associated pulmonary embolism occurred. The preoperative and first three postoperative days are in shaded boxes, to indicate that these data should be censored in the interpretation of platelet counts in HIT. In this patient, the abrupt fall in platelet count from 227 to 98 (day 0) is expected (heart surgery). This patient was treated successfully with danaparoid sodium (D.S.), with longer-term anticoagulation with warfarin. The patient's clinical course is also shown in Fig. 3B in Chap. 12.

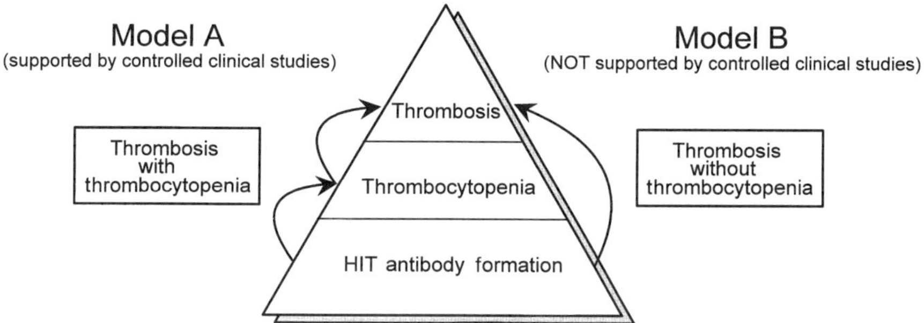

Figure 4 "Iceberg" model of HIT: Model A indicates that thrombosis occurs in patients who develop HIT antibody formation and thrombocytopenia. This model is supported by clinical data. In contrast, model B indicates the possibility of HIT antibody formation contributing to thrombosis without the intermediary process of thrombocytopenia. Although anecdotal experience suggests occasional patients consistent with model B, controlled studies indicate that HIT antibody formation without thrombocytopenia does not have an increased frequency of thrombosis, compared with controls (Warkentin et al., 1995a, b). Note that thrombocytopenia is broadly defined, and includes patients with large relative falls in the platelet count, even if the platelet nadir is $> 150 \times 10^9/L$. (From Warkentin, 1999.)

required for the platelet count to reach a stable plateau. In patients with very severe HIT, the platelet count may take 2 weeks or more to recover. Unlike nonimmune heparin-associated thrombocytopenia, the platelet count will generally not recover in patients with HIT unless the heparin is discontinued.

III. THROMBOSIS

A. The HIT Paradox: Thrombosis but not Hemorrhage

Table 1 summarizes the clinical spectrum and approximate frequency of clinical sequelae associated with HIT. Spontaneous hemorrhage is not characteristic of HIT, and petechiae are not typically observed, even in those occasional patients whose platelet count is less than $10 \times 10^9/L$ (Fig. 5). Bleeding complications were not increased over controls in two prospective studies of HIT (Cipolle et al., 1983; Warkentin et al., 1995a).

Rule 4

Petechiae and other signs of spontaneous bleeding are not clinical features of HIT, even in patients with very severe thrombocytopenia.

The explanation for this clinical feature is unknown, but could be related to unique pathophysiological aspects of HIT, such as in vivo platelet activation

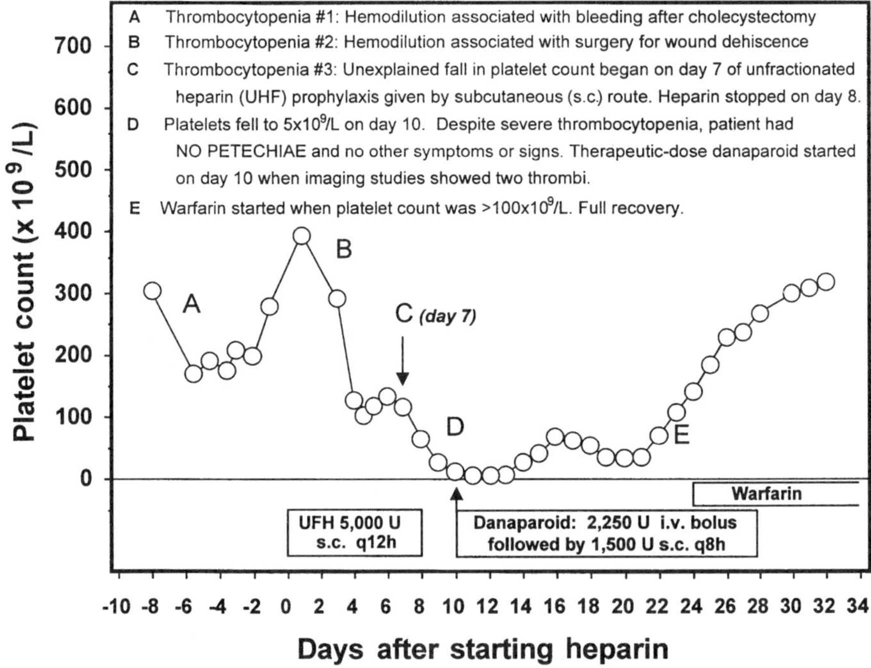

Figure 5 HIT with very severe thrombocytopenia: A 50-year-old woman developed a platelet count fall to a nadir of 4×10^9/L. The platelet count began to fall about 1 week after receiving blood transfusions as well as starting heparin prophylaxis. Despite the very severe thrombocytopenia, and recent treatment with UFH, no petechiae were observed. Platelet-specific alloantibodies were not present, but strong HIT antibodies, by serotonin release assay, were readily detectable. Two venous thrombi were shown by duplex ultrasonography (right internal jugular vein thrombosis at intravascular catheter site; left saphenous vein thrombosis). The patient was treated successfully with therapeutic-dose danaparoid given by subcutaneous injections, although it took more than 3 weeks before platelet recovery to a stable plateau occurred. In vitro cross-reactivity of HIT antibodies for danaparoid was not present, despite the slow platelet count recovery observed. (From Warkentin, 1998a.)

and generation of procoagulant, platelet-derived microparticles (Warkentin et al., 1994b).

B. HIT Is a Hypercoagulable State

A large controlled study (Warkentin et al., 1995a,b) concluded that HIT is independently associated with thrombosis, even in a patient population at high

Table 3 The Prothrombotic Nature of HIT: Comparison with Other Hypercoagulable States

Hypercoagulable state	Odds ratio for thrombosis
Heparin-induced thrombocytopenia:	
Platelet count $< 150 \times 10^9$/L	36.9
Platelet fall > 50% beginning ≥ 5 days of heparin	12.4
Platelet fall > 50%, but platelet count remains $> 150 \times 10^9$/L	6.0
Factor V Leiden	6.6
Congenital protein C deficiency	14.4
Congenital protein S deficiency	10.9
Congenital antithrombin deficiency	24.1
Dysfibrinogenemia	11.3
Lupus anticoagulant	5.4

Source: Warkentin et al. 1995; 1995a,b.

baseline risk for thrombosis (postoperative orthopedic patients). Moreover, both venous and arterial thrombosis was seen. Thus, HIT can be considered a *hypercoagulable state* (Table 3), a designation consistent with increased in vivo thrombin generation seen in almost all patients with HIT (Warkentin et al., 1997).

C. Timing of Thrombotic Complications

Thrombosis occurs in association with HIT in at least four ways. Only the last three situations are conventionally considered as HIT-associated thrombosis. First, thrombosis can precede heparin treatment, for which it usually represents the initial indication for heparin therapy. Second, HIT can be the presenting clinical manifestation of HIT, often occurring early during the platelet count fall. Indeed, new thrombosis is the initial clinical manifestation in about half of all HIT patients (Warkentin and Kelton, 1996; Greinacher et al., 1999; see Fig. 1A).

Third, thrombosis can occur during the period of thrombocytopenia or early platelet count recovery, even despite discontinuation of the heparin (discussed subsequently). Finally, thrombosis can occur following platelet count recovery (Gallus et al., 1987; Warkentin and Kelton, 1996). In these patients, it is possible that subclinical thrombosis occurred during the thrombocytopenia, but became clinically evident only later. The term, *heparin-induced thrombocytopenia–thrombosis (syndrome)*, also known as HITT or HITTS, is sometimes used to describe patients with HIT-associated thrombosis.

Natural History of "Isolated HIT"

There is a high probability of subsequent thrombosis even when heparin administration is stopped because of thrombocytopenia caused by HIT. A retrospective cohort study (Warkentin and Kelton, 1996) identified 62 patients with serologically confirmed HIT in whom the diagnosis was clinically suspected because of thrombocytopenia alone, and not because of signs and symptoms indicative of possible new thrombosis. Thus, this cohort was identified without an apparent recognition bias caused by symptomatic thrombosis. Nevertheless, the 30-day thrombosis event rate was about 50% (see Fig. 2 in Chap. 4). This high frequency of thrombosis occurred whether the heparin administration was simply stopped, or substituted by warfarin. Prospective treatment cohort studies also found a high initial thrombotic event rate after stopping heparin therapy, about 5–10% per day, before beginning alternative anticoagulant therapy with lepirudin (Greinacher et al., 1999; see Fig. 3 in Chap. 15).

Rule 5

> HIT is associated with a high frequency of thrombosis despite discontinuation of heparin therapy with or without substitution by coumarin: the initial rate of thrombosis is about 5–10% per day over the first 1–2 days; the 30-day cumulative risk is about 50%.

About 5% of patients (3 of 62) in the largest study died suddenly, two with proved or probable pulmonary embolism (Warkentin and Kelton, 1996). This experience supports the recommendation that further anticoagulation be considered for patients in whom isolated HIT has been diagnosed (Hirsh et al., 1998; Warkentin et al., 1998; see Chap. 13).

D. Clinical Factors in the Pathogenesis of HIT-Associated Thrombosis

Clinical factors help determine the location of thrombosis in HIT. For example, Makhoul and colleagues (1986) observed prior vessel injury (e.g., recent angiography) in 19 of 25 patients with lower limb HIT-associated thrombosis. Similarly, central venous catheters are crucial for the occurrence of an upper limb deep vein thrombosis (DVT) in patients with HIT (Warkentin and Hong, 1998).

Prospective studies of HIT in medical patients show that venous and arterial thrombotic events occur in approximately equal numbers; in contrast, there is a marked predominance of venous thrombosis when HIT occurs in surgical patients (see Table 4 in Chap. 4). In a retrospective study, Boshkov and colleagues (1993) found that HIT patients with cardiovascular disease were more likely to develop arterial thrombosis, whereas venous thrombosis was strongly associated with the postoperative state.

Rule 6

Localization of thrombosis in patients with HIT is strongly influenced by independent acute and chronic clinical factors, such as the postoperative state, atherosclerosis, or the location of intravascular catheters in central veins or arteries.

E. Venous Thrombosis

Large case series suggest that venous thrombotic complications predominate in HIT (Warkentin and Kelton, 1996; Nand et al., 1997; see Table 4 in Chap. 4). Indeed, pulmonary embolism occurs more often than all arterial thrombotic events combined. Furthermore, the strength of association between HIT and venous thromboembolism increases in relation to the severity of thrombosis, as follows: distal DVT < proximal DVT < bilateral DVT (proximal or distal) < bilateral proximal DVT < pulmonary embolism (Table 4). Thus:

Table 4 Association of HIT and Thrombosis

Thrombotic event	Patients with HIT (n = 9)	Controls (n = 656)	Odds ratio (95% CI)	p Value
Any venous or arterial thrombosis	8	117	36.9 (4.8–1638)[a]	<0.001
Arterial thrombosis	1	2	40.9 (0.6–831)	0.04
Any venous thromboembolic event	7	115	16.5 (3.1–163)	<0.001
Distal DVT without proximal extension	2	84	1.9 (0.3–10.4)	0.74
Bilateral DVT (distal or proximal)[b]	3	18	17.7 (2.6–89.9)	0.002
Proximal DVT	5	29	27.0 (5.4–141)	<0.001
Bilateral proximal DVT	2	4	46.6 (3.5–380)	0.002
Pulmonary embolism	2	2	93.4 (5.7–1374)	<0.001

HIT is defined as a platelet count fall to fewer than 150×10^9/L. The data show a stronger association (by odds ratio) between progressively more severe venous thrombosis and HIT (see clinical rule 7).

[a] Using a more sensitive definition for HIT (50% platelet count fall from postoperative peak), the odds ratio for any thrombosis was 12.4 (95% CI, 4.0–45.2; $p < 0.001$), based on the data, 13/18 vs. 112/647. Analyzing the data for only the subgroup with a platelet count fall > 50% that remained more than 150×10^9/L, the odds ratio for any thrombosis was 6.0 (1.26–30.46; $p = 0.011$), based on the data, 5/9 vs. 112/647.

[b] At least one proximal DVT was observed in each of the three HIT patients with bilateral DVT; in contrast, 12 of 18 bilateral DVTs in the non-HIT patients involved distal veins only.

Source: Modified from Warkentin et al., 1995a.

Rule 7

In patients receiving heparin, the more unusual or severe a subsequent thrombotic event, the more likely the thrombosis is caused by HIT.

Regardless of the severity of thrombosis, in any patient who develops a symptomatic venous or arterial thrombosis while receiving heparin, the platelet count should be measured to evaluate whether HIT could be present.

Lower Limb DVT

Lower limb DVT is the most frequent thrombotic manifestation of HIT. Many venous thrombi are extensive, and are often bilateral (see Table 4). There is a slight left-sided predominance: we found that 76/137 (56%) of lower limb DVT complicating HIT involved the left lower limb (Warkentin and Hong, 1998), a similar proportion as in control patients (57%). A slight left-sided predominance (~55 vs. ~45%) for lower limb DVT has also been noted in non-HIT populations (Kerr et al., 1990; Markel et al., 1992). This is attributed to the left iliac vein crossing the left iliac artery, causing an increase in left-sided lower limb venous pressures. Pregnancy amplifies further this phenomenon, thus explaining the marked predominance (> 95%) of left lower limb DVT in pregnancy (Ginsberg et al., 1992).

Upper Limb DVT

Upper limb DVT is relatively common in HIT, occurring in about 5% of patients with HIT (Warkentin and Hong, 1998). Notably, in these patients, the upper limb DVT occurred at the site of a current or recent central venous catheter. Most (86%) of the patients therefore had right upper limb DVT complicating HIT, reflecting strong physician preference to using the right neck veins for insertion of central lines. This study suggests that a systemic hypercoagulable state (HIT) interacts with a local factor (location of central lines) to result in clinical events (upper limb DVT).

Recurrence of Venous Thromboembolism

Gallus and colleagues (1987) identified HIT as a significant risk factor for recurrence of venous thromboembolism in a prospective treatment study: 3 of the 9 patients with HIT developed recurrent venous thromboembolism, compared with 12 of the 223 patients in whom HIT was not diagnosed (odds ratio, 8.8; $p < 0.01$).

Warfarin-Induced Venous Limb Gangrene

Venous limb gangrene is one of two clinical syndromes associated with HIT in which coumarin anticoagulation paradoxically plays an important pathogenic role (Fig. 6). Venous limb gangrene is defined as acral (extremity) necrosis that occurs in a limb affected by DVT. Additional features include (1) absence of large artery occlusion (palpable or doppler-identifiable pulses); (2) extensive thrombotic occlusion of large and small veins, as well as venules; and (3) the characteristic hallmark of a *supra*therapeutic international normalized ratio (INR), generally > 4.0.

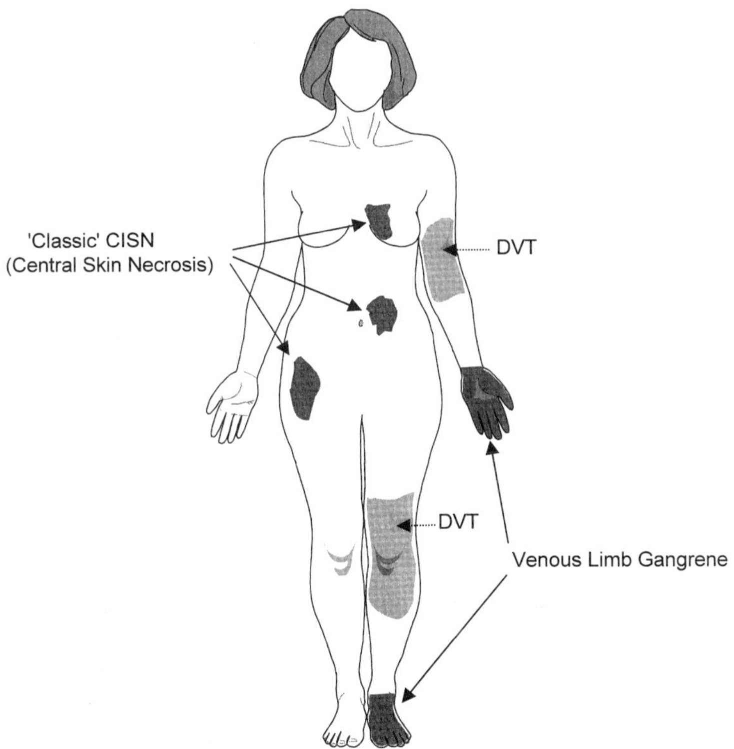

Figure 6 Coumarin-induced skin necrosis (CISN): HIT is associated with two forms of CISN: (1) venous limb gangrene, affecting extremities with active deep vein thrombosis, and (2) "classic" CISN, which involves central (nonacral) tissues, such as breast, abdomen, thigh, flank, and leg, among other tissue sites. CISN complicating HIT typically manifests as venous limb gangrene (~90%) (Warkentin et al., 1997, 1999), whereas CISN in other settings most commonly affects central tissues (~90%) (Cole et al., 1988). (From Warkentin, 1996b.)

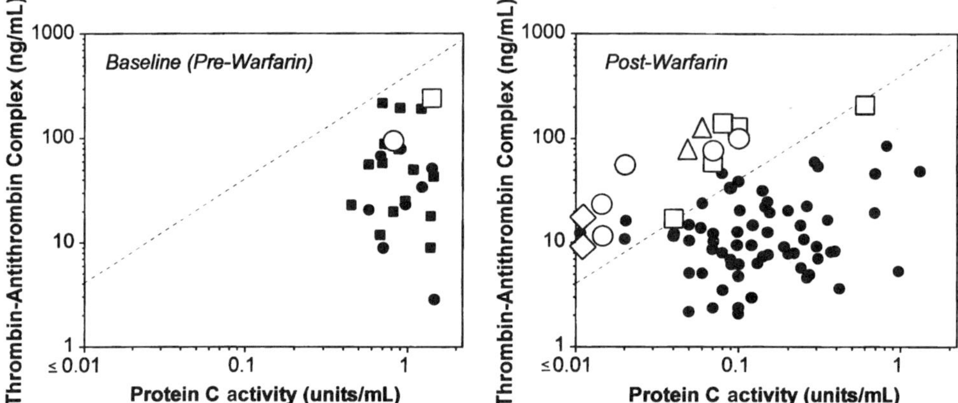

Figure 7 Thrombin–antithrombin (TAT) complexes compared with protein C activity in patients with HIT: Each data point represents TAT complexes and protein C activity per single treatment day per patient. In both panels, the open symbols represent three patients with warfarin-induced venous limb gangrene, and one patient with phlegmasia cerulea dolens (open squares). The diagonal line represents an arbitrary ratio of TAT complex to protein C of 400. (Left) Results when HIT was first diagnosed, and before warfarin therapy. Control samples included 8 patients (closed circles) who subsequently received warfarin for DVT without developing venous limb gangrene, and 14 patients without DVT who did not later receive warfarin. (Right) Results in 16 patients who were receiving warfarin for HIT, including 4 patients (open symbols) who developed venous limb gangrene/phlegmasia, and 12 patients (closed circles) who received warfarin without developing venous limb gangrene. The data suggest that patients who develop venous limb gangrene or phlegmasia have a higher ratio of TAT to protein C, consistent with a disturbance in procoagulant–anticoagulant balance during warfarin treatment of HIT. (From Warkentin et al., 1997.)

Anticoagulation with warfarin, phenprocoumon, or other coumarins is a crucial factor to explain the progression of DVT to venous limb gangrene (Warkentin, 1996b; Warkentin et al., 1997). A case–control study of 8 patients with HIT-associated venous limb gangrene found a higher median INR, compared with 58 control HIT patients treated with warfarin for DVT who did not develop venous gangrene (5.8 vs. 3.1; $p < 0.001$). Laboratory studies showed a characteristic hemostatic profile for patients with venous gangrene: persisting in vivo thrombin generation (elevated thrombin–antithrombin complex levels), together with reduced protein C activity (Fig. 7). The high INR is a surrogate marker for severely reduced protein C (through parallel coumarin-induced reduction in factor VII). Thus, venous limb gangrene appears to result from a profound disturbance in procoagulant–anticoagulant balance.

The association between venous limb gangrene and HIT was first reported by Towne and colleagues (1979). They noted a prodrome of ''phlegmasia cerulea dolens'' (i.e., an inflamed, blue, painful limb) before progression to distal gangrene (information on possible coumarin treatment was not given). Other reports of venous limb gangrene complicating HIT, however, do suggest that warfarin had been used during the evolution to necrosis (Thomas and Block, 1992; Hunter et al., 1993; Kaufman et al., 1998).

Patients have also developed venous limb gangrene during combined treatment with both ancrod and warfarin (Warkentin et al., 1997; Gupta et al., 1998); because thrombin generation *increases* during treatment of HIT with ancrod (Warkentin, 1998b), ancrod could predispose to a greater risk for venous gangrene during warfarin treatment. In contrast, venous limb gangrene has not been observed in patients who have received coumarin anticoagulants during combined treatment with an agent that reduces thrombin generation or inhibits thrombin (e.g., danaparoid, lepirudin, argatroban) (Warkentin et al., 1998).

Rule 8

> Venous limb gangrene is characterized by (1) in vivo thrombin generation associated with acute HIT; (2) active DVT in the limb(s) affected by venous gangrene; and (3) a supratherapeutic INR during coumarin anticoagulation. This syndrome can be prevented by delaying coumarin use in acute HIT until therapeutic anticoagulation is achieved with an agent that reduces thrombin generation (e.g., danaparoid) or that inhibits thrombin directly (e.g., lepirudin).

Venous limb gangrene may be a more frequent cause of limb loss in HIT patients than arterial occlusion (Warkentin et al., 1997).

Cerebral Dural Sinus Thrombosis

Thrombosis of the dural venous sinuses is an unusual cause of stroke in HIT patients that was first reported by Stevenson (1976). Often, there is a second hypercoagulable state, such as pregnancy (Van der Weyden et al., 1983; Calhoun and Hesser, 1987) or myeloproliferative disease (Kyritsis et al., 1990), that may have interacted with HIT to cause this complication. Platelet-rich ''white clots'' were identified in the superior sagittal venous sinus in one necropsy study (Meyer-Linderberg et al., 1997). Clinicians should have a high index of suspicion for dural sinus thrombosis when a patient develops progressive focal neurological signs, decreased level of consciousness, seizures, or headache during heparin treatment. Treatment includes immediate discontinuation of heparin, use of an alternative anticoagulant, and possibly, intravenous gammaglobulin (see Chap. 13).

Adrenal Hemorrhagic Infarction

Clinicians should suspect bilateral adrenal hemorrhagic infarction when thrombocytopenic patients develop abdominal pain and hypotension in association with heparin treatment (Arthur et al., 1985; Dahlberg et al., 1990; Ernest and Fisher, 1991; Delhumeau and Granry, 1992; Bleasel et al., 1992). Fever and hyponatremia occur in some patients. These patients require corticosteroid replacement to prevent death from acute or chronic adrenal failure. Unilateral adrenal hemorrhagic infarction typically presents with ipsilateral flank pain without signs of adrenal failure (Warkentin, 1996a).

This hemorrhagic manifestation of HIT is caused by thrombosis of adrenal veins leading to hemorrhagic necrosis of the glands. Other hypercoagulable states associated with adrenal necrosis include disseminated intravascular coagulation (DIC) complicating meningococcemia (Waterhouse-Friderichsen syndrome) and the antiphospholipid antibody syndrome (McKay, 1965; Carette and Jobin, 1989).

DIC and Acquired Anticoagulant Deficiency

Although increased thrombin generation occurs in most patients with HIT, *decompensated DIC*, defined as reduced fibrinogen levels, is relatively uncommon, occurring in about 5–10% of patients (Natelson et al., 1969; Klein and Bell, 1974; Zalcberg et al., 1983; Castaman et al., 1992). Protein C consumption also is well-compensated, as protein C levels are usually within the normal range when HIT is diagnosed (Warkentin et al., 1997).

Nevertheless, acquired natural anticoagulant failure from DIC could contribute to thrombosis in some patients with HIT. Markedly reduced antithrombin levels were found in a young woman with three-limb DVT and bilateral adrenal infarction complicating HIT; following recovery, antithrombin levels were normal (unpublished observations of the author). This hypothesis implies that plasmapheresis could benefit patients by correcting acquired anticoagulant deficiency; if so, the replacement fluid must be plasma, rather than albumin, to correct antithrombin and other natural anticoagulant deficiencies.

Congenital Hypercoagulability and HIT-Associated Thrombosis

Gardyn and associates (1995) reported a patient with fatal HIT and widespread microvascular thrombosis. The investigators identified heterozygous factor V Leiden in this patient, and they speculated that this contributed to the severe clinical course. However, the complications may also have been related to the treatment with low molecular weight heparin (LMWH) and warfarin.

The interaction between factor V Leiden and thrombotic sequelae of HIT was formally investigated in a study of 165 patients with HIT, 16 (9.7%) of whom had factor V Leiden (Lee et al., 1998). No increase in the number or severity of venous or arterial thrombosis was seen. This result is not surprising, as thrombosis occurs in about 50–75% of patients with HIT (Warkentin and Kelton, 1996). Thus, even if the most common congenital hypercoagulable disorders, factor V Leiden and the prothrombin 20210 A mutation (each occurring in about 5% of the population), were strongly associated with increased risk for thrombosis in HIT, only a few HIT-associated thromboses could thereby be explained.

F. Arterial Thrombosis

Lower limb artery thrombosis was the first recognized complication of HIT (Weismann and Tobin, 1958; Roberts et al., 1964; Rhodes et al., 1973, 1977). Arterial thrombosis most commonly involves the distal aorta (e.g., saddle embolism) or the large arteries of the lower limbs, leading to acute limb ischemia with absent pulses. Sometimes, platelet-rich thromboemboli from the left heart or proximal aorta explain acute lower limb arterial ischemia (Vignon et al., 1996). Other arterial thrombotic complications that are relatively common in HIT include acute thrombotic stroke and myocardial infarction. The relative frequency of arterial thrombosis in HIT by location, namely, lower limb artery occlusion $\gg$ stroke syndrome $>$ myocardial infarction (Benhamou et al., 1985; Kappa et al., 1987; Warkentin and Kelton, 1996; Nand et al., 1997), is reversed from that observed in the non-HIT population (myocardial infarction $>$ stroke syndrome $\gg$ lower limb artery occlusion).

Uncommon but well-described arterial thrombotic events in HIT include mesenteric artery thrombosis (bowel infarction), brachial artery thrombosis (upper limb gangrene), and renal artery thrombosis (renal infarction). Multiple arterial thrombotic events are quite common, as are recurrences following surgical thromboembolectomy, especially if further heparin is given during or after surgery. Occasionally, microembolization of thrombus originating from the heart or aorta causes foot or toe necrosis with palpable arterial pulses.

Angiographic Appearance

Lindsey and colleagues (1979) reported a distinct angiographic appearance of heparin-induced thromboembolic lesions, described as "broad-based, isolated, gently lobulated excrescences which produced 30–95% narrowing of the arterial lumen. The abrupt appearance of such prominent luminal contour deformities in arterial segments that were otherwise smooth and undistorted was unexpected and impressive. . . . In each case, the lesions were located proximal to sites of arterial occlusion." The radiologic and surgical experience described suggests that distal embolization of "white" clots composed of "platelet-fibrin aggregates" accounted for the limb ischemia.

G. Graft, Prosthetic Device, and Extracorporeal Circuit Thrombosis

Heparin-induced thrombocytopenia predisposes to thrombosis of blood in contact with native or prosthetic grafts or vascular fistulae, valve or other intravascular prostheses, as well as extracorporeal circuits (Towne et al., 1979; Silver et al., 1983; Bernasconi et al., 1988; AbuRahma et al., 1991; Lipton and Gould, 1992; Hall et al., 1992). This presents serious management problems in certain situations, such as renal hemodialysis (see Chap. 16). Clinicians should check for unexpected platelet count declines, and test for HIT antibodies, in patients who develop thrombosis of grafts, prostheses, or other devices during heparin treatment.

IV. MISCELLANEOUS COMPLICATIONS OF HIT

A. Heparin-Induced Skin Lesions at Subcutaneous Injection Sites

Clinical Picture

Skin lesions that occur at the site(s) of subcutaneous heparin injection are a manifestation of the HIT syndrome. For unknown reasons, only 10–20% of patients who form HIT antibodies during subcutaneous UFH or LMWH treatment develop these lesions. Furthermore, about 75% of patients who develop heparin-induced skin lesions do not develop thrombocytopenia, even though heparin-dependent, platelet-activating HIT antibodies are readily detectable (Warkentin, 1996a, 1997).

The skin abnormalities range in appearance from indurated, erythematous nodules or plaques to frank necrotizing lesions that start 5 or more days (median, day 8 after beginning heparin injections (Hasegawa 1984; MacLean et al., 1990; Wütschert et al., 1999). The lesions can occur earlier if there was recent treatment with heparin given by another route that resulted in formation of HIT antibodies. Some erythematous plaques have an eczematous appearance. Necrotic lesions typically consist of a central black eschar surrounded by a cuff of induration and erythema (Fig. 8). Complex skin lesions can result; for example, several discrete areas of necrosis (each lesion corresponding to a different heparin injection site), each with a surrounding violaceous halo, with all circumscribed by a diffuse erythema. Even the least severe forms of heparin-induced skin lesions usually cause pain or pruritus.

Both UFH and LMWH can cause these reactions. Patients who develop UFH-induced skin lesions generally will develop further lesions if LMWH is substituted for the UFH (Bircher et al., 1990). In contrast, it is uncommon for danaparoid to cause skin lesions in these patients.

Histopathology

Lymphocyte infiltration of the upper and middermis that can extend into the epidermis characterizes the erythematous plaque (Bircher et al., 1990). Dermal and

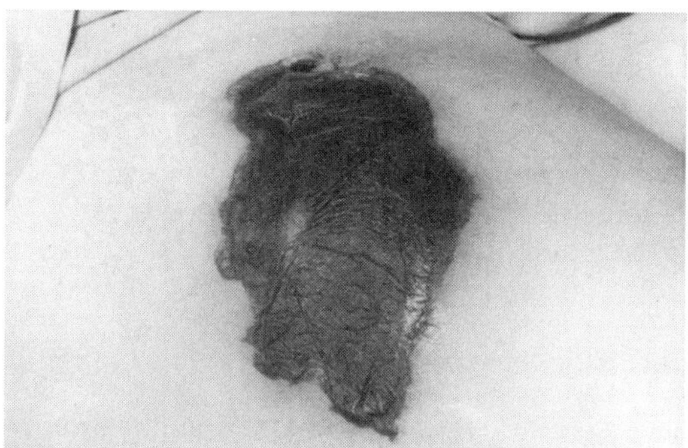

Figure 8 Heparin-induced skin necrosis: UFH injections into the right anterior thigh led to skin necrosis: a large black eschar with irregular borders is surrounded by a narrow band of erythema. The platelet count fell to 32×10^9/L; despite stopping heparin, the patient developed symptomatic proximal DVT 10 days later.

epidermal edema (spongiosis) is observed in lesions that appear eczematous. The T lymphocytes of helper–suppressor (CD4+) phenotype predominate, together with CD1+/DR+ dendritic (Langerhans) cells, consistent with a type IV delayed hypersensitivity immune response. Cytokine synthesis by activated CD4 cells could explain the peripheral blood eosinophilia that has been reported in a few patients (Bircher et al., 1994). In contrast, histopathology of lesions associated with cutaneous necrosis usually shows intravascular thrombosis of dermal vessels, with or without perivascular inflammation and red cell extravasation of variable degree (Hall et al., 1980; Kearsley et al., 1982; Cohen et al., 1988; MacLean et al., 1990; Balestra et al., 1994).

Management

Heparin-induced skin lesions should be considered a marker for the HIT syndrome. Platelet count monitoring, if not already being performed, should be initiated and continued for several days, even after stopping heparin administration. The reason is that some patients develop a fall in platelet count, together with thrombosis (often affecting limb arteries), that begins several days after stopping the heparin (Warkentin, 1996a, 1997). An alternative anticoagulant, such as danaparoid or lepirudin, should be given, particularly in patients whose original indication for anticoagulation still exists, or who develop progressive thrombocytopenia. The skin lesions themselves should be managed conservatively whenever possible, although some patients require debridement of necrotic tissues followed by skin grafting (Hall et al., 1980).

Rule 9

Erythematous or necrotizing skin lesions at heparin injection sites should be considered dermal manifestations of the HIT syndrome, irrespective of the platelet count, unless proved otherwise. Patients who develop thrombocytopenia in association with heparin-induced skin lesions are at increased risk for venous and, especially, arterial thrombosis.

B. Classic Coumarin-Induced Skin Necrosis

Classic coumarin-induced skin necrosis (CISN) is a very rare complication of oral anticoagulant therapy (Comp, 1993). In its classic form, it is characterized by dermal necrosis, usually in a central (nonacral) location, such as breast, abdomen, thigh, or leg, that begins 3–6 days after starting therapy with warfarin or other coumarin anticoagulants (see Fig. 6). Initially, there is localized pain, induration, and erythema that progresses over hours to central purplish-black skin discoloration and blistering, ultimately evolving to well-demarcated, full-thickness necrosis involving skin and subdermal tissues. Some patients require surgical debridement. Case reports suggest that congenital deficiency of natural anticoagulant proteins, especially protein C, is sometimes a pathogenic factor (Broekmans et al., 1983; Comp, 1993).

There is evidence that HIT also predisposes to classic CISN (Celoria et al., 1988; Cohen et al., 1989; Warkentin et al., 1999). Theoretically, this could result from increased consumption of anticoagulant factors, thereby leading to greater reduction in protein C in the setting of increased thrombin generation in HIT (Tans et al., 1991; Warkentin et al., 1997). However, central lesions of CISN seem less likely to complicate HIT than the related syndrome of coumarin-induced venous limb gangrene (Warkentin et al., 1997, 1999). Perhaps, active DVT in HIT localizes the progressive microvascular thrombosis to acral tissues already affected by extensive venous thrombosis.

C. Other Heparin-Associated Skin Lesions

Skin Necrosis in the Absence of Coumarin Therapy

Other patients have developed skin lesions during *intravenous* heparin therapy, or at locations otherwise distant from subcutaneous injection sites, in the absence of coumarin therapy. Hartman and colleagues (1988) reported a man who received intravenous heparin for saphenous vein thrombosis: the platelet count fell from 864 to 44 $\times$ 10^9/L (day 10). On day 7, when the platelet count had fallen by 33% to 575 $\times$ 10^9/L, progressive necrosis of skin in the thigh at the region of the thrombosed vein occurred, necessitating surgical excision. Thrombosis of veins and capillaries, with arterial sparing, was noted. Balestra et al. (1994) reported a patient who developed thrombocytopenia (75×10^9/L) and skin necrosis of the thigh on day 9 of subcutaneous injections of LMWH given into the lower abdominal wall. A skin biopsy showed small vessel thrombosis with a mild inflammatory reaction.

Other Skin Lesions Associated with Heparin Treatment

Livedo Reticularis The bluish, reticulated (network-like), mottled appearance of livedo reticularis was reported in a patient with HIT complicating intravenous UFH given for atrial fibrillation after heart surgery (Gross et al., 1993). This patient also had DIC, microangiopathic peripheral blood abnormalities, and fibrin thrombi noted within small dermal vessels. The livedo appearance results from microvascular thrombosis, with slowing of blood flow and dilation of the horizontally oriented dermal venous drainage channels (Copeman, 1975).

Urticaria and Other Miscellaneous Lesions Other dermatological consequences of heparin treatment do not appear to be related to HIT. These range from common lesions (ecchymosis) to rare effects of intravenous heparin, such as vasculitis (Jones and Epstein, 1987) and cutaneous necrosis with hemorrhagic bullae (Kelly et al., 1981). Some patients have developed widespread urticarial lesions, sometimes accompanied by angioedema, during treatment with subcutaneous or intravenous heparin (Odeh and Oliven, 1992; Patriarca et al., 1994). In one patient, skin testing suggested a generalized reaction against the preservative, chlorbutol (Dux et al., 1981).

D. Acute Systemic Reactions Following an Intravenous Heparin Bolus

Acute systemic reaction (ASR) refers to a variety of symptoms and signs that characteristically begin 5–30 min after an intravenous heparin bolus is given to a patient with circulating HIT antibodies (Nelson et al., 1978; Warkentin et al., 1992, 1994a; Ling and Warkentin, 1998; Popov et al., 1997; Table 5). Only about one-quarter of at-risk patients who receive a heparin bolus develop such a reaction. The most common signs and symptoms are fever and chills, hypertension, and tachycardia. Less common are flushing, headache, chest pain, dyspnea, tachypnea, and large-volume diarrhea. In some patients, severe dyspnea is the predominant sign, termed ''pseudo-pulmonary embolism'' by Popov and colleagues (1997); multiple small perfusion defects on radionuclide lung scans can be shown (Nelson et al., 1978; Ling and Warkentin, 1998). Fatal cardiac and respiratory arrest has been reported (Ansell et al., 1986; Platell and Tan, 1986; Hewitt et al., 1998).

An abrupt fall in the platelet count invariably accompanies these reactions. However, the platelet count drop is transient (see Fig. 1A in Chap. 4). Thus,

Table 5 Clinical Features of Acute Systemic Reactions Following Intravenous Heparin Bolus

Timing: onset 5–30 min after intravenous heparin bolus
Clinical context: recent use of heparin (past 5–100 days)
Laboratory features: abrupt, reversible fall in the platelet count
Signs and symptoms:
Inflammatory: chills, rigors, fever, flushing
Cardiorespiratory: tachycardia, hypertension, tachypnea, dyspnea, chest pain or tightness, cardiopulmonary arrest (rare)
Gastrointestinal: nausea, vomiting, diarrhea
Neurological: headache, transient global amnesia (rare)

physicians should determine the platelet count immediately on suspecting the diagnosis, and test for HIT antibodies. Heparin must be discontinued, as further use can lead to fatal complications (Ling and Warkentin, 1998).

Rule 10

Any inflammatory, cardiopulmonary, or other unexpected acute event that begins 5–30 minutes after an intravenous heparin bolus should be considered acute HIT unless proved otherwise. The postbolus platelet count should be measured promptly, and compared with prebolus levels, because the platelet count fall is abrupt and often transient.

The clinical features of postheparin bolus ASR are *not* typical of IgE-mediated anaphylaxis (i.e., urticaria, angioedema, and hypotension are not seen). Rather, the syndrome resembles febrile transfusion reactions commonly observed after platelet transfusions, suggesting a common pathogenesis of proinflammatory cytokines associated with cellular activation (Heddle et al., 1994). Moreover, there are similarities between ASR and the administration of ADP in humans, including acute dyspnea, tachycardia, and transient thrombocytopenia (Davey and Lander, 1964).

A few patients have developed acute, transient impairment of anterograde memory (i.e., the ability to form new memories) following an intravenous heparin bolus in association with acute HIT (Warkentin et al., 1994a). This syndrome resembles that of transient global amnesia, a well-characterized neurological syndrome of uncertain pathogenesis.

E. Heparin Resistance

Difficulty in maintaining therapeutic anticoagulation despite increasing heparin dosage, or heparin resistance, is a common finding in patients with HIT-associated thrombosis (Rhodes et al., 1977; Silver et al., 1983). Possible explanations include neutralization of heparin by PF4 released from activated platelets (Padilla et al., 1992), or pathophysiological consequences of platelet-derived microparticles (Bode et al., 1991). Heparin resistance is not specific for HIT, however, and occurs in many patients with extensive thrombosis of various etiologies (e.g., cancer).

V. SPECIAL CLINICAL SITUATIONS

A. Cardiac and Neurological Complications of HIT

Although HIT can affect almost any organ system, some clinical specialties observe a wider spectrum of thrombotic and other sequelae of HIT. Table 6 lists complications encountered in cardiology and neurology.

B. HIT in Pregnancy

Heparin-induced thrombocytopenia has complicated UFH treatment given for venous thromboembolism complicating pregnancy (Van der Weyden et al., 1983; Meytes et al., 1986; Copplestone and Oscier, 1987; Greinacher et al., 1992) or the postpartum period (Calhoun and Hesser, 1987). HIT seems to be rare in this patient population; no pregnant patients have been diagnosed with HIT over a 15-year period in Hamilton. Plasma glycosaminoglycans are increased during pregnancy (Andrew et al., 1992), which could contribute to lower frequency or pathogenicity of HIT antibodies. HIT antibodies cross the placenta (Greinacher et al., 1993), so it is at least theoretically possible that a heparin-treated newborn delivered from a mother with acute HIT could develop this drug reaction.

Pregnant patients with HIT have developed unusual events, such as cerebral dural sinus thrombosis (Van der Weyden et al., 1983; Calhoun and Hesser, 1987). A treatment option for pregnant patients with life-threatening thrombosis is danaparoid, as this drug does not cross the placenta (see Chap. 14). The more benign syndrome of heparin-induced skin lesions without thrombocytopenia has also been reported in pregnant patients (Drouet et al., 1992).

C. HIT in Children and Neonates

There are anecdotal reports of HIT occurring in children, some as young as 3 months of age (Laster et al., 1987; Oriot et al., 1990; Potter et al., 1992; Murdoch et al., 1993; Klement et al., 1996; Butler et al., 1997). However, not all of these patients underwent confirmatory testing with specific diagnostic assays. HIT in children has a similar, oftentimes dramatic, clinical course as seen in adults. The frequency of HIT in the pediatric population is unknown.

The frequency and clinical import of HIT in neonates receiving heparin in

Table 6 Cardiological and Neurological Complications of HIT

Cardiological complications
- Myocardial infarction (Rhodes et al., 1973; Van der Weyden et al., 1983)
- Intra-atrial thrombus (left and right[a] heart chambers) (Scheffold et al., 1995)
- Intraventricular thrombus (left and right[a] heart chambers) (Commeau et al., 1986; Dion et al., 1989; Vignon et al., 1996)
- Prosthetic valve thrombosis (Bernasconi et al., 1988)
- Right heart failure secondary to massive pulmonary embolism
- Cardiac arrest postintravenous heparin bolus (Ansell et al., 1986; Platell and Tan, 1986; 1986; Hewitt et al., 1998)

Neurological complications
- Stroke syndrome
  - In situ thrombosis
  - Progressive stroke in patients receiving heparin for treatment of stroke (Ramirez-Lassepas et al., 1984)
  - Cardiac embolization (Scheffold et al., 1995)
  - Cerebral vein (dural venous sinus) thrombosis (Van der Weyden et al., 1983; Kyritsis et al., 1990; Meyer-Lindenberg et al., 1997); complicating pregnancy (Calhoun et al., 1987)
- Ischemic lumbosacral plexopathy (Jain, 1986)
- Paraplegia, transient (Maurin et al., 1991) or permanent (Feng et al., 1993), associated with distal aortic thrombosis
- Transient global amnesia (Warkentin et al., 1994a)
- Headache[b]

[a] Although adherent thrombi that likely developed in situ have been reported (Dion et al., 1989), emboli originating from limb veins can explain right-sided intra-atrial or intraventricular clots.

[b] Headache as a feature of HIT is suggested by (1) its occurrence in patients with acute systemic reactions post-heparin bolus (see Fig. 1A; Chap. 4) and (2) its concurrence with onset of thrombocytopenia in several patients who developed HIT in a clinical trial (unpublished observations of the author).

intensive care settings is controversial. Spadone and colleagues (1992) investigated 34 newborn infants (average gestational age, 29 weeks) who developed thrombocytopenia or thrombosis, beginning an average of 22 days after starting heparin therapy. Platelet aggregation studies suggested the presence of HIT antibodies in 41% of these neonates. Aortic thrombosis complicating umbilical artery catheter use was the most common complication. Another group (Butler et al., 1997), also using platelet aggregation studies, reported a neonate who may have developed fatal HIT shortly after birth. More specific activation or antigen assays were not performed in either study, however, and confirmation of these studies is required.

D. HIT in Bone Marrow Transplantation

Given the widespread use of heparin to maintain patency of indwelling catheters, it is surprising that there are few reports of HIT in patients undergoing intensive anticancer chemotherapy. Two reports describe patients with apparent HIT complicating allogeneic or autologous marrow or stem cell transplantation (Tezcan et al., 1994; Sauer et al., 1998). Subclavian vein thrombosis occurred in one patient. It is possible that the combination of intensive chemotherapy and treatment-induced thrombocytopenia reduces the likelihood of HIT antibody formation or clinical expression of HIT.

REFERENCES

AbuRahma AF, Boland JP, Witsberger T. Diagnostic and therapeutic strategies of white clot syndrome. Am J Surg 162:175–179, 1991.

Anderson KC, Kihajda FP, Bell WR. Diagnosis and treatment of anticoagulant-related adrenal hemorrhage. Am J Hematol 11:379–385, 1981.

Andrew M, Mitchell L, Berry L, Paes B, Delorme M, Ofosu F, Burrows R, Khambalia B. An anticoagulant dermatan sulfate proteoglycan circulates in the pregnant woman and her fetus. J Clin Invest 89:321–326, 1992.

Ansell JE, Clark WP Jr, Compton CC. Fatal reactions associated with intravenous heparin [letter]. Drug Intell Clin Pharm 20:74–75, 1986.

Arthur CK, Grant SJB, Murray WK, Isbister JP, Stiel JN, Lauer CS. Heparin-associated acute adrenal insufficiency. Aust NZ J Med 15:454–455, 1985.

Balestra B, Quadri P, Demarmels Biasiutti F, Furlan M, Lämmle B. Low molecular weight heparin-induced thrombocytopenia and skin necrosis distant from injection sites. Eur J Haematol 53:61–63, 1994.

Benhamou AC, Gruel Y, Barsotti J, Castellani L, Marchand M, Guerois C, Leclerc MH, Delahousse B, Griguer P, Leroy J. The white clot syndrome or heparin-associated thrombocytopenia and thrombosis (WCS or HATT). Int Angiol 4:303–310, 1985.

Bernasconi F, Metivet F, Estrade G, Garnier D, Donatien Y. Thrombose d'une prosthèse valvulaire mitrale au cours d'une thrombopénie induite par l'héparine. Traitement fibrinolytique. Presse Méd 17:1366, 1988.

Bircher AJ, Flückiger R, Buchner SA. Eczematous infiltrated plaques to subcutaneous heparin: a type IV allergic reaction. Br J Dermatol 123:507–514, 1990.

Bircher AJ, Itin PH, Büchner SA. Skin lesions, hypereosinophilia, and subcutaneous heparin [letter]. Lancet 343:861, 1994.

Bleasel JF, Rasko JEJ, Rickard KA, Richards G. Acute adrenal insufficiency secondary to heparin-induced thrombocytopenia–thrombosis syndrome. Med J Aust 157:192–193, 1992.

Bode AP, Castellani WJ, Hodges ED, Yelverton S. The effect of lysed platelets on neutralization of heparin in vitro with protamine as measured by the activated coagulation time (ACT). Thromb Haemost 66:213–217, 1991.

Boshkov LK, Warkentin TE, Hayward CPM, Andrew M, Kelton JG. Heparin-induced thrombocytopenia and thrombosis: clinical and laboratory studies. Br J Haematol 84:322–328, 1993.

Broekmans AW, Bertina RM, Loeliger EA, Hofmann V, Klingemann HG. Protein C and the development of skin necrosis during anticoagulant therapy [letter]. Thromb Haemost 49:251, 1983.

Brushwood DB. Hospital liable for allergic reaction to heparin used in injection flush. Am J Hosp Pharm 49:1491–1492, 1992.

Butler TJ, Sodoma LJ, Doski JJ, Cheu HW, Berg ST, Stokes GN, Lancaster KJ. Heparin-associated thrombocytopenia and thrombosis as the cause of a fatal thrombus on extracorporeal membrane oxygenation. J Pediatr Surg 32:768–771, 1997.

Calhoun BC, Hesser JW. Heparin-associated antibody with pregnancy: discussion of two cases. Am J Obstet Gynecol 156:964–966, 1987.

Carette S, Jobin F. Acute adrenal insufficiency as a manifestation of the anticardiolipin syndrome? Ann Rheum Dis 48:430–431, 1989.

Castaman G, Ruggeri M, Girardello R, Rodeghiero F. An unusually prolonged case of heparin-induced thrombocytopenia and disseminated intravascular coagulation. Haematologica 77:174–176, 1992.

Celoria GM, Steingart RH, Banson B, Friedmann P, Rhee SW, Berman JA. Coumarin skin necrosis in a patient with heparin-induced thrombocytopenia—a case report. Angiology 39:915–920, 1988.

Cipolle RJ, Rodvoid KA, Seifert R, Clarens R, Ramirez-Lassepas M. Heparin-associated thrombocytopenia: a prospective evaluation of 211 patients. Ther Drug Monit 5: 205–211, 1983.

Cohen GR, Hall JC, Yeast JD, Field-Kriese D. Heparin-induced cutaneous necrosis in a postpartum patient. Obstet Gynecol 72:498–499, 1988.

Cohen DJ, Briggs R, Head HD, Acher CW. Phlegmasia cerulea dolens and its association with hypercoagulable states: case reports. Angiology 40:498–500, 1989.

Cole MS, Minifee PK, Wolma FJ. Coumarin necrosis—a review of the literature. Surgery 103:271–277, 1988.

Commeau P, Grollier G, Charbonneau P, Troussard X, Lequerrec A, Bazin C, Potier JC. Thrombopénie immuno-allergique induite par l'héparine responsable d'une thrombose intraventriculaire gauche. Therapie 41:345–347, 1986.

Comp PC. Coumarin-induced skin necrosis. Incidence, mechanisms, management and avoidance. Drug Safety 8:128–135, 1993.

Copeman PWM. Livedo reticularis. Signs in the skin of disturbance of blood viscosity and of blood flow. Br J Dermatol 93:519–522, 1975.

Copplestone A, Oscier DG. Heparin-induced thrombocytopenia in pregnancy [letter]. Br J Haematol 65:248, 1987.

Dahlberg PJ, Goellner MH, Pehling GB. Adrenal insufficiency secondary to adrenal hemorrhage. Two case reports and a review of cases confirmed by computed tomography. Arch Intern Med 150:905–909, 1990.

Davey MG, Lander H. Effect of adenosine diphosphate on circulating platelets in man. Nature 201:1037–1039, 1964.

Delhumeau A, Granry JC. Heparin-associated thrombocytopenia [letter]. Crit Care Med 20:1192, 1992.

Dion D, Dumesnil JG, LeBlanc P. In situ right ventricular thrombus secondary to heparin induced thrombocytopenia. Can J Cardiol 5:308–310, 1989.

Drouet M, Le Pabic F, Le Sellin J, Bonneau JC, Sabbah A. Allergy to heparin. Special problems set by pregnant women. Allergol Immunopathol 20:225–229, 1992.

Dux S, Pitlik S, Perry G, Rosenfeld JB. Hypersensitivity reaction to chlorbutol-preserved heparin [letter]. Lancet 1:149, 1981.

Ernest D, Fisher MM. Heparin-induced thrombocytopaenia complicated by bilateral adrenal haemorrhage. Intensive Care Med 17:238–240, 1991.

Feng WC, Singh AK, Bert AA, Sanofsky SJ, Crowley JP. Perioperative paraplegia and multiorgan failure from heparin-induced thrombocytopenia. Ann Thorac Surg 55: 1555–1557, 1993.

Gallus AS, Goodall KT, Tillett J, Jackaman J, Wycherley A. The relative contributions of antithrombin III during heparin treatment, and of clinically recognisable risk factors, to early recurrence of venous thromboembolism. Thromb Res 46:539–553, 1987.

Ganzer D, Gutezeit A, Mayer G, Greinacher A, Eichler P. Thromboembolieprophylaxe als Auslöser thrombembolischer Komplikationen. Eine Untersuchung zur Inzidenz der Heparin-induzierten Thrombozytopenie (HIT) Typ II. Z Orthop Ihre Grenzgeb 1997; 135:543–549.

Gardyn J, Sorkin P, Kluger Y, Kabili S, Klausner JM, Zivelin A, Eldor A. Heparin-induced thrombocytopenia and fatal thrombosis in a patient with activated protein C resistance. Am J Hematol 50:292–295, 1995.

Ginsberg JS, Brill-Edwards P, Burrows RF, Bona R, Prandoni P, Büller HR, Lensing A. Venous thrombosis during pregnancy: leg and trimester of presentation. Thromb Haemost 67:519–520, 1992.

Greinacher A, Michels I, Mueller-Eckhardt C. Heparin-associated thrombocytopenia: the antibody is not heparin specific. Thromb Haemost 67:545–549, 1992.

Greinacher A, Eckhardt T, Mussmann J, Mueller-Eckhardt C. Pregnancy complicated by heparin associated thrombocytopenia: management by a prospectively in vitro selected heparinoid (Org 10172). Thromb Res 71:123–126, 1993.

Greinacher A, Völpel H, Janssens U, Hach-Wunderle V, Kemkes-Matthes B, Eichler P, Mueller-Velten HG, Pötzsch B, for the HIT Investigators Group. Recombinant hirudin (lepirudin) provides safe and effective anticoagulation in patients with heparin-induced thrombocytopenia: a prospective study. Circulation 99:73–80, 1999.

Gross AS, Thompson FL, Arzubiaga MC, Graber SE, Hammer RD, Schulman G, Ellis DL, King LE Jr. Heparin-associated thrombocytopenia and thrombosis (HATT) presenting with livedo reticularis. Int J Dermatol 32:276–279, 1993.

Gruel Y, Lang M, Darnige L, Pacouret G, Dreyfus X, Leroy J, Charbonnier B. Fatal effect of reexposure to heparin after previous heparin-associated thrombocytopenia and thrombosis [letter]. Lancet 336:1077–1078, 1990.

Gupta AK, Kovacs MJ, Sauder DN. Heparin-induced thrombocytopenia. Ann Pharmacother 32:55–59, 1998.

Hach-Wunderle V, Kainer K, Krug B, Müller-Berghaus G, Pötzsch B. Heparin-associated thrombosis despite normal platelet counts [letter]. Lancet 344:469–470, 1994.

Hall AV, Clark WF, Parbtani A. Heparin-induced thrombocytopenia in renal failure. Clin Nephrol 38:86–89, 1992.

Hall JC, McConahay D, Gibson D. Heparin necrosis. An anticoagulation syndrome. JAMA 244:1831–1832, 1980.

Hartman AR, Hood RM, Anagnostopoulos CE. Phenomenon of heparin-induced thrombocytopenia associated with skin necrosis. J Vasc Surg 7:781–784, 1988.

Hasegawa GR. Heparin-induced skin lesions. Drug Intell Clin Pharm 18:313–314, 1984.

Heddle NM, Klama L, Singer J, Richards C, Fedak P, Walker I, Kelton JG. The role of the plasma from platelet concentrates in transfusion reactions. N Engl J Med 331: 625–628, 1994.

Hewitt RL, Akers DL, Leissinger CA, Gill JI, Aster RH. Concurrence of anaphylaxis and acute heparin-induced thrombocytopenia in a patients with heparin-induced antibodies. J Vasc Surg 28:561–565, 1998.

Hirsh J, Warkentin TE, Raschke R, Granger C, Ohman EM, Dalen JE. Heparin and low-molecular-weight heparin. Mechanisms of action, pharmacokinetics, dosing considerations, monitoring, efficacy, and safety. Chest 114(suppl):489S–510S, 1998.

Hunter JB, Lonsdale RJ, Wenham PW, Frostick SP. Heparin-induced thrombosis: an important complication of heparin prophylaxis for thromboembolic disease in surgery. Br Med J 307:53–55, 1993.

Jain A. Ischemic lumbosacral plexus neuropathy secondary to possible heparin-induced thrombosis following aortoiliac bypass [abstr]. Arch Phys Med Rehabil 67:680, 1986.

Jones BF, Epstein MT. Cutaneous heparin necrosis associated with glomerulonephritis. Australas J Dermatol 28:117–118, 1987.

Kappa JR, Fisher CA, Berkowitz HD, Cottrell ED, Addonizio VP Jr. Heparin-induced platelet activation in sixteen surgical patients: diagnosis and management. J Vasc Surg 5:101–109, 1987.

Kaufman BR, Zoldos J, Bentz M, Nyström NÅ. Venous gangrene of the upper extremity. Ann Plast Surg 40:370–377, 1998.

Kearsley JH, Jeremy RW, Coates AS. Leukocytoclastic vasculitis and skin necrosis following subcutaneous heparin calcium. Aust NZ J Med 12:288–289, 1982.

Kelly RA, Gelfand JA, Pincus SH. Cutaneous necrosis caused by systemically administered heparin. JAMA 246:1582–1583, 1981.

Kerr TM, Cranley JJ, Johnson JR, Lutter KS, Riechmann GC, Cranley RD, True MA, Sampson M. Analysis of 1084 consecutive lower extremities involved with acute venous thrombosis diagnosed by duplex scanning. Surgery 108:520–527, 1990.

King DJ, Kelton JG. Heparin-associated thrombocytopenia. Ann Intern Med 100:535–540, 1984.

Klein HG, Bell WR. Disseminated intravascular coagulation during heparin therapy. Ann Intern Med 80:477–481, 1974.

Klement D, Rammos S, von Kries R, Kirschke W, Kniemeyer HW, Greinacher A. Heparin as a cause of thrombus progression. Heparin-associated thrombocytopenia is an important differential diagnosis in paediatric patients even with normal platelet counts. Eur J Pediatr 155:11–14, 1996.

Kyritsis AP, Williams EC, Schutta HS. Cerebral venous thrombosis due to heparin-induced thrombocytopenia. Stroke 21:1503–1505, 1990.

Laster J, Cikrit D, Waler N, Silver D. The heparin-induced thrombocytopenia syndrome: an update. Surgery 102:763–770, 1987.

Lee DH, Warkentin TE, Denomme GA, Lagrotteria DD, Kelton JG. Factor V Leiden and thrombotic complications in heparin-induced thrombocytopenia. Thromb Haemost 79:50–53, 1998.

Lindsey SM, Maddison FE, Towne JB. Heparin-induced thromboembolism: angiographic features. Radiology 131:771–774, 1979.

Ling E, Warkentin TE. Intraoperative heparin flushes and acute heparin-induced thrombocytopenia. Anesthesiology 89:1567–1569, 1998.

Lipton ME, Gould D. Case report: heparin-induced thrombocytopenia—a complication presenting to the vascular radiologist. Clin Radiol 45:137–138, 1992.

MacLean JA, Moscicki R, Bloch KJ. Adverse reactions to heparin. Ann Allerg 65:254–259, 1990.

Makhoul RG, Greenberg CS, McCann RL. Heparin-associated thrombocytopenia and thrombosis: a serious clinical problem and potential solution. J Vasc Surg 4:522–528, 1986.

Markel A, Manzo RA, Bergelin RO, Strandness DE Jr. Pattern and distribution of thrombi in acute venous thrombosis. Arch Surg 127:305–309, 1992.

Maurin N, Biniek R, Heintz B. Kierdorf H. Heparin-induced thrombocytopenia and thrombosis with spinal ischaemia—recovery of platelet count following a change to a low molecular weight heparin [letter]. Intensive Care Med 17:185–186, 1991.

McKay DG. Late manifestations of intravascular coagulation—tissue necrosis. In: McKay DG, ed. Disseminated Intravascular Coagulation. An Intermediary Mechanism of Disease. New York: Harper & Row, 1965:392–471.

Meyer-Lindenberg A, Quenzel E-M, Bierhoff E, Wolff H, Schindler E, Biniek R. Fatal cerebral venous sinus thrombosis in heparin-induced thrombotic thrombocytopenia. Eur Neurol 37:191–192, 1997.

Meytes D, Ayalon H, Virag I, Weisbort Y, Zakut H. Heparin-induced thrombocytopenia and recurrent thrombosis in pregnancy. A case report. J Reprod Med 31:993–996, 1986.

Muntean W, Finding K, Gamillscheg A, Zenz W. Multiple thromboses and coumarin-induced skin necrosis in a young child with antiphospholipid antibodies. Thromb Haemorrh Disord 5:43–45, 1992.

Murdoch IA, Beattie RM, Silver DM. Heparin-induced thrombocytopenia in children. Acta Paediatr 82:495–497, 1993.

Nand S, Wong W, Yuen B, Yetter A, Schmulbach E, Gross Fisher S. Heparin-induced thrombocytopenia with thrombosis: incidence, analysis of risk factors, and clinical outcomes in 108 consecutive patients treated at a single institution. Am J Hematol 56:12–16, 1997.

Natelson EA, Lynch EC, Alfrey CP Jr, Gross JB. Heparin-induced thrombocytopenia. An unexpected response to treatment of consumption coagulopathy. Ann Intern Med 71:1121–1125, 1969.

Nelson JC, Lerner RG, Goldstein R, Cagin NA. Heparin-induced thrombocytopenia. Arch Intern Med 138:548–552, 1978.

Odeh M, Oliven A. Urticaria and angioedema induced by low-molecular-weight heparin [letter]. Lancet 340:972–973, 1992.

Olinger GN, Hussey CV, Olive JA, Malik MI. Cardiopulmonary bypass for patients with previously documented heparin-induced platelet aggregation. J Thorac Cardiovasc Surg 87:673–677, 1984.

Oriot D, Wolf M, Wood C, Brun P, Sidi D, Devictor D, Tchernia G, Huault G. Thrombopénie sévère induite par l'héparine chez un nourrisson porteur d'une myocardite aiguë. Arch Fr Pediatr 47:357–359, 1990.

Padilla A, Gray E, Pepper DS, Barrowcliffe TW. Inhibition of thrombin generation by heparin and low molecular weight (LMW) heparins in the absence and presence of platelet factor 4 (PF4). Br J Haematol 82:406–413, 1992.

Patriarca G, Rossi M, Schiavino D, Schinco G, Fais G, Varano C, Schiavello R. Rush desensitization in heparin hypersensitivity: a case report. Allergy 49:292–294, 1994.

Pedersen-Bjergaard U, Andersen M, Hansen PB. Drug-induced thrombocytopenia: clinical data on 309 cases and the effect of corticosteroid therapy. Eur J Clin Pharmacol 52:183–189, 1997.

Pfueller SL, David R, Firkin BG, Bilston RA, Cortizo F. Platelet aggregating IgG antibody to platelet surface glycoproteins associated with thrombosis and thrombocytopenia. Br J Haematol 74:336–341, 1990.

Phelan BK. Heparin-associated thrombosis without thrombocytopenia. Ann Intern Med 99:637–638, 1983.

Platell CFE, Tan EGC. Hypersensitivity reactions to heparin: delayed onset thrombocytopenia and necrotizing skin lesions. Aust NZ J Surg 56:621–623, 1986.

Popov D, Zarrabi MH, Foda H, Graber M. Pseudopulmonary embolism: acute respiratory distress in the syndrome of heparin-induced thrombocytopenia. Am J Kidney Dis 29:449–452, 1997.

Potter C, Gill JC, Scott JP, McFarland JG. Heparin-induced thrombocytopenia in a child. J Pediatr 121:135–138, 1992.

Ramirez-Lassepas M, Cipolle RJ, Rodvold KA, Seifert RD, Strand L, Taddeini L, Cusulos M. Heparin-induced thrombocytopenia in patients with cerebrovascular disease. Neurology 34:736–740, 1984.

Rhodes GR, Dixon RH, Silver D. Heparin-induced thrombocytopenia with thrombotic and hemorrhagic manifestations. Surg Gynecol Obstet 136:409–416, 1973.

Rhodes GR, Dixon RH, Silver D. Heparin induced thrombocytopenia: eight cases with thrombotic–hemorrhagic complications. Ann Surg 186:752–758, 1977.

Roberts B, Rosato FE, Rosato EF. Heparin—a cause of arterial emboli? Surgery 55:803–808, 1964.

Sauer M, Gruhn B, Fuchs D, Altermann W, Zintl F. Heparin-induzierte Thrombozytopenie Typ II im Rahmen einer Hochdosis-Chemotherapie mit anschließender Stammzellrescue. Klin Pädiatr 210:102–105, 1998.

Scheffold N, Greinacher A, Cyran J. Intrakardiale Thrombenbildung bei Heparin-assoziierter Thrombozytopenie Typ II. Dtsch Med Wochenschr 120:519–522, 1995.

Silver D, Kapsch DN, Tsoi EKM. Heparin-induced thrombocytopenia, thrombosis, and hemorrhage. Ann Surg 198:301–306, 1983.

Solomon SA, Cotton DWK, Preston FE, Ramsay LE. Severe disseminated intravascular coagulation associated with massive ventricular mural thrombus following acute myocardial infarction. Postgrad Med J 64:791–795, 1988.

Spadone D, Clark F, James E, Laster J, Hoch J, Silver D. Heparin-induced thrombocytopenia in the newborn. J Vasc Surg 15:306–312, 1992.

Stevenson MM. Thrombocytopenia during heparin therapy [letter]. N Engl J Med 295: 1200–1201, 1976.

Tans G, Rosing J, Thomassen MC, Heeb MJ, Zwaal RF, Griffin JH. Comparison of anticoagulant and procoagulant activities of stimulated platelets and platelet-derived microparticles. Blood 77:2641–2648, 1991.

Tezcan AZ, Tezcan H, Gastineau DA, Armitage JO, Haire WD. Heparin-induced thrombocytopenia after bone marrow transplantation: report of two cases. Bone Marrow Transplant 14:487–490, 1994.

Thode U, Greinacher A, Overdick K, Anlauf M. Life-threatening anaphylactic reaction following parathyroidectomy in a dialysis patient with heparin-induced thrombocytopenia. Nephrol Dial Transplant 12:2750–2755, 1997.

Thomas D, Block AJ. Thrombocytopenia, cutaneous necrosis, and gangrene of the upper and lower extremities in a 35-year-old man. Chest 102:1578–1580, 1992.

Towne JB, Bernhard VM, Hussey C, Garancis JC. White clot syndrome. Peripheral vascular complications of heparin therapy. Arch Surg 114:372–377, 1979.

Van der Weyden MB, Hunt H, McGrath K, Fawcett T, Fitzmaurice A, Sawers RJ, Rosengarten DS. Delayed-onset heparin-induced thrombocytopenia. A potentially malignant syndrome. Med J Aust 2:132–135, 1983.

Vignon P, Guéret P, François B, Serhal C, Fermeaux V, Bensaid J. Acute limb ischemia and heparin-induced thrombocytopenia: the value of echocardiography in eliminating a cardiac source of arterial emboli. J Am Soc Echocardiogr 9:344–347, 1996.

Warkentin TE. Hemostasis and atherosclerosis. Can J Cardiol 11(suppl C):29C–34C, 1995.

Warkentin TE. Heparin-induced skin lesions. Br J Haematol 92:494–497, 1996a.

Warkentin TE. Heparin-induced thrombocytopenia: IgG-mediated platelet activation, platelet microparticle generation, and altered procoagulant/anticoagulant balance in the pathogenesis of thrombosis and venous limb gangrene complicating heparin-induced thrombocytopenia. Transfusion Med Rev 10:249–258, 1996b.

Warkentin TE. Heparin-induced thrombocytopenia, heparin-induced skin lesions, and arterial thrombosis. Thromb Haemost 77(suppl):562, 1997.

Warkentin TE. Clinical presentation of heparin-induced thrombocytopenia. Semin Hematol 35(suppl 5):9–16, 1998a.

Warkentin TE. Limitations of conventional treatment options for heparin-induced thrombocytopenia. Semin Hematol 35(suppl 5):17–25, 1998b.

Warkentin TE. Heparin-induced thrombocytopenia: a clinicopathologic syndrome. Thromb Haemost 82(suppl):439–447, 1999.

Warkentin TE, Hong AP. Frequency of upper limb deep venous thrombosis (UL-DVT) in relation to central venous catheter (CVC) use in patients with heparin-induced thrombocytopenia (HIT): evidence for interaction of systemic (HIT) and local (CVC) prothrombotic risk factors [abstr]. Blood 92(suppl 1):500a–501a, 1998.

Warkentin TE, Kelton JG. Interaction of heparin with platelets, including heparin-induced thrombocytopenia. In: Bounameaux H, ed. Low-Molecular-Weight Heparins in Prophylaxis and Therapy of Thromboembolic Diseases. New York: Marcel Dekker, 1994, pp 75–127.

Warkentin TE, Kelton JG. A 14-year study of heparin-induced thrombocytopenia. Am J Med 101:502–507, 1996.

Warkentin TE, Kelton JG. Timing of heparin-induced thrombocytopenia (HIT) in relation to previous heparin use: absence of an anamnestic immune response, and implications for repeat heparin use in patients with a history of HIT. Blood 92(suppl 1): 182a, 1998.

Warkentin TE, Soutar RL, Panju A, Ginsberg JS. Acute systemic reactions to intravenous bolus heparin therapy: characterization and relationship to heparin-induced thrombocytopenia [abstr]. Blood 80(suppl 1):160a, 1992.

Warkentin TE, Hirte HW, Anderson DR, Wilson WEC, O'Connell GJ, Lo RC. Transient global amnesia associated with acute heparin-induced thrombocytopenia. Am J Med 97:489–491, 1994a.

Warkentin TE, Hayward CPM, Boshkov LK, Santos AV, Sheppard JI, Bode AP, Kelton JG. Sera from patients with heparin-induced thrombocytopenia generate platelet-derived microparticles with procoagulant activity: an explanation for the thrombotic complications of heparin-induced thrombocytopenia. Blood 84:3691–3699, 1994b.

Warkentin TE, Levine MN, Hirsh J, Horsewood P, Roberts RS, Gent M, Kelton JG. Heparin-induced thrombocytopenia in patients treated with low-molecular-weight heparin or unfractionated heparin. N Engl J Med 332:1330–1335, 1995a.

Warkentin TE, Levine MN, Hirsh J, Klama LN, Kelton JG. Formation of heparin-induced thrombocytopenia IgG without thrombocytopenia: analysis of a clinical trial [abstr]. Blood 86(suppl 1):537a, 1995b.

Warkentin TE, Elavathil LJ, Hayward CPM, Johnston MA, Russett JI, Kelton JG. The pathogenesis of venous limb gangrene associated with heparin-induced thrombocytopenia. Ann Intern Med 127:804–812, 1997.

Warkentin TE, Chong BH, Greinacher A. Heparin-induced thrombocytopenia: towards consensus. Thromb Haemost 79:1–7, 1998.

Warkentin TE, Sikov WM, Lillicrap DP. Multicentric warfarin-induced skin necrosis complicating heparin-induced thrombocytopenia. Am J Med 62:44–48, 1999.

Weismann RE, Tobin RW. Arterial embolism occurring during systemic heparin therapy. Arch Surg 76:219–227, 1958.

Wütschert R, Piletta P, Bounameaux H. Adverse skin reactions to low molecular weight heparins: frequency, management and prevention. Drug Safety 20:515–525, 1999.

Zalcberg JR, McGrath K, Dauer R, Wiley SJ. Heparin-induced thrombocytopenia with associated disseminated intravascular coagulation. Br J Haematol 54:655–660, 1983.

4
Frequency of Heparin-Induced Thrombocytopenia

David H. Lee
Queen's University, Kingston, Ontario, Canada

Theodore E. Warkentin
McMaster University and Hamilton Health Sciences Corporation, Hamilton, Ontario, Canada

I. INTRODUCTION

Thrombocytopenia is a common problem encountered in hospitalized patients. For patients receiving heparin, there are three general explanations for thrombocytopenia: (1) heparin-induced thrombocytopenia (HIT), (2) nonidiosyncratic heparin-induced platelet activation (see Chap. 5), and—perhaps most often—(3) an unrelated clinical problem, either common (e.g., hemodilution, septicemia) or rare (e.g., posttransfusion purpura, drug-induced immune thrombocytopenic purpura) (see Chaps. 2 and 12). The availability of sensitive and specific laboratory assays (e.g., enzyme immunoassay [EIA] and serotonin release assay [SRA]) for pathogenic HIT antibodies means that patients with HIT can usually be readily distinguished from the other conditions (see Chap. 11). However, the role of heparin in causing thrombocytopenia because of nonimmune platelet activation cannot readily be separated from other common medical problems encountered in hospitalized patients, either on clinical or laboratory criteria. Furthermore, these two conditions can coexist (Chong and Castaldi, 1986). Thus, the term ''nonimmune heparin-associated thrombocytopenia'' (nonimmune HAT) has been recommended to describe patients who develop thrombocytopenia during heparin treatment in which a role for HIT antibodies cannot be implicated (Warkentin et al., 1998a).

Unfortunately, many early studies of HIT frequency either did not perform laboratory testing, or used relatively insensitive or nonspecific assays, to diagnose

HIT. In contrast, more recent studies have used one, or even two, sensitive and complementary assays. Perhaps for this reason, the understanding of the frequency and clinical import of HIT has shifted over the years. Formerly, the range of views on immune-mediated HIT were divergent: it was considered both nonexistent (Bell, 1988) and common (Kelton, 1986). Nevertheless, both viewpoints acknowledged that thrombosis resulting from HIT was very uncommon. Today's perspective on HIT is very different. The frequency of HIT is now shown to be *variable*, partly depending on patient population and type of heparin used. For example, the frequency ranges from less than 1% (cardiac medical patients) to 5% (orthopedic surgical patients) receiving unfractionated heparin (UFH); HIT antibody formation following UFH use ranges from 2% (cardiac medical patients) to 15% (orthopedic surgical patients) to 50% (cardiac surgical patients). Most importantly, however, it is now becoming clear that the risk for thrombosis in patients who develop HIT is 33–50%, a frequency that is far greater than in control patients who do not develop HIT (Warkentin et al., 1995a).

The biological basis for this variability in frequency of HIT and HIT antibody formation is now apparent. The HIT antigen is a cryptic autoantigen, or neoantigen, on platelet factor 4 (PF4) that is formed when PF4 binds to heparin (see Chaps. 6–8). Only stoichiometric concentrations of heparin and PF4 will form the antigen. Thus, it can be hypothesized that the frequency of HIT antibody formation will be influenced not only by heparin dose and composition, but also by circulating PF4 levels. Conditions associated with fluctuating, but at times high, circulating PF4 and heparin levels (e.g., cardiac surgery) might be ideal for immunization to the HIT antigen. Thus, real differences in HIT frequency observed among prospective studies can be understood in a biologically plausible context.

The key role of the pathogenic HIT antibodies, and the availability of sensitive and specific assays for their detection, suggest that HIT should be considered a *clinicopathologic syndrome*. Consequently, this chapter will focus on studies that have used in vitro testing to evaluate HIT antibodies. However, other features known to be useful to diagnose HIT, such as the timing of the onset of thrombocytopenia in typical HIT, and the rapid platelet count fall on heparin rechallenge, will also be used (see Chap. 3). The importance of confirmatory laboratory testing should not be underestimated: prospective (Greinacher et al., 1994; Lee et al., 1996) and retrospective (Look et al., 1997) studies suggest that only 25–55% of sera referred for evaluation test positive for HIT antibodies. Furthermore, systematic analysis of a large clinical trial of heparin treatment (Warkentin et al., 1995a,b) revealed several patients in whom unusual clinical events subsequently linked to HIT were initially attributed to other problems (Fig. 1a,b).

Table 1 lists various biological and technical explanations that underlie the reported variability in frequency of HIT among the prospective studies. We will begin our discussion by summarizing an important technical problem in many studies (i.e., the failure to exclude patients with early, nonimmune HAT).

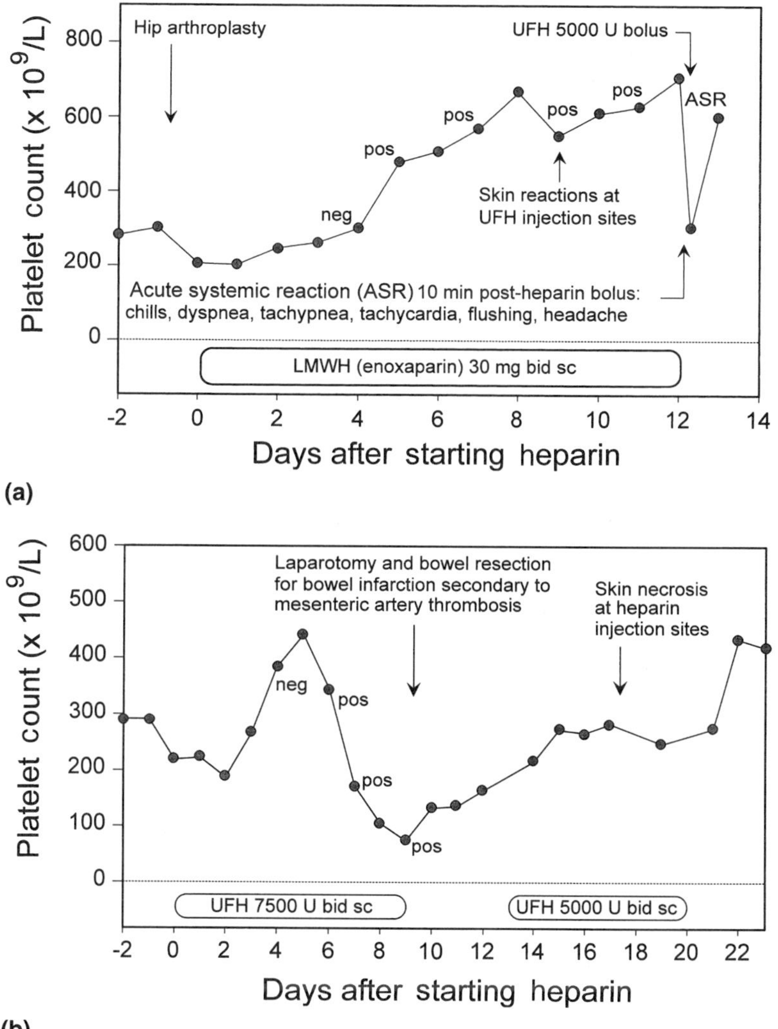

Figure 1 Initially unrecognized HIT during prospective studies: (a) A 57-year-old man developed skin lesions at the sites of LMWH (enoxaparin) injections on day 9. An acute systemic reaction (ASR; see Chap. 3) developed after a 5000 U intravenous UFH bolus. This patient was recognized as having had the HIT syndrome only following systematic testing for HIT antibodies performed later (Warkentin et al., 1995a,b). (b) A 73-year-old woman developed bowel infarction necessitating resection while receiving UFH prophylaxis after hip replacement surgery. The thrombocytopenia was initially attributed to "sepsis." However, the patient was later recognized as having the HIT syndrome following systematic testing for HIT antibodies performed later (Warkentin et al., 1995a,b).

Table 1 Explanations for Variable Frequency of HIT Among Prospective Studies

Biological explanations
1. Patient population studied (frequency of HIT antibody formation may differ among patient populations, possibly because of differences in platelet activation and PF4 release)
2. Type of heparin used (UFH more immunogenic than LMWH; bovine lung heparin more immunogenic than porcine mucosal heparin; possibly, lot-to-lot variability in immunogenicity of heparin)
3. Variable duration of heparin treatment (HIT typically begins between days 5 and 10)
4. Dose of heparin used (dose-dependent thrombocytopenia)

Technical explanations
1. Variable definition of thrombocytopenia used
2. Differing baseline platelet counts permitted for study entry
3. Requirement to repeat platelet count testing to confirm thrombocytopenia
4. Variable intensity of platelet count surveillance
5. Variable intensity of surveillance for thrombotic events
6. Failure to exclude nonimmune heparin-associated thrombocytopenia
   a. Lack of use of in vitro test for HIT antibodies
   b. Use of insensitive or nonspecific HIT antibody assays
   c. Inclusion of patients with ''early'' thrombocytopenia
   d. Failure to exclude patients whose platelet count recovered during continued heparin treatment
   e. Failure to exclude patients with other explanations for thrombocytopenia

II. EARLY- VERSUS LATE-ONSET THROMBOCYTOPENIA

The distinction between thrombocytopenia that begins early (within 4 days) or late (5 or more days after beginning heparin treatment) is a simple clinical feature that is useful to distinguish nonimmune HAT, which begins early, from (immune) HIT, which begins late. For this assessment, the first day of heparin use is considered day 0 (see Table 2 in Chap. 3). There is an important exception to this rule of timing for HIT: a rapid fall in platelet count on starting heparin therapy can represent acute HIT, but usually only if a patient already has circulating HIT antibodies, usually the result of a recent heparin exposure. HIT antibodies are transient, and retrospective data suggest that acute HIT in patients who did not receive heparin within the past 100 days is very rare (Warkentin and Kelton, 1998) (see Chap. 3).

Typically, nonimmune HAT begins 1–2 days after starting heparin administration and resolves during continued heparin therapy (Johnson et al., 1984; Chong and Berndt, 1989; Warkentin and Kelton, 1994; Warkentin et al., 1995a;

Greinacher, 1995). The platelet count fall is usually mild, with a nadir between 75 and 150 × 10^9/L. This early platelet count fall may be the result of a direct activating effect of heparin on platelets (Chong and Ismail, 1989; Chong and Castaldi, 1986), or to comorbid clinical factors.

Early nonimmune HAT occurs in up to 30% of patients receiving heparin (Bell et al., 1976; Nelson et al., 1978; Warkentin et al., 1995a). Systematic serological investigation of patients with early thrombocytopenia was performed in one study comparing UFH with low molecular weight heparin (LMWH) for postoperative antithrombotic prophylaxis in patients who underwent hip replacement surgery (Warkentin et al., 1995a). With 150 × 10^9/L as a platelet count threshold, early thrombocytopenia was observed in 189/665 (28%) of patients; however, HIT antibodies were not detected in any of the 98 patients tested, and platelet count recovery to more than 150 × 10^9/L within 3 days occurred despite continuing the heparin (Warkentin et al., 1995a). No difference in the frequency of early thrombocytopenia was observed between patients who received UFH (28%) and those who received LMWH (29%). This suggests that unrelated clinical factors, such as perioperative hemodilution with fluid and blood products, were primarily responsible. In contrast, the onset of late thrombocytopenia (i.e., between days 5 and 10 of heparin treatment) was strongly associated with the formation of HIT antibodies, and occurred significantly more frequently in the patients who received UFH (discussed subsequently).

III. FREQUENCY OF IMMUNE HIT

Tables 2 and 3 list the prospective studies of the frequency of HIT that either employed in vitro testing for HIT antibodies, or were studies in which the likelihood of HIT could be judged based on information provided, especially the timing of the onset of thrombocytopenia. Relevant variables influencing the frequency of HIT include the type of heparin used and the patient population.

A. Frequency of HIT in Medical Patients and Normal Volunteers: Comparison of UFH of Bovine Versus Porcine Origin

Five randomized trials (Bell and Royall, 1980; Green et al., 1984; Powers et al., 1984; Ansell et al., 1985; Bailey et al., 1986) and one nonrandomized study (Cipolle et al., 1983; Ramirez-Lassepas et al., 1984) compared the frequency of HIT during treatment with UFH that was derived either from bovine lung or porcine intestinal mucosa. In addition, the frequency of HIT was evaluated in normal volunteers in one randomized (Schwartz et al., 1985) and one nonrandomized prospective study (Saffle et al., 1980) involving porcine and bovine heparins.

Table 2 The Frequency of HIT: Prospective Studies of HIT in Medical Patients Using In Vitro Testing of Patient Serum/Plasma for HIT Antibodies, or Indicating a High Likelihood of HIT Based on Timing of Platelet Count Fall

Study	Major indication for heparin	In vitro test	Route, dose	Frequency of (immune) HIT (%) Bovine UFH	Porcine UFH	LMWH	Timing of platelet fall reported?	Definition of thrombocytopenia ($\times 10^9$/L)
Comparisons between bovine UFH and porcine UFH (studies and data in **bold** are randomized, controlled trials (RCTs)								
Ansell et al., 1980 (RCT)	VTE	PRP(SR)	iv ther	**4/21 (19.0)**	**0/22 (0)**		Yes	< 150
Green et al., 1984 (RCT)	VTE	HIPA	iv ther	**2/45 (4.4)**	**0/44 (0)**		Yes	< 150
Powers et al., 1984 (RCT)	VTE	SRA[a]	iv ther	**2/65[a] (3.1)**	**0/66 (0)**		Yes	< 150
Bailey et al., 1986 (RCT)	VTE, ATE	no test	iv ther	**1/21 (4.8)**	**0/22 (0)**		Yes	< 100
Cipolle et al., 1983; Ramirez-Lassepas et al., 1984 [stroke subgroup]	VTE, ATE [stroke subgroup]	PRP	iv ther	6/100[b] (6.0) [3/54] (5.6)	1/111 (0.9) (1/83) (1.2)		Yes	< 100
Predominant treatment for venous (VTE) or arterial (ATE) thromboembolism								
Bell et al., 1976; Alving et al., 1977	VTE, ATE	PRP/SRA[c]	iv ther	3/52[c] (5.8)			Yes	< 100
Powers et al., 1979	VTE	no test	iv ther		2/120[d] (1.7)		Yes[d]	< 150
Gallus et al., 1980	VTE	PRP	iv ther		3/166[e] (1.8)		Yes	< 100
			sc proph		0/5 (0)			
Holm et al., 1980	VTE	no test	iv ther		0/90[f] (0)		Yes	< 100
Monreal et al., 1989	VTE	no test	iv ther		2/89 (2.2)		Low platelets day 8	< 100
			sc proph		0/49 (0)	0/43 (0)		
Kakkasseril et al., 1985	VTE, ATE	PRP	iv ther	4/142[g] (2.8)			No	< 100
Malcolm et al., 1979	Multiple indications	PRP	iv ther		1/66[h] (1.5)		Yes	< 100
			sc proph		0/38 (0)			
Rao et al., 1989	Multiple indications	PRP(SR)	iv ther		0/94 (0)		NA	< 100
			sc proph		0/99 (0)			
Predominant treatment for myocardial infarction or acute coronary syndromes (MI/ACS)								
Kappers-Klunne et al., 1997	MI/ACS	HIPA, EIA	iv ther		1/358 (0.3)		Yes	< 60 and > 50% fall
					2/358 (0.6)			(< 120)
Romeril et al., 1982	MI/ACS	PRP	sc proph		0/45 (0)		NA	< 150
Weitberg et al., 1982	MI/ACS	No test	sc proph		0/50 (0)		NA	< 150
Johnson et al., 1984	MI/ACS	No test	sc proph		0/66 (0)		Yes	< 150

Hemodialysis							
Yamamoto et al., 1996	New-onset hemodialysis	EIA, PRP	iv ther		6/154 (3.9) 3/154 (1.9)	Yes	Clotting and > 20% fall (> 50% fall)
Healthy volunteers							
Saffle et al., 1980	—	PRP	sc proph	0/25 (0)	0/14 (0)	NA	< 150
Schwartz et al., 1985	—	No test	Bolus iv ther	3/20 (15.0)	0/10 (0)	Yes	< 150

HIT was excluded if the platelet count rose during continued heparin after an early fall (e.g., Johnson et al., 1984). Also, where uncertainty existed as to the number of patients with probable HIT, the lower number was indicated in the table, to avoid overestimating the number of patients with HIT (contrast the analysis shown in Table 4). Some data relating to Cipolle et al. (1983) were obtained by personal communication, as reported (Warkentin and Kelton, 1991). The study by Gallus et al. (1980) was excluded because the source of heparin was not specified. Some reports (e.g., Nelson et al., 1978) were excluded because timing of thrombocytopenia was not reported.

Abbreviations: ATE, arterial thromboembolism; EIA, PF4–heparin enzyme-linked immunosorbent assay; HIPA, heparin-induced platelet activation test (aggregation of washed platelets); iv ther, intravenous therapeutic-dose heparin; LMWH, low molecular weight heparin; MI/ACS, myocardial infarction/acute coronary syndromes; PRP, HIT assay using citrated platelet-rich plasma (PRP/SR, with serotonin release); sc proph, subcutaneous prophylactic-dose heparin; RCT, randomized controlled trial; SRA, serotonin release assay using washed platelets; UFH, unfractionated heparin; VTE, venous thromboembolism.

[a] Powers et al. (1984) described five patients who developed thrombocytopenia during bovine UFH use (none during porcine UFH use); two patients whose platelet counts fell beginning on day 7 (to nadir of 41×10^9/L) and on day 8 (to nadir of 53×10^9/L) had positive testing for HIT antibodies by SRA; test results are not available for one patient whose platelet count fell on day 5 (excluded from Table 2, but included in Table 4); one patient with proved HIT developed progression of deep venous thrombosis, as indicated in Table 4 (laboratory records of Dr. J. G. Kelton).

[b] Cipolle et al. (1983) described ten patients who received bovine UFH who may have had HIT; only six are included here, all of whom developed a platelet count fall between days 7 and 10. Ramirez-Lassepas et al. (1984) examined the subgroup with underlying cerebrovascular disease and reported six patients who developed thrombocytopenia after receiving bovine heparin. Only the three who developed late thrombocytopenia are reported here.

[c] Only 8 of 16 thrombocytopenia patients underwent PRP testing (all negative) and only 5 underwent SRA testing. The 3 who developed late thrombocytopenia (HIT) had negative PRP testing, but did not have SRA testing.

[d] Information on timing of platelet count fall to determine the likelihood of HIT was obtained by personal communication, as described (Warkentin and Kelton, 1991).

[e] Origin of heparin is uncertain and may have used mucosal heparin from sheep; at least 3, and as many as 5, patients appeared to have HIT based on in vitro testing and timing of platelet count fall.

[f] One case of early thrombocytopenia due to DIC reported in original paper was excluded.

[g] At least four, and as many as 9, patients appeared to have HIT; the four that tested positive for HIT antibodies are included here.

[h] One patient appeared to have HIT based on positive heparin rechallenge, despite negative in vitro HIT test.

Table 3 The Frequency of HIT: Prospective Studies of Surgical Patients Using Confirmatory In Vitro Laboratory Testing of Patient Serum or Plasma, or Indicating a High Likelihood of HIT Based on Timing of Platelet Count Fall

Study	Major indication for heparin	In vitro test	Route, dose	Frequency of (immune) HIT			Timing of platelet fall reported?	Definition of thrombocytopenia ($\times 10^9$/L)
				Bovine UFH	Porcine UFH	LMWH		
Comparisons between porcine UFH and LMWH								
Leyvraz et al., 1991	orthopedic	PRP	sc proph		2/204 (1.0)	0/205 (0)	Yes	< 100, > 40% fall
Warkentin et al., 1995a,b	orthopedic	SRA	sc proph		9/332 (2.7) 16/332 (4.8)	0/333 (0) 2/333 (0.6)	Yes	< 150 >50% fall
Other studies								
Louridas, 1991	Vascular	PRP[a]	iv ther, sc proph		5/114[b] (4.4)		Yes	< 100
Warkentin et al., 1998b	Orthopedic	SRA/EIA	sc proph			2/246 (0.8)	Yes	< 150 or > 50% fall
Ganzer et al., 1997	Orthopedic	HIPA	sc proph		15/307 (4.9)		Yes	> 50% fall
Trossaert et al., 1998	Cardiac	PRP/EIA	sc proph		0/51 (0)		Yes	Not stated
Warkentin et al., 1999	Cardiac	SRA	sc proph		1/100 (1.0)		Yes	> 50% fall
Pouplard et al., 1999	Cardiac	SRA, EIA	sc proph		6/157 (3.8)	0/171 (0)	No	< 100 or > 40% fall

Abbreviations: EIA, PF4–heparin enzyme-linked immunosorbent assay; HIPA, heparin-induced platelet activation test (aggregation of washed platelets); LMWH, low molecular weight heparin; PRP, HIT assay using citrated platelet-rich plasma; sc proph, subcutaneous prophylactic-dose heparin; SRA, serotonin release assay using washed platelets; UFH, unfractionated heparin.

[a] Ineffective testing was used (platelet aggregation without heparin).

[b] Of seven patients with thrombocytopenia reported, two were excluded because of early onset of thrombocytopenia.

The study of Bell and Royall (1980) has been excluded from primary analysis because neither laboratory testing for HIT antibodies nor data on the timing of onset of thrombocytopenia were provided.

Taken together, the four randomized controlled trials in medical patients strongly suggest that bovine UFH is more likely to cause HIT than porcine UFH, as all nine patients with HIT had received UFH of bovine origin ($p = 0.0059$ by Mantel-Haenszel; see Table 2). Similarly, an increased frequency of HIT in patients receiving bovine lung heparin was suggested in the nonrandomized comparison by Cipolle and colleagues (1983) (6/100, 6% vs. 1/111, 0.9%; $p = 0.055$), as well as in the study of Bell and Royall (1980) (26% vs. 8%; $p < 0.005$), although this latter study probably included patients with nonimmune HAT.

A higher frequency of immune HIT with bovine lung heparin is biologically plausible. Bovine heparin has a higher sulfate/disaccharide ratio than does porcine heparin (Casu et al., 1983), and it is better able to activate platelets in vitro (Barradas et al., 1987). These properties could lead to greater platelet activation in vivo and, consequently, greater potential for PF4 release. Moreover, the bovine heparin chains would be expected to better form the large multimolecular complexes that compose the target antigen for HIT antibodies.

Lot-to-lot variability within heparin of a particular animal source could also contribute to variable frequency of HIT. Stead and co-workers (1984) reported a striking cluster of six patients with pulmonary embolism complicating HIT identified within a few weeks at one institution. A particular lot of bovine lung heparin in use in the operating room was linked to these events: patient serum-induced platelet aggregation occurred in the presence of this particular lot of heparin, but not when other lots of bovine lung heparin from the same manufacturer were used.

B. Frequency of HIT in Medical Patients Treated with Porcine Mucosal UFH

Table 2 also lists the frequency of HIT observed in several prospective studies that have evaluated medical patients receiving intravenous, therapeutic-dose UFH, usually for venous thromboembolism (VTE). Excluding a study of hemodialysis, an overall frequency of HIT of slightly less than 1% is suggested (7/992; 95% CI, 0.3–1.4%). This is a relatively low number, particularly when one considers that, paradoxically, the frequency appears to be much higher in postoperative surgical patients who received lower (prophylactic) doses of porcine heparin (discussed subsequently).

In contrast, HIT seemed to occur more often in a prospective study of acute hemodialysis patients receiving porcine UFH (Yamamoto et al., 1996). Whether this is a real difference that reflects increased platelet activation (and PF4 release) during hemodialysis, or reflects a more sensitive definition of thrombocytopenia (any platelet count fall associated with line clotting) requires further investigation.

C. Frequency of HIT in Surgical Patients Treated with Porcine Mucosal UFH

Two large prospective studies suggest that HIT is an important problem in orthopedic patients receiving UFH (Warkentin et al., 1995a,b; Ganzer et al., 1997). When using a definition of a 50% fall in platelet count that began on or after day 5 of heparin treatment, and that was confirmed by serologic testing for HIT antibodies, both studies observed a frequency of HIT of about 5% (see Table 3). Each study used porcine mucosal heparin, derived from a different manufacturer, that was given by the subcutaneous route, at a dosage of 15,000 U/day. Thrombocytopenia that was likely attributable to HIT has also been observed in several other clinical trials of patients receiving UFH following orthopedic surgery (see Warkentin et al., 1995a for discussion), but only one study (Leyvraz et al., 1991) reported confirmatory in vitro testing.

There is little prospective information of the frequency of HIT in other postoperative surgical populations treated with UFH (see Table 3). Three studies have been performed on postoperative cardiac surgical patients who also received postoperative UFH in addition to high doses of heparin during preceding cardiopulmonary bypass (Trossaert et al., 1998; Warkentin et al., 1999; Pouplard et al., 1999; see Table 3). Pooling the three studies, about 2.3% of the patients developed serologically confirmed HIT. Interestingly the frequency of HIT in this population appears to be lower than in orthopedic patients receiving UFH, even though the cardiac surgical patients appear to have a higher frequency of formation of HIT antibodies (Warkentin et al., 1999).

D. HIT Is Less Frequent in Orthopedic Patients Receiving LMWH Compared with UFH Prophylaxis

Anecdotal reports indicate that HIT can occur during treatment with LMWH (Ball et al., 1989; Tardy et al., 1990; de Raucourt et al., 1996; Plath et al., 1997; Elalamy et al., 1996; Warkentin, 1998). Clinical trial data suggest that the frequency is low, however. Using a sensitive definition for HIT (> 50% fall on or after day 5 and confirmed by positive HIT antibodies), two studies in Hamilton found an overall frequency of only 4/439 (0.9%; 95% CI, 0.25–2.32%) for HIT complicating use of LMWH given for postoperative orthopedic patients (Warkentin et al., 1995a,b, 1998b). In contrast, using the same definition of HIT, patients who received UFH had a much higher frequency of HIT, 16/332 (4.8%; 95% CI, 2.78–7.71%) (Warkentin et al., 1995a,b). A similar high frequency of UFH-induced HIT was observed in a German study, 15/307 (4.9%; 95% CI, 2.76–7.93) (Ganzer et al., 1997).

The strongest evidence that LMWH is indeed associated with a lower frequency of HIT was provided by a randomized trial that directly compared the frequency of HIT between the two types of heparin (Warkentin et al., 1995a,b). The frequency of HIT in patients treated with the LMWH preparation, enoxaparin (itself derived from porcine mucosal heparin), was lower than that seen in patients treated with porcine UFH, irrespective of whether a standard definition (platelet fall to $< 150 \times 10^9$/L on or after day 5 of heparin treatment) or a more sensitive definition ($>$ 50% platelet count fall) of thrombocytopenia was used. The frequency of HIT antibody formation also differed between the two patient groups, using either the serotonin release assay (Warkentin et al., 1995a) or the PF4–heparin enzyme-linked immunoassay. Thrombocytopenia also appeared to be infrequent in other clinical efficacy trials of LMWH (Simonneau et al., 1997; ENOXACAN study group, 1997; Warkentin et al., 1995a).

E. Role of Incidental UFH Flushes in the Frequency of HIT

There are two ways that incidental exposure to heparin by ''flushing'' of intravascular catheters can affect the frequency or clinical effect of HIT. First, such minor heparin exposures can trigger formation of HIT antibodies (Ling and Warkentin, 1998; Warkentin et al., 1998b). And second, in patients who have already formed potent HIT antibodies for any reason, any ongoing or recurrent heparin exposure—including small-dose exposure—could lead to recurrence or exacerbation of thrombocytopenia. Indeed, several patients have been reported in whom severe HIT occurred while only small amounts of heparin were being given as flushes to maintain the patency of intravascular catheters (Kappa et al., 1987; Doty et al., 1986; Heeger and Backstrom 1986; Rama et al., 1991; Brushwood, 1992).

In most of the reports of patients developing HIT during LMWH treatment, recent prior exposure to UFH was not excluded. Indeed, incidental exposure to UFH by intraoperative invasive catheters could lead to formation of HIT antibodies that are inappropriately attributed to later postoperative LMWH prophylaxis (Shumate, 1995). However, if true, it would suggest that the apparent difference in immunogenicity between UFH and LMWH could be even greater than initially reported (Warkentin et al., 1995a,b,c).

To address this issue, a randomized, double-blind clinical trial was performed to test the hypothesis that incidental exposure to UFH by intraoperative invasive lines, rather than postoperative LMWH antithrombotic prophylaxis, was the predominant explanation for postoperative HIT antibody formation (Warkentin et al., 1998b). Patients were randomized to receive either UFH or normal saline flushes during surgery. However, the data obtained essentially ruled out the hypothesis: the frequency of HIT antibodies was not higher in the patients who were randomized to receive UFH flushes (2.2% vs. 2.7%; $p = 0.73$). Rather, the results suggested that postoperative LMWH prophylaxis administered to both groups was the predominant factor in causing HIT antibody formation. However, HIT antibody formation occurred in two patients who received UFH flushes, but who subsequently were given warfarin anticoagulation. Because intraoperative UFH flushes occasionally result in formation of high levels of HIT antibodies that can lead to life-threatening, acute HIT if therapeutic-dose UFH is administered a few weeks later (Ling and Warkentin, 1998), and because there is no clinical benefit to flushing intravascular catheters with UFH (Warkentin et al., 1998b), it seems reasonable to recommend that normal saline flushes be considered for routine flushing of intravascular catheters used during surgery.

F. HIT and Heparin-Coated Devices

Heparin can be bonded to artificial surfaces (Larsson et al., 1987), either through ionic attachment, as used for pulmonary artery catheters (Eldh and Jacobsson, 1974), or by end-linked covalent bonding (e.g., Carmeda BioActive Surface, or CBAS) (Larm et al., 1983). CBAS has been used for cardiopulmonary bypass circuits and filters (Borowiec et al., 1992a,b, 1993), extracorporeal membrane oxygenation (ECMO) devices (Koul et al., 1992), and coronary stents (Serruys et al., 1996). During use in patients, ionically attached heparin is displaced by albumin from the catheter surface, where it could contribute to HIT (discussed subsequently). End-linked heparin is an effective and longer-lasting anticoagulant, as the immobilized, but flexible, heparin chains are able to interact with fluid-phase antithrombin and thrombin (Elgue et al., 1993). Nevertheless, the end-linked, but relatively unconstrained, heparin is capable of interacting with PF4 (Suh et al., 1998). Therefore, it is theoretically possible that covalent heparin-bonded devices could result in formation of HIT antibodies, or could cause HIT in a patient who has formed antibodies. Alternatively, even covalently bonded heparin might ''leach'' into blood by proteolytic mechanisms, thereby contributing in a more conventional way to the pathogenesis of HIT (Almeida et al., 1998a).

Use of heparin-coated pulmonary catheters in contributing to HIT has been implicated by Laster and Silver (1988). These workers reported ten patients with HIT whose platelet counts did not rise until the removal of their heparin-coated pulmonary catheters, despite discontinuing all other sources of heparin. Incubation of the heparin-coated catheters with platelets in the presence of patient sera resulted in ''catheter-induced'' platelet aggregation. Based on the identification of four such cases, during which time 1112 heparin-coated catheters had been used, they estimated the frequency of catheter-associated HIT to be 0.4%.

G. HIT Caused by Other Sulfated Polysaccharides

The cryptic HIT autoantigen comprises conformationally altered PF4 when it forms a multimolecular complex with heparin. Other negatively charged polysaccharides can interact with PF4 to produce the HIT antigen (Wolf et al., 1983; Greinacher et al., 1992a,b,c; Anderson 1992; see Chap. 8). These considerations explain why a number of high-sulfated polysaccharides, ten or more subunits in length, have been reported to cause a syndrome of thrombocytopenia and thrombosis that essentially mimics HIT. These drugs include the semisynthetic 5-carbon subunit-based "heparinoid," pentosan polysulfate (Gouault-Heilman et al., 1985; Vitoux et al., 1985; Follea et al., 1986; Goad et al., 1994; Tardy-Poncet et al., 1994), as well as polysulfated chondroitin sulfate (Bouvier, 1980; Wolf et al., 1983; Greinacher et al., 1992a). The frequency of immune-mediated thrombocytopenia, with or without thrombosis, after exposure to these compounds is unknown, but may be high.

H. Variable Duration of Heparin Treatment

As HIT typically begins 5–10 days after starting therapy with heparin, it follows that the length of heparin treatment can influence the risk for HIT (e.g., a 10-day course is far more likely to produce clinical HIT than a 3-day treatment period). On the other hand, there is evidence that the risk of HIT begins to decrease after 10 days of uninterrupted heparin use (see Fig. 1C, Chap. 3). In a large study of postoperative orthopedic surgical patients receiving postoperative heparin prophylaxis, no patient developed HIT antibodies after day 10, even though many patients received heparin for up to 14 days (Warkentin et al., 1995a). These data are consistent with a "point exposure" model for risk of HIT in this patient population, such as a brief time shortly after surgery, when high circulating PF4 levels coincide with the first few subcutaneous heparin injections. However, even if HIT antibody formation occurs during the day 5- to 10-window period, thrombocytopenia itself can occur somewhat later, particularly if a larger dose of heparin is given, or UFH is substituted for LMWH (see Fig. 1A). The characteristic timing of HIT should assist clinicians in focusing their platelet count monitoring for HIT during the critical time period, so that the early diagnosis of HIT is improved (discussed subsequently).

I. Heparin Dose-Dependence in HIT

Analysis of individual patients with HIT often shows dose-dependence; that is, mild thrombocytopenia during subcutaneous heparin prophylaxis is followed by a marked drop in platelet count if the patient then receives therapeutic-dose heparin (Figs. 1A and B; see Fig. 5A in Chap. 11).

However, dose-dependence of HIT is not readily apparent when reviewing prospective studies of HIT (see Tables 2 and 3). However, this could be explained by differences in frequency of HIT among different patient populations that confounds the influence of heparin dose. For example, among medical patients, porcine UFH is more likely to result in HIT when given in therapeutic, rather than prophylactic, doses (0.7 vs. 0%; see Table 2). This difference, if real, could reflect dose-dependence of heparin in HIT. On the other hand, the relatively high frequency of HIT in surgical patients (up to 5%) receiving ''only'' prophylactic-dose porcine UFH more likely reflects differences in risk related to this patient population.

IV. FREQUENCY OF THROMBOSIS COMPLICATING HIT

Ironically, although thrombosis was the first manifestation of the HIT syndrome first recognized 40 years ago (Weismann and Tobin, 1958; Roberts et al., 1964), widespread recognition that thrombosis was a common complication of HIT did not occur until recently. Indeed, until 1995, no study of HIT had compared the frequency of thrombosis with a matched control population (Warkentin et al., 1995a). This study quantitated the strength of the association between HIT and thrombosis, and noted that the more unusual the thrombotic event (e.g., bilateral deep venous thrombosis, pulmonary embolism), the stronger the association with HIT (see Chap. 3).

Table 4 summarizes the thrombotic events that have been observed during prospective studies of HIT. The major observation is that thrombosis is relatively common in HIT patients, occurring in approximately one-third of medical patients, and about one-half of postoperative surgical patients. The data also support findings from a prior retrospective study (Boshkov et al., 1993) that found the type of thrombotic event complicating HIT was influenced by the patient population. Table 4 suggests that the ratio of arterial/venous thrombosis is about 1:1 in medical patients, many of whom might have had arterial disease as their basis for hospitalization. Additionally, the therapeutic-dose heparin used in many of these studies may have partially protected from venous thromboembolic complications, although it may not have prevented platelet-mediated arterial occlusion. In contrast, there appears to be a strong predisposition to venous thromboembolism in postoperative surgical patients who have developed HIT (ratio, venous/arterial, at least 14:1; see Table 4).

The retrospective identification of patients with serologically confirmed HIT permits analysis of large groups of HIT patients (Table 5). This provides an alternative assessment of the spectrum of thrombotic complications in HIT. Two large studies (Warkentin and Kelton, 1996; Nand et al., 1997) showed a predominance of venous thrombosis complicating HIT. Indeed, pulmonary embolism was even more frequent than all types of arterial thromboses combined.

In contrast, a different spectrum of thrombotic complications was reported by investigators at the University of Missouri–Columbia Health Sciences Center (Silver et al., 1983; Laster et al., 1987; Almeida et al., 1998b). Arterial, rather than venous, thromboembolism predominates in these patient series. Because this work is from the perspective of a vascular surgery service, it is possible that patients with arterial thrombosis are either more likely to be recognized as having HIT, or greater numbers of patients with preexisting arteriopathy are treated with heparin, and thus at higher risk for developing arterial thrombosis if HIT develops.

Another pattern that emerges from the Missouri series is a progressively decreasing frequency of reported thrombotic or hemorrhagic complications, from 61% in 1983, to 23% in 1987, then to 7.4% in 1998. The authors believe this to be the result of earlier recognition of HIT. A reduction in mortality associated with HIT has also been reported (see Table 5). Although HIT-associated mortality may be reduced by effective alternative anticoagulation (Greinacher et al., 1999), deaths for reasons unrelated to HIT are relatively common in HIT (Greinacher et al., 1999; Warkentin and Kelton, 1996).

It is possible that nonthrombotic mortality may be higher than expected by chance in patients with HIT. This speculation is based on the observation that only a minority of patients who form HIT antibodies develop HIT (discussed subsequently); a corollary to this statement is that comorbid factors that tend to result in increased pathogenicity of HIT antibodies may also independently contribute to increased patient morbidity and mortality (i.e., patients with septicemia or multisystem organ failure may be more likely to have platelet activation in the presence of HIT antibodies than ''well'' patients). Future comparative trials will be required to determine to what extent HIT-associated mortality can be influenced by antithrombotic or other treatment for HIT.

A. Natural History of Isolated HIT

Isolated HIT is defined as the initial recognition of HIT because of thrombocytopenia alone, rather than because symptoms or signs of thrombosis draw attention to the possibility of underlying HIT. A large retrospective cohort study (Warkentin and Kelton, 1996) suggests that the subsequent frequency of new, progressive, or recurrent thrombosis is relatively high in such a patient population with serologically confirmed HIT (Fig. 2). Although these data are retrospective, the investigators attempted to minimize bias. First, the date that the HIT assay was ordered was used as an objective marker of first suspicion of the diagnosis of HIT. Second, patients were excluded from analysis if there was any evidence in the medical records to suggest the possibility of new signs or symptoms of thrombosis that may have caused the physician to suspect HIT. In other words, efforts were made to identify patients in whom HIT was suggested because of thrombocytopenia alone. Finally, only objectively documented new, progressive, or recurrent thrombotic events were analyzed.

The study identified 62 patients who met the definition of isolated thrombocytopenia. The 30-day cumulative risk for thrombosis in this study was 52.8%

Table 4 Proportion of Patients with HIT Developing HIT-Associated Thrombosis in Prospective Studies Employing In Vitro Laboratory Testing or in Which Data on Timing of Platelet Count Fall Were Reported

Study	Major indication for heparin	In vitro test	Number treated	Definition of thrombocytopenia ($\times 10^9$/L)	Patients with HIT (using more sensitive definition of HIT)	Thrombotic complication of HIT	
						Venous	Arterial
Medical patients (only intravenous therapeutic-dose or hemodialysis included in table)							
Ansell et al., 1980	VTE	PRP(SR)	43	< 150	4	0	0
Green et al., 1984; Green, 1986	VTE	HIPA	89	< 150	2	1	1
Powers et al., 1984	VTE	SRA	65	< 150	3	1	0
Bailey et al., 1986	VTE, ATE	no test	43	< 100	1	0	1
Cipolle et al., 1983; Ramirez-Lassepas et al., 1984	Cerebrovascular ischemia	PRP	137[a]	< 100 (> 40% fall)	5 (16)	0 Not stated	1 (6)
Powers et al., 1979	VTE	no test	120	< 150	2	1	1
Gallus et al., 1980	VTE	PRP	166	< 100	5	1	0
Monreal et al., 1989	VTE	no test	89	< 100	2	1	0
Kakkasseril et al., 1985	VTE, ATE	PRP	142	< 100	9	2	2
Malcolm et al., 1979	Multiple	PRP	66	< 100	1	1	0
Kappers-Klunne et al., 1997	Acute coronary syndromes	HIPA, EIA	358	< 120, > 30% fall (< 60 or > 50% fall)	2 (1)	1 (1)	0 (0)
Yamamoto et al., 1996	Hemodialysis	PRP, EIA	154	Clotting, platelet fall	5	0	1
Total medical: Venous/arterial thrombosis ratio = 9/7 = 1.3			1472		41	9	7

Orthopedic surgical patients (total joint arthroplasty)							
Warkentin et al., 1995a,b	Hip	SRA	332	< 150 (> 50% fall)	9 (18)	7 (12)	1 (1)
Warkentin et al., 1998b	Hip, knee	SRA	246	< 150, > 50%	2	0	0
Ganzer et al., 1997	Hip, knee	HIPA	307	> 50% fall	15	5[c]	0
Leyvraz et al., 1991	Hip	PRP	175	< 100, > 40% fall	2	2	0
Total orthopedic: Venous/arterial thrombosis ratio = 14/1 = 14.0			1060		28 (37)	14 (19)	1 (1)
Surgical, other							
Louridas, 1991	Vascular	PRP[b]	114	< 100	5	0	0

Where there was uncertainty over the numbers of patients with HIT, the higher estimated value was indicated in the table, to minimize the bias toward a high frequency of HIT-associated thrombosis (contrast analysis shown in Table 2).

Abbreviations: ATE, arterial thromboembolism; EIA, PF4–heparin enzyme-linked immunosorbent assay; HIPA, heparin-induced platelet activation test (aggregation of washed platelets); LMWH, low molecular weight heparin; MI/ACS, myocardial infarction or acute coronary syndromes; PRP, HIT assay using citrated platelet-rich plasma (PRP/SR, with serotonin release); SRA, serotonin release assay using washed platelets; UFH, unfractionated heparin; VTE, venous thromboembolism.

[a] Detailed clinical data on thrombosis were available only on the subset of patients with cerebrovascular disease ($n = 137$).

[b] Ineffective testing was used (platelet aggregation without heparin).

[c] Another five patients developed venous thrombosis in association with a positive HIPA assay, but the platelet count did not fall by > 50%.

Table 5 Frequency of Thrombosis Complicating HIT in Retrospective Treatment Cohort Studies

Study	Patients with HIT	Mean platelet count nadir ($\times 10^9$/L)	Patients with thrombosis (%)	Ratio of venous/arterial thrombosis	Number of deaths (%)
Warkentin and Kelton, 1996	127	59[a]	97 (76%)	4.3	26 (20%)
Subgroup with "isolated" thrombocytopenia	62	57	32 (52%)[b]	4	13 (21%)
Nand et al., 1997	108	58	32 (29%)	2.5	5 (5%)[c]
Silver et al., 1983	62	Range: 5–83	38 (61%)	0.6	20 (32%)[d]
Laster et al., 1987	169	57	30 (18%)	0.5	20 (12%)
Almeida et al., 1998b	94[e]	>108	7 (7%)	0.6[f]	0 (0%)

[a] The *mean* platelet count nadir for 127 patients with HIT and platelet count $< 150 \times 10^9$/L, and the *median* platelet count nadir for all 142 patients diagnosed with HIT (including those whose platelet count nadir was $\geq 150 \times 10^9$/L), were both 59×10^9/L (Warkentin, 1998a; see Fig. 3 in Chap. 3).

[b] The cumulative 30-day frequency of new thrombosis in patients with isolated thrombocytopenia following recognition of HIT was 52.8% by Kaplan-Meier analysis.

[c] Only deaths in patients who developed thrombosis were reported. Total number of deaths in the HIT cohort was not reported.

[d] Fourteen of the 20 deaths were judged to be caused by HIT-associated thrombosis.

[e] Of 100 consecutive patients with positive in vitro testing, 6 were previously known to have heparin-dependent antibodies and were not subsequently reexposed to heparin.

[f] Two thromboses of arteriovenous grafts were excluded from classification into arterial or venous thrombosis.

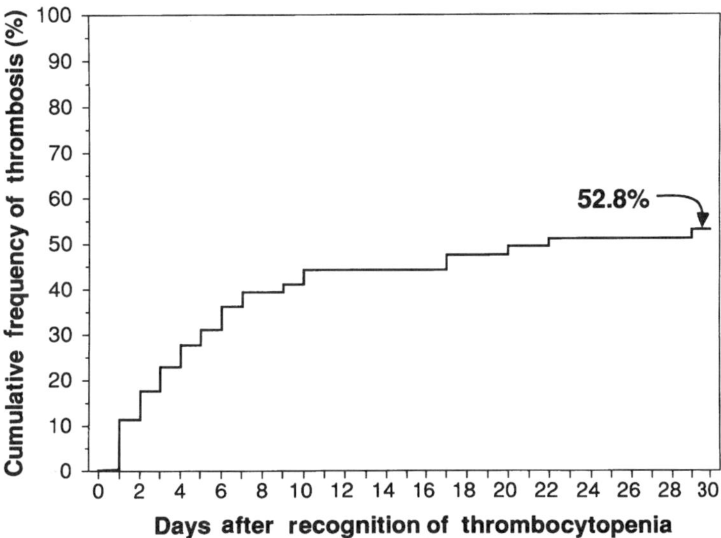

Figure 2 Cumulative frequency of thrombosis in HIT patients presenting with isolated thrombocytopenia. Approximately 50% of HIT patients initially recognized with isolated thrombocytopenia developed objective evidence for thrombosis during the subsequent 30-day period. The 1- and 2-day thrombotic event rates were approximately 10 and 18%, respectively. (From Warkentin and Kelton, 1996.)

(see Fig. 2). This risk did not differ whether the heparin had been discontinued, or whether warfarin had been substituted for the heparin. Similar findings were reported from a much smaller earlier study performed in Europe (Boon et al., 1994). This high risk for thrombosis in HIT is also supported by a prospective study (Warkentin et al., 1995a), in which five of six HIT patients either developed thrombosis on the first day that their platelet count fell below 150 × 10^9/L, or within the next few days despite the discontinuation of heparin.

B. Summary of Observations from Prospective and Retrospective Studies

Observations emerging from these studies include the following:

1. The risk of thrombosis in patients with HIT is higher than previously recognized (up to 50%), and remains high despite the discontinuation of heparin. Mortality in patients with HIT is significant, although it

remains uncertain what proportion is related to HIT-associated thrombosis, and whether these can be prevented by effective treatment.

2. Most thrombotic events are venous, rather than arterial, although this predominance may not be observed in patient populations at high risk for arterial disease. Pulmonary embolism may be the most frequent life-threatening manifestation of HIT.

V. POPULATION-BASED STUDIES OF HIT ANTIBODY SEROCONVERSION

Usually, serological investigation for HIT antibodies is performed on patients who develop thrombocytopenia during heparin treatment. Since 1995, however, nine studies have performed systematic studies of HIT antibody seroconversion, using sensitive assays (EIA, SRA, or both), irrespective of whether or not thrombocytopenia occurred. Some interesting insights into the pathogenesis of HIT have emerged from these reports (Warkentin et al., 1995a,b, 1998b, 1999; Amiral et al., 1996; Visentin et al., 1996; Kappers-Klunne et al., 1997; Bauer et al., 1997; Trossaert et al., 1998; Pouplard et al., 1999).

As shown in Table 6, three general types of patient population have been investigated: medical patients receiving therapeutic-dose UFH; orthopedic patients receiving UFH or LMWH; and cardiac surgical patients receiving UFH or LMWH. There appear to be distinct frequencies of HIT antibody formation, as well as varying risks of ''breakthrough'' of HIT, among these different populations (Fig. 3). Several observations emerge from these studies:

1. The prevalence of seroconversion depends on the diagnostic assay used. PF4–heparin EIA is more sensitive than the SRA for the detection of HIT antibodies (Bauer et al., 1997; Warkentin et al., 1999; Pouplard et al., 1999); however, this increase in sensitivity does not necessarily translate into greater predictive value for clinical HIT (see Chap. 11).
2. With use of PF4–heparin EIA, the frequency of seroconversion following cardiac surgery approaches 50% in three of the studies (Visentin et al., 1996; Bauer et al., 1997; Warkentin et al., 1999). A high frequency of seroconversion (13–20%) was also observed using the SRA. Despite the highest frequency of HIT seroconversion reported in this patient population, the likelihood of developing HIT appears to be less than in another patient population also treated with postoperative UFH (orthopedic surgery).
3. Seroconversion occurs frequently without thrombocytopenia or thrombosis. Indeed, most patients who form HIT antibodies do not develop

HIT. The proportion who develop HIT, however, is highest among the patients who have a positive SRA. This suggests that HIT antibodies ''strong'' enough to activate platelets are more likely to be clinically significant. Patient-dependent factors also must be important, however, because the probability of a positive SRA indicating clinical HIT ranges from about < 10% (cardiac surgery) to approximately 50% (orthopedic surgery).

4. Regardless of which diagnostic assay is used, new seroconversion occurs more frequently after exposure to UFH than LMWH (Warkentin et al., 1995a,b, 1999; Amiral et al., 1996).

A. HIT in Patients Undergoing Cardiac Surgery

Three prospective studies have evaluated the frequency of HIT in postoperative cardiac surgical patients who also have received postoperative antithrombotic prophylaxis with UFH (Trossaert et al., 1998; Pouplard et al., 1999; Warkentin et al., 1998). Pooling the data, the frequency of HIT appears to be about 2% (7/307 = 2.3%). This frequency is consistent with a number of retrospective studies (Glock et al., 1988; Walls et al., 1992a,b; Singer et al., 1993) that reported a frequency of HIT of up to 5%, but overall, also noted a frequency of about 2% (Table 7). Furthermore, HIT was associated with a risk of thrombosis of 38–81%, and with an overall mortality of 18–43% in these studies. In contrast to the orthopedic patient population, the predominant thrombotic event appears to be arterial, in keeping with the increased risk of associated arterial vasculopathy in this patient population.

VI. VARIABLE FREQUENCY OF HIT: IMPLICATIONS FOR PLATELET COUNT MONITORING

Until recently, studies of HIT frequency have yielded seemingly confusing and inconsistent results. However, as argued in this chapter, by taking into consideration (1) type of heparin used, (2) patient population treated, and (3) laboratory and clinical evidence to distinguish (immune) HIT from nonimmune HAT, distinct profiles for HIT antibody seroconversion, HIT itself, and HIT-associated thrombosis can be discerned (see Fig. 3). New research questions will be generated in the search for the biological basis for these intriguing differences in HIT risk. But perhaps the most important insight to emerge from these collective studies is the simple and clinically relevant observation that new, progressive, or recurrent thrombosis occurs in about 33–50% of patients who develop proven HIT. This underscores the need for prompt recognition and urgent therapy in all patients suspected of having this adverse drug reaction.

Table 6 Studies Describing Systematic Screening for HIT Antibodies Using Sensitive Assays in Patients Receiving Heparin

Study	Trial design	Heparin (porcine UFH used unless otherwise indicated)	HIT assay used	Number of patients	Patients with HIT antibodies (%)	Patients with HIT (%)
Medical patients						
Amiral et al., 1996	Retrospective	iv ther UFH	EIA-IgM/A/G EIA-IgG	109	19 (17.4) 3 (2.8)	1 (0.9)[a]
Kappers-Klunne et al., 1997	Prospective	iv ther UFH	EIA-IgG HIPA	358	9 (2.5) 30 (8.4)	2 (0.6) 0 (0)
Hemodialysis patients						
Greinacher et al., 1996	Prevalence study	iv ther UFH	HIPA	165	7 (4.2%)	0 (0)
de Sancho et al., 1996	Prevalence study	iv ther UFH	EIA-IgM/A/G	45	0 (0)	0 (0)
		iv ther UFH	EIA-IgM/G EIA-IgG	128	4 (3.1) 3 (2.3)	0 (0)[b]
Boon et al., 1996	Prevalence study					
		LMWH	EIA-IgM/G EIA-IgG	133	1 (0.8) 1 (0.8)	0 (0)[b]
Luzzatto et al., 1998	Prevalence study	iv ther UFH	EIA-IgG	50	6 (12.0)	0 (0)
Orthopedic postoperative surgical patients						
		sc proph UFH	EIA-IgG SRA	205	29 (14.1) 19 (9.3)	10 (4.9)
Warkentin et al., 1995a,b; 1999	Substudy of RCT					
		sc proph LMWH	EIA-IgG SRA	182	11 (6.0) 5 (2.7)[c]	2 (1.1)
Warkentin et al., 1999	Prospective	sc proph LMWH	EIA-IgG SRA	257	22 (8.6) 9 (3.5)[c]	2 (0.8)
Amiral et al., 1996	Retrospective	sc proph LMWH	EIA-IgM/A/G EIA-IgG	100	8 (8.0) 2 (2.0)	0 (0)

Cardiac postoperative surgical patients (all received porcine UFH at cardiopulmonary bypass except where otherwise stated)						
Visentin et al., 1996	Retrospective	CPB: UFH	EIA-IgM/G		27 (61.4)[d]	0 (0)
		No postoperative heparin	EIA-IgG	44	23 (52.3)	
Bauer et al., 1997	Prospective	CPB: bovine UFH	EIA-IgM/A/G		57 (51.4)[e]	0 (0)
		(no postoperative heparin)	SRA	111	23 (52.3)	
Trossaert et al., 1998	Retrospective	CPB: UFH	EIA-IgM/A/G		14 (27.5)[f]	
		sc proph UFH	EIA-IgG	51	9 (17.6)	0 (0)
			PRP		2 (3.9)	
			EIA-IgM/A/G		46 (29.3)	
Pouplard et al., 1999	Prospective	sc proph UFH	EIA-IgG	157	24 (15.3)	6 (3.8)
			SRA		6 (3.8)	
			EIA-IgM/A/G		37 (21.6)	
		sc proph LMWH	EIA-IgG	171	24 (14.0)	0 (0)
			SRA		2 (1.2)	
Warkentin et al., 1999	Prospective	CPB: UFH	EIA-IgG	100	50 (50.0)	1 (1.0)
		sc proph UFH	SRA		20 (20.0)	
Vascular surgical patients						
Jackson et al., 1998	Prospective	iv ther UFH	EIA-IgM/G	54	3 (5.6)[g]	

Although Romeril et al. (1982) were the first to report the systematic testing of all patients, this study was excluded because the test used was insensitive.

Abbreviations: CPB, cardiopulmonary bypass; EIA, PF4–heparin enzyme-linked immunosorbent assay (-IgM/A/G, one or more of IgM, IgA, and IgG antibodies present; -IgG, IgG antibodies only present); iv ther, intravenous therapeutic-dose heparin; LMWH, low molecular weight heparin; MI, myocardial infarction; RCT, randomized controlled trial; sc proph, subcutaneous prophylactic-dose heparin; SRA, serotonin release assay using washed platelets; UFH, unfractionated heparin; VTE, venous thromboembolism.

[a] Thrombocytopenia defined as platelet count fall > 50% from baseline.

[b] Two patients with HIT antibodies had mild thrombocytopenia, but a causal relation to heparin was not stated.

[c] 20% serotonin release used in Warkentin et al. (1999) rather than 50% serotonin release cutoff used in Warkentin et al. (1995a).

[d] Ten patients had HIT-IgG preoperatively: incidence of new seroconversion was 17/44 (38.6%).

[e] Incidence of new seroconversion was 43% for EIA and 9% for SRA.

[f] Two patients had HIT-IgG preoperatively: incidence of new seroconversion was 12/51 (23.5%) for EIA-IgM/A/G and 7/51 (13.7%) for EIA-IgG. None had a positive aggregation assay preoperatively.

[g] Two patients had HIT-IgG preoperatively: incidence of new seroconversion was 1/54 (1.9%).

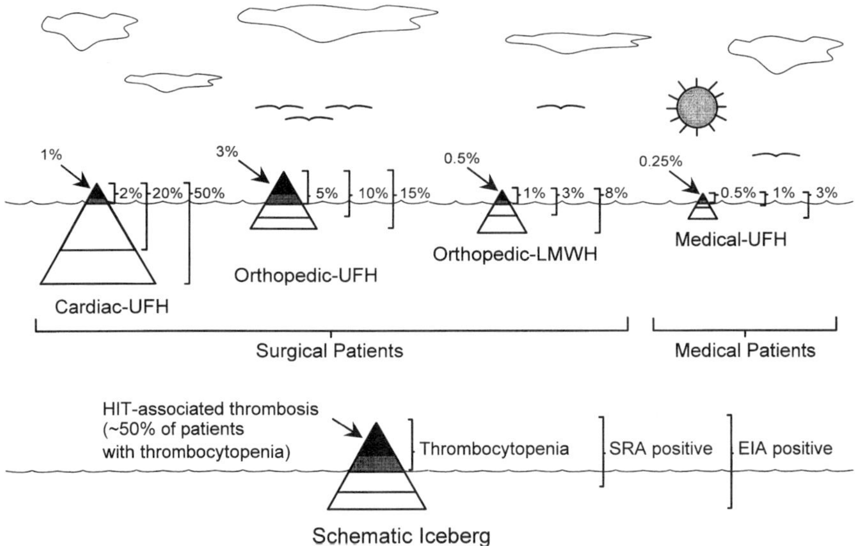

Figure 3 Variable frequency of HIT antibody formation and clinical HIT among different patient populations treated with unfractionated heparin (UFH) or low molecular weight heparin (LMWH). A schematic "iceberg," shown on lower line, illustrates the relation among HIT-associated thrombosis, thrombocytopenia, HIT antibodies detected by serotonin release assay (SRA), and HIT antibodies detected by enzyme-immunoassay (EIA). The size of the iceberg reflects the relative frequency of HIT antibody formation by EIA (i.e., the cardiac–UFH iceberg is about six times larger than the orthopedic–LMWH iceberg [50 vs. 8% frequency of HIT antibody formation]. Noteworthy aspects include the observation that HIT-associated thrombosis is most common in orthopedic–UFH patients, even though HIT antibody formation is most common in cardiac–UFH patients, and the observation that orthopedic–LMWH has a higher frequency of thrombosis than does medical–UFH.

Practically, these findings suggest strategies for platelet count monitoring in patients receiving heparin. Many physicians are reluctant to institute regular platelet count monitoring for HIT. One explanation is the almost ubiquitous use of heparin in hospitalized patients. Thus, a requirement that regular, perhaps even daily, platelet count monitoring be performed seems excessive. Additionally, there is no convincing evidence that regular platelet count monitoring can prevent the thrombotic complications of HIT. Indeed, a prospective study (Warkentin et al., 1995a) that employed daily platelet count monitoring, and in which heparin administration was generally stopped when the platelet count fell to less than

Table 7 Frequency of HIT and Thrombosis in Retrospective Studies of HIT in Cardiovascular Surgery Patients

Study	Patients at risk *n*	Patients with HIT *n* (%)	Patients with HIT and thrombosis *n* (%)	Ratio of venous: arterial thrombosis	Total deaths in patients with HIT *n* (%)
Walls et al., 1992a	4261	82 (1.9)	31 (38)	0.3:1	23 (28)
Walls et al., 1992b	764	35 (4.5)	17 (49)	0.3:1	15 (43)
Visentin et al., 1996	51	0 (0)	—	—	—
Glock et al., 1988	—	21	17 (81)	0.7:1	8 (38)
Singer et al., 1993	1500	11 (0.75)	7 (64)[a]	0.3:1[b]	2 (18)

[a] In seven patients, 17 thrombotic events occurred.

[b] Precise number of arterial and venous events is unclear from the published data. For this analysis, of six limb amputations associated with intravascular catheters or devices, five were assumed to be arterial and one venous, based on the type of intravascular catheter or device that was associated with the amputated limb.

150×10^9/L, observed thrombosis in eight of nine patients who met this platelet count definition for HIT.

These comments notwithstanding, marked differences in risk for HIT are apparent among different patient populations. Thus, it seems prudent to recommend that patients at the highest risk of HIT, and for HIT-associated thrombosis (e.g., postoperative patients receiving UFH, or any patient receiving bovine lung UFH) should have platelet counts monitored regularly, ranging from at least three times per week to daily testing. For patients whose risk for HIT appears to be 1% or less (e.g., medical patients receiving UFH, surgical patients receiving LMWH), many physicians probably feel that regular monitoring is unnecessary. Since HIT is unlikely to occur before day 5, or after day 10, the monitoring could be performed on days 4, 6, 8, and 10 (every-other-day monitoring), or daily from days 4 to 10. Most patients have frequent complete blood counts performed on the first few days of hospitalization, so comparative platelet count results for days 0–3 are usually available.

Regardless of the intensity of surveillance, all physicians who monitor platelet counts need to understand how to distinguish HIT from nonimmune HAT, because diagnostic confusion may lead to inappropriate decisions to discontinue heparin therapy in patients with nonimmune HAT who otherwise require anticoagulation because of high risk for thrombosis. Irrespective of whether platelet count monitoring is being performed, HIT should be considered promptly in the differential diagnosis of any patient who develops symptoms or signs of new, progressive, or recurrent thrombosis during, or within a few days of discontinuing, heparin treatment.

ACKNOWLEDGMENTS

Studies described in this chapter were supported by grants from the Heart and Stroke Foundation of Ontario, and were performed when Dr. Warkentin was a Research Scholar of the Heart and Stroke Foundation of Canada. Dr. Lee was supported by a Research Fellowship from the Heart and Stroke Foundation of Canada.

REFERENCES

Almeida JI, Liem TK, Silver D. Heparin-bonded grafts induce platelet aggregation in the presence of heparin-associated antiplatelet antibodies. J Vasc Surg 27:896–901, 1998a.

Almeida JI, Coats R, Liem TK, Silver D. Reduced morbidity and mortality rates of the heparin-induced thrombocytopenia syndrome. J Vasc Surg 27:309–316, 1998b.

Alving BM, Shulman NR, Bell WR, Evatt BL, Tack KM. In vitro studies of heparin-induced thrombocytopenia. Thromb Res 11:827–834, 1977.

Amiral J, Peynaud-Debayle E, Wolf M, Bridey F, Vissac A-M, Meyer D. Generation of antibodies to heparin-PF4 complexes without thrombocytopenia in patients treated with unfractionated or low-molecular-weight heparin. Am J Hematol 52:90–95, 1996.

Anderson GP. Insights into heparin-induced thrombocytopenia. Br J Haematol 80:504–508, 1992.

Ansell J, Slepchuk N Jr, Kumar R, Lopez A, Southard L, Deykin D. Heparin-induced thrombocytopenia: a prospective study. Thromb Haemost 43:61–65, 1980.

Ansell JE, Price JM, Shah S, Beckner RR. Heparin-induced thrombocytopenia: What is its real frequency? Chest 88:878–882, 1985.

Bailey RT Jr, Ursick JA, Heim KL, Hilleman DE, Reich JW. Heparin-associated thrombocytopenia: a prospective comparison of bovine lung heparin, manufactured by new process, and porcine intestinal heparin. Drug Intell Clin Pharm 20:374–378, 1986.

Ball A, L'Huillier AM, Dreyfuss L, Porte JL, Barthel JC. Thrombopénie à la Fraxiparine. Une observation. Presse Méd 18:1254–1255, 1989.

Barradas MA, Mikhailidis DP, Epemolu O, Jeremy JY, Fonseca V, Dandona P. Comparison of the platelet proaggregatory effect of conventional unfractionated heparins and a low molecular weight heparin fraction (CY 222). Br J Haematol 67:451–457, 1987.

Bauer TL, Arepally G, Konkle BA, Mestichelli B, Shapiro SS, Cines DB, Poncz M, McNulty S, Amiral J, Hauck WW, Edie RN, Mannion JC. Prevalence of heparin-associated antibodies without thrombosis in patients undergoing cardiopulmonary bypass surgery. Circulation 95:1242–1246, 1997.

Bell WR. Heparin-associated thrombocytopenia and thrombosis. J Lab Clin Med 111: 600–605, 1988.

Bell WR, Royall RM. Heparin-associated thrombocytopenia: a comparison of three heparin preparations. N Engl J Med 303:902–907, 1980.

Bell WR, Tomasulo PA, Alving FM, Duffy TP. Thrombocytopenia occurring during the administration of heparin. A prospective study in 52 patients. Ann Intern Med 85: 155–160, 1976.

Boon DMS, Michiels JJ, Stibbe J, van Vliet HHDM, Kappers-Klunne MC. Heparin-induced thrombocytopenia and antithrombotic therapy [letter]. Lancet 344:1296, 1994.

Boon DMS, van Vliet HHDM, Zietse R, Kappers-Klunne MC. The presence of antibodies against a PF4–heparin complex in patients on haemodialysis [letter]. Thromb Haemost 76:480, 1996.

Borowiec J, Thelin S, Bagge L, Hultman J, Hansson H-E. Decreased blood loss after cardiopulmonary bypass using heparin-coated circuit and 50% reduction of heparin dose. Scand J Thorac Cardiovasc Surg 26:177–185, 1992a.

Borowiec J, Thelin S, Bagge L, Nilsson L, Venge P, Hansson HE. Heparin-coated circuits reduce activation of granulocytes during cardiopulmonary bypass. A clinical study. J Thorac Cardiovasc Surg 104:642–667, 1992b.

Borowiec JW, Bylock A, van der Linden J, Thelin S. Heparin coating reduces blood cell adhesion to arterial filters during coronary bypass: a clinical study. Ann Thorac Surg 55:1540–1545, 1993.

Boshkov LK, Warkentin TE, Hayward CPM, Andrew M, Kelton JG. Heparin-induced thrombocytopenia and thrombosis: clinical and laboratory studies. Br J Haematol 84:322–328, 1993.

Bouvier C. In: Van Aken WG. Thrombocytopenia (and consumption coagulopathy) induced by heparin. A case report [discussion]. Scand J Haematol 25(suppl 36):85–90, 1980.

Brushwood DB. Hospital liable for allergic reaction to heparin used in injection flush. Am J Hosp Pharm 49:1491–1492, 1992.

Casu B, Johnson EA, Mantovani M, Mulloy B, Oreste P, Pescador R, Prino G, Torri G, Zoppetti G. Correlation between structure, fat-clearing and anticoagulant properties of heparins and heparan sulphates. Arzneimittal, forschung Drug Res 33:135–142, 1983.

Chong BH, Castaldi PA. Platelet proaggregating effect of heparin: possible mechanism for nonimmune heparin-associated thrombocytopenia. Aust NZ J Med 16:715–716, 1986.

Chong BH, Berndt MC. Heparin-induced thrombocytopenia. Blut 58:53–57, 1989.

Chong BH, Ismail F. The mechanism of heparin-induced platelet aggregation. Eur J Haematol 43:245–251, 1989.

Cipolle RJ, Rodvoid KA, Seifert R, Clarens R, Ramirez-Lassepas M. Heparin-associated thrombocytopenia: a prospective evaluation of 211 patients. Ther Drug Monit 5: 205–211, 1983.

de Raucourt E, Vinsonneau C, Juvin K, Fischer AM, Meyer G. Heparin-induced thrombocytopenia with thrombotic complications during prophylactic treatment with low-molecular-weight heparin. Blood Coagul Fibrinolysis 7:786–788, 1996.

de Sancho M, Lema MG, Amiral J, Rand J. Frequency of antibodies directed against heparin–platelet factor 4 in patients exposed to heparin through chronic hemodialysis [letter]. Thromb Haemost 75:695–696, 1996.

Doty JR, Alving BM, McDonnell DE, Ondra SL. Heparin-associated thrombocytopenia in the neurosurgical patient. Neurosurgery 19:69–72, 1986.

Elalamy I, Potevin F, Lecrubier C, Bara L, Marie JP, Samama MM. A fatal low-molecular-weight heparin-associated thrombocytopenia after hip surgery: possible usefulness of PF4–heparin ELISA test. Blood Coagul Fibrinolysis 7:665–671, 1996.

Eldh P, Jacobsson B. Heparinized vascular catheters: a clinical trial. Radiology 111:289–292, 1974.

Elgue G, Blombäck M, Olsson P, Riesenfeld J. On the mechanism of coagulation inhibition on surfaces with end point immobilized heparin. Thromb Haemost 70:289–293, 1993.

ENOXACAN Study Group. Efficacy and safety of enoxaparin versus unfractionated heparin for prevention of deep vein thrombosis in elective cancer surgery: a double-blind randomized multicentre trial with venographic assessment. Br J Surg 84: 1099–1103, 1997.

Follea G, Hamandijan I, Trzeciak MC, Nedey C, Streichenberger R, Dechavanne M. Pentosane polysulfate associated thrombocytopenia. Thromb Res 42:413–418, 1986.

Gallus AS, Goodall KT, Beswick W, Chesterman CN. Heparin-associated thrombocytopenia: case report and prospective study. Aust NZ J Med 10:25–31, 1980.

Ganzer D, Gutezeit A, Mayer G, Greinacher A, Eichler P. Thromboembolieprophylaxe als auslöser thrombembolischer Komplicationen. Eine Untersuchung zur inzidenz der Heparin-induzierten Thrombozytopenie (HIT) Typ II. Z Orthop 135:543–549, 1997.

Glock Y, Szmil E, Boudjema B, Boccalon H, Fournial G, Cerene AL, Puel P. Cardiovascular surgery and heparin-induced thrombocytopenia. Int Angiol 7:238–245, 1988.

Goad KE, Horne MK III, Gralnick HR. Pentosan-induced thrombocytopenia: support for an immune complex mechanism. Br J Haematol 88:803–808, 1994.

Gouault-Heilman M, Payen D, Contant G, Intrator L, Huet Y, Schaeffer A. Thrombocytopenia related to synthetic heparin analogue therapy [letter]. Thromb Haemost 54: 557, 1985.

Green D. Heparin-induced thrombocytopenia. Med J Aust 144(suppl):HS37–HS39, 1986.

Green D, Martin GJ, Shoichet SH, DeBacker N, Bomalaski JS, Lind RN. Thrombocytopenia in a prospective, randomized, double-blind trial of bovine and porcine heparin. Am J Med Sci 288:60–64, 1984.

Greinacher A. Antigen generation in heparin-associated thrombocytopenia: the nonimmunologic type and the immunologic type are closely linked in their pathogenesis. Semin Thromb Hemostas 21:106–116, 1995.

Greinacher A, Michels I, Schäfer M, Kiefel V, Muller-Eckhardt C. Heparin-associated thrombocytopenia in a patient treated with polysulphated chondroitin sulphate: evidence for immunological crossreactivity between heparin and polysulphated glycosaminoglycan. Br J Haematol 81:252–254, 1992a.

Greinacher A, Drost W, Michels I, Leitl J, Gottsmann M, Kohl HG, Glaser M, Mueller-Eckhardt C. Heparin-associated thrombocytopenia successfully treated with the

heparinoid Org 10172 in a patient showing cross-reaction to LMW heparins. Ann Haematol 64:40–42, 1992b.
Greinacher A, Michels I, Muller-Eckardt C. Heparin-associated thrombocytopenia: the antibody is not heparin-specific. Thromb Haemost 67:545–549, 1992c.
Greinacher A, Amiral J, Dummel V, Vissac A, Keifel V, Mueller-Eckhardt C. Laboratory diagnosis of heparin-associated thrombocytopenia and comparison of platelet aggregation test, heparin-induced platelet activation test, and platelet factor 4/heparin enzyme-linked immunosorbent assay. Transfusion 34:381–385, 1994.
Greinacher A, Zinn S, Wizemann, Birk UW. Heparin-induced antibodies as a risk factor for thromboembolism and haemorrhage in patients undergoing chronic haemodialysis [letter]. Lancet 348:764, 1996.
Greinacher A, Völpel H, Janssens U, Hach-Wunderle V, Kemkes-Matthes B, Eichler P, Mueller-Velten HG, Pötzsch B. Recombinant hirudin (lepirudin) provides effective and safe anticoagulation in patients with the immunologic type of heparin-induced thrombocytopenia. Circulation 99:73–80, 1999.
Heeger PS, Backstrom JT. Heparin flushes and thrombocytopenia [letter]. Ann Intern Med 105:143, 1986.
Holm HA, Eika C, Laake K. Thrombocytoes and treatment with heparin from porcine mucosa. Scand J Haematol 36(suppl):81–84, 1980.
Jackson MR, Gillespie DL, Chang AS, Longenecker EG, Peat RA, Alving B. The incidence of heparin-induced antibodies in patients undergoing vascular surgery: a prospective study. J Vasc Surg 28:439–445, 1998.
Johnson RA, Lazarus KH, Henry DH. Heparin-induced thrombocytopenia: a prospective study. Am J Hematol 17:349–353, 1984.
Kakkasseril JS, Cranley JJ, Panke T, Grannan K. Heparin-induced thrombocytopenia: a prospective study of 142 patients. J Vasc Surg 2:382–384, 1985.
Kappa JR, Fisher CA, Berkowitz HD, Cottrell ED, Addonizio VP Jr. Heparin-induced platelet activation in sixteen surgical patients: diagnosis and management. J Vasc Surg 5:101–109, 1987.
Kappers-Klunne MC, Boon DMS, Hop WCJ, Michiels JJ, Stibbe J, van der Zwaan C, Koudstaal PJ, van Vliet HHDM. Heparin-induced thrombocytopenia and thrombosis: a prospective analysis of the incidence in patients with heart and cerebrovascular diseases. Br J Haematol 96:442–446, 1997.
Kelton JG. Heparin-induced thrombocytopenia. Haemostasis 16:173–186, 1986.
Koul B, Vesterqvist O, Egberg N, Steen S. Twenty-four–hour heparin-free veno–right ventricular ECMO: an experimental study. Ann Thorac Surg 53:1046–1051, 1992.
Larm O, Larsson R, Olsson P. A new non-thrombogenic surface prepared by selective covalent binding of heparin via a modified reducing terminal residue. Biomater Med Devices Artif Organs 11:161–173, 1983.
Larsson R, Larm O, Olsson P. The search for thromboresistance using immobilized heparin. Ann NY Acad Sci 516:102–115, 1987.
Laster J, Silver D. Heparin-coated catheters and heparin-induced thrombocytopenia. J Vasc Surg 7:667–672, 1988.
Laster J, Cikrit D, Walker N, Silver D. The heparin-induced thrombocytopenia syndrome: an update. Surgery 102:763–770, 1987.
Lee DH, Warkentin TE, Denomme GA, Hayward CPM, Kelton JG. A diagnostic test for

heparin-induced thrombocytopenia: detection of platelet microparticles using flow cytometry. Br J Haematol 95:724–731, 1996.

Leyvraz PF, Bachmann F, Hoek J, Büller HR, Postel M, Samama M, Vandenbroek MD. Prevention of deep vein thrombosis after hip replacement: randomised comparison between unfractionated heparin and low molecular weight heparin. Br Med J 303: 543–548, 1991.

Ling E, Warkentin TE. Intraoperative heparin flushes and subsequent acute heparin-induced thrombocytopenia. Anesthesiology 89:1567–1569, 1998.

Look KA, Sahud M, Flaherty S, Zehnder JL. Heparin-induced platelet aggregation vs platelet factor 4 enzyme-linked immunosorbent assay in the diagnosis of heparin-induced thrombocytopenia–thrombosis. Am J Clin Pathol 108:78–82, 1997.

Louridas G. Heparin-induced thrombocytopenia. S Afr J Surg 29:50–52, 1991.

Luzzatto G, Bertoli M, Cella G, Fabris F, Zaia B, Girolami A. Platelet count, anti-heparin/platelet factor 4 antibodies and tissue factor pathway inhibitor plasma antigen level in chronic dialysis. Thromb Res 89:115–122, 1998.

Malcolm ID, Wigmore TA, Steinbrecher UP. Heparin-associated thrombocytopenia: low frequency in 104 patients treated with heparin of intestinal mucosal origin. Can Med Assoc J 120:1086–1088, 1979.

Monreal M, Lafoz, E, Salvador R, Roncales J, Navarro A. Adverse effects of three different forms of heparin therapy: thrombocytopenia, increased transaminases, and hyperkalemia. Eur J Clin Pharmacol 37:415–418, 1989.

Nand S, Wong W, Yuen B, Yetter A, Schmulbach E, Gross Fisher S. Heparin-induced thrombocytopenia with thrombosis: incidence, analysis of risk factors, and clinical outcomes in 108 consecutive patients treated at a single institution. Am J Hematol 56:12–16, 1997.

Nelson JC, Lerner RG, Goldstein R, Cagin NA. Heparin-induced thrombocytopenia. Arch Intern Med 138:548–552, 1978.

Plath J, Schulze R, Barz D, Krammer B, Steiner M, Anders O, Mach J. Necrotizing skin lesions induced by low-molecular-weight heparin after total knee arthroplasty. Arch Orthop Trauma Surg 116:443–445, 1997.

Pouplard C, May MA, Iochmann S, Amiral J, Vissac AM, Marchand M, Gruel Y. Antibodies to platelet factor 4-heparin after cardiopulmonary bypass in patients anticoagulated with unfractionated heparin or a low-molecular-weight heparin: clinical implications for heparin-induced thrombocytopenia. Circulation 99:2530–2536, 1999.

Powers PJ, Cuthbert D, Hirsh J. Thrombocytopenia found uncommonly during heparin therapy. JAMA 241:2396–2397, 1979.

Powers PJ, Kelton JG, Carter CJ. Studies on the frequency of heparin-associated thrombocytopenia. Thromb Res 33:439–443, 1984.

Rao AK, White GC, Sherman L, Colman R, Lan G, Ball AP. Low incidence of thrombocytopenia with porcine mucosal heparin. A prospective multicentre study. Arch Intern Med 149:1285–1288, 1989.

Rama BN, Haake RE, Bander SJ, Ghasem-Zadeh A, Gorla C. Heparin-flush associated thrombocytopenia-induced hemorrhage: a case report. Nebr Med J 76:392–394, 1991.

Ramirez-Lassepas M, Cipolle RJ, Rodvold KA, Seifert RD, Strand L, Taddeini L, Cusulos M. Heparin-induced thrombocytopenia in patients with cerebrovascular ischemic disease. Neurology 34:736–740, 1984.

Roberts B, Rosato FE, Rosato EF. Heparin—a cause of arterial emboli? Surgery 55:803–808, 1964.

Romeril KR, Hickton CM, Hamer JW, Heaton DC. Heparin-induced thrombocytopenia: case reports and a prospective study. NZ Med J 95:267–269, 1982.

Saffle JR, Russon J Jr, Dukes GE, Warden GD. The effect of low-dose heparin therapy on serum platelet and transaminase levels. J Surg Res 28:297–305, 1980.

Schwartz KA, Royer G, Kaufman DB, Penner JA. Complications of heparin administration in normal individuals. Am J Hematol 19:355–363, 1985.

Serruys PW, Emanuelsson H, van der Giessen W, Lunn AC, Kiemeney F, Macaya C, Rutsch W, Heyndrickx G, Suryapranata H, Legrand V, Goy JJ, Materne P, Bonnier H, Morice M-C, Fajadet J, Belardi J, Colombo A, Garcia E, Ruygrok P, de Jaegere P, Morel M-A, on behalf of the Benestent-II Study Group. Heparin-coated Palmaz-Schatz stents in human coronary arteries. Early outcome of the Benestent-II pilot study. Circulation 93:412–422, 1996.

Shumate MJ. Heparin-induced thrombocytopenia [letter]. N Engl J Med 333:1006–1007, 1995.

Silver D, Kapsch DN, Tsoi EK. Heparin-induced thrombocytopenia, thrombosis, and hemorrhage. Ann Surg 198:301–306, 1983.

Simonneau G, Sors H, Charbonnier B, Page Y, Laaban JP, Azarian R, Lauent M, Hirsch JL, Ferrari E, Bosson JL, Mottier D, Beau B. A comparison of low-molecular-weight heparin with unfractionated heparin for acute pulmonary embolism. N Engl J Med 337:663–669, 1997.

Singer RL, Mannion JD, Bauer TL, Armenti FR, Edie RN. Complications from heparin-induced thrombocytopenia in patients undergoing cardiopulmonary bypass. Chest 104:1436–1440, 1993.

Stead RB, Schafer AI, Rosenberg RD, Handin RI, Josa M, Khuri SF. Heterogeneity of heparin lots associated with thrombocytopenia and thromboembolism. Am J Med 77:185–188, 1984.

Suh JS, Aster RH, Visentin GP. Antibodies from patients with heparin-induced thrombocytopenia/thrombosis recognize different epitopes on heparin:platelet factor 4. Blood 91:916–922, 1998.

Tardy-Poncet B, Tardy B, Grelac F, Reynaud J, Mismetti P, Bertrand JC, Guyotat D. Pentosan polysulfate-induced thrombocytopenia and thrombosis. Am J Hematol 45: 252–257, 1994.

Tardy B, Page Y, Tardy-Poncet B, Comtet C, Zeni F, Bertrand JC. Thrombopénie induite par une héparine de bas poids moléculaire [letter]. Therapie 45:453, 1990.

Trossaert M, Gaillard A, Commin PL, Amiral J, Vissac AM, Fressinaud E. High incidence of anti-heparin/platelet factor 4 antibodies after cardiopulmonary bypass. Br J Haematol 101:653–655, 1998.

Visentin GP, Malik M, Cyganiak KA, Aster RH. Patients treated with unfractionated heparin during open heart surgery are at high risk to form antibodies reactive with heparin:platelet factor 4 complexes. J Lab Clin Med 128:376–383, 1996.

Vitoux JF, Roncato M, Hourdbaigt P, Aiach M, Fiessinger J-N. Heparin-induced thrombocytopenia and pentosan polysulfate: treatment with a low molecular weight heparin despite in vitro platelet aggregation [letter]. Thromb Hemost 55:294–295, 1985.

Walls JT, Curtis JJ, Silver D, Boley TM, Schmaltz RA, Nawarawong W. Heparin-induced thrombocytopenia in open heart surgical patients: sequelae of late recognition. Ann Thorac Surg 53:787–791, 1992a.

Walls JT, Boley TM, Curtis JJ, Silver D. Heparin-induced thrombocytopenia in patients undergoing intra-aortic balloon pumping after open heart surgery. ASAIO J 38: M574–M576, 1992b.

Warkentin TE. Limitations of conventional treatment options for heparin-induced thrombocytopenia. Semin Hematol 35(suppl 4):17–25, 1998.

Warkentin TE, Kelton JG. Heparin-induced thrombocytopenia. Prog Hemost Thromb 10: 1–34, 1991.

Warkentin TE, Kelton JG. Interaction of heparin with platelets, including heparin-induced thrombocytopenia. In: Bounameaux H, ed. Low-Molecular-Weight Heparins in Prophylaxis and Therapy of Thromboembolic Diseases. New York: Marcel Dekker, 1994, pp 75–127.

Warkentin TE, Kelton JG. A 14-year study of heparin-induced thrombocytopenia. Am J Med 101:502–507, 1996.

Warkentin TE, Kelton JG. Timing of heparin-induced thrombocytopenia (HIT) in relation to previous heparin use: absence of an anamnestic immune response, and implications for repeat heparin use in patients with a history of HIT [abstr]. Blood 92(suppl 1):182a, 1998.

Warkentin TE, Levine MN, Hirsh J, Horsewood P, Roberts RS, Gent M, Kelton JG. Heparin-induced thrombocytopenia in patients treated with low-molecular weight heparin or unfractionated heparin. N Engl J Med 332:1330–1335, 1995a.

Warkentin TE, Levine MN, Hirsh J, Klama LN, Kelton JG. Formation of heparin-induced thrombocytopenia IgG without thrombocytopenia: analysis of a clinical trial [abstr]. Blood 86(suppl 1):537a, 1995b.

Warkentin TE, Hirsh J, Kelton JG. Heparin-induced thrombocytopenia [letter]. N Engl J Med 333:1007, 1995c.

Warkentin TE, Chong BH, Greinacher A. Heparin-induced thrombocytopenia: towards consensus. Thromb Haemost 79:1–7, 1998a.

Warkentin TE, Ling E, Ho A, Sheppard JI. ''Incidental'' unfractionated heparin (UFH) vs normal saline (NS) flushes for intraoperative invasive catheters and the frequency of formation of heparin-induced thrombocytopenia IgG antibodies (HIT-IgG): a randomized, controlled trial [abstr]. Blood 92(suppl 1):91b, 1998b.

Warkentin TE, Simpson PJ, Sheppard JI, Moore JC, Horsewood P, Kelton JG. Importance of patient population in the frequency of HIT: a comparison of activation and antigen assays [abstr]. Thromb Haemost 82(suppl):363–364, 1999.

Weismann RE, Tobin RW. Arterial embolism occurring during systemic heparin therapy. Arch Surg 76:219–227, 1958.

Weitberg AB, Spremulli E, Cummings FJ. Effect of low-dose heparin on the platelet count. South Med J 75:190–192, 1982.

Wolf H, Nowak H, Wick G. Detection of antibodies interacting with glycosaminoglycans polysulfate in patients treated with heparin or other polysulfated glycosaminoglycans. Int Arch Allergy Appl Immunol 70:157–163, 1983.

Yamamoto S, Koide M, Matsuo M, Suzuki S, Ohtaka M, Saika S, Matsuo T. Heparin-induced thrombocytopenia in hemodialysis patients. Am J Kidney Dis 28:82–85, 1996.

5

Nonimmune Heparin–Platelet Interactions: Implications for the Pathogenesis of Heparin-Induced Thrombocytopenia

McDonald K. Horne III
Warren G. Magnuson Clinical Center, National Institutes of Health, Bethesda, Maryland

I. INTRODUCTION

Almost as soon as heparin was introduced into clinical medicine, the new drug was reported to cause immediate small, but consistent, reductions in platelet count (Sappington, 1939). Later it was also found to produce platelet dysfunction (Heiden et al., 1977), accounting for at least some of its hemorrhagic risk (Hirsh, 1984; John et al., 1993). These effects, which most likely result from direct contact between the sulfated glycosaminoglycans and platelets, are distinct from the role heparin plays in immune-mediated heparin-induced thrombocytopenia (HIT). However, direct heparin–platelet binding is critical in the pathogenesis of HIT as well (Horne and Hutchison, 1998). Therefore, the various ''nonimmune'' heparin–platelet interactions will be reviewed.

II. HEPARIN BINDING TO PLATELETS

Appreciation of the functional effects of heparin on platelets led to studies of heparin binding to these cells, which is specific and saturable (Sobel and Adelman, 1988; Horne, 1988; Horne and Chao, 1989). No unique heparin or platelet

Table 1 Platelet Binding Parameters for Heparin Fractions of Different Molecular Mass

Heparin M_r range (Da)	Sulfate/ carboxylate (mol/mol)	Dissociation constant		Binding capacity	
		(mg/L)	(nM)	(mg/10^{15} cells)	(molecules/cell)
14,000–16,000	2.0 ± 0.29[a]	4.6 ± 1.1	310 ± 73	66 ± 2.5	2600 ± 100
9,500–10,500	1.8 ± 0.26	3.9 ± 2.1	390 ± 210	56 ± 8.4	3400 ± 500
4,500–5,500	1.9 ± 0.15	3.2 ± 1.0	640 ± 200	23 ± 5.7	2800 ± 680
2,700–3,300	1.7 ± 0.25	4.0 ± 2.0	1300 ± 650	10 ± 5.4	2000 ± 1100

[a] Values are means ± 1 standard deviation.
Source: Horne and Chao, 1990.

structures have been identified as critical for binding. The negative charge density of the ligand largely determines its binding specificity (Horne, 1988). Polysaccharide molecules with various primary structures can displace heparin from platelets if they are sufficiently charged (Horne, 1988; Greinacher et al., 1993; Table 1). Other than providing a complementary positive charge, the platelet-binding sites for heparin seem to have few distinguishing features. The major platelet membrane glycoprotein complexes IIb/IIIa and Ib/IX do not appear to be involved (Horne, 1988, 1991).

Next to negative charge density, molecular size has the greatest effect on polysaccharide binding to platelets. Heparin molecular weight, for example, affects both its platelet-binding affinity and capacity (Horne and Chao, 1990). As medicinal heparin is polydisperse (i.e., comprises a mixture of molecules varying in mass from about 1000–30,000 Da), the mass of a mole of heparin (approximately 6×10^{23} molecules) depends on the mean size of the molecules in the sample. The maximum number of molecules bound per platelet is approximately the same for heparin species with molecular weights between about 15,000 and 5,000 Da (see Table 1). However, larger molecules bring more glycosaminoglycan mass to the platelet surface than smaller molecules (Fig. 1). Therefore, when heparin-binding capacity is expressed in terms of mass, rather than moles or molecules, the capacity of larger heparins is greater than that of smaller heparins.

Similar distinctions apply to the parameters of binding affinity. Longer heparin molecules contain more potential platelet-binding domains than shorter molecules. Therefore, a large heparin species can half-saturate platelets at a lower molar concentration (K_d) than a smaller heparin species, although the concentration of platelet-binding domains in the suspension is the same for both species at half-saturation (Horne and Chao, 1990).

Because of its high charge density, as well as the high linear flexibility conferred by its constituent L-iduronic acid residues, heparin binds readily to a

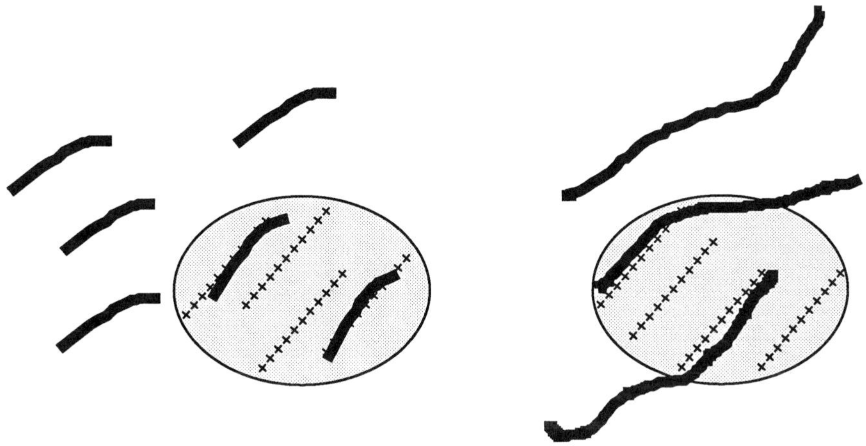

Heparin		
Mr	5000	15,000
Platelet-binding domains per molecule	1	2
Bound Heparin	2 molecules 10,000 daltons	2 molecules 30,000 daltons
Binding Capacity	4 molecules 20,000 daltons	4 molecules 60,000 daltons
Heparin Concentration at Half-Saturation (Kd)	6 platelet-binding domains/volume 6 molecules/volume 30,000 daltons/volume	6 platelet-binding domains/volume 3 molecules/volume 45,000 daltons/volume

Figure 1 Schematic binding of heparin to platelets comparing heparin of M_r 5000 with heparin of M_r 15,000. Each "platelet-binding domain" of heparin is hypothesized to have $M_r > 3000$, whereas heparin binding sites on the platelets (indicated as ++++) can bind 7000 Da of heparin. Therefore, each binding site is not quite filled with M_r 5000 heparin, but is too occupied to allow binding of a second heparin molecule. In contrast, M_r 15,000 heparin has adequate length to occupy two binding sites, but physical constraints, such as limited heparin flexibility and spacial distribution of binding sites, allow it to occupy only one site at a time. The scheme is consistent with the binding parameters shown in Table 1.

variety of basic plasma proteins, which theoretically could compete with platelets for heparin (Casu et al., 1988; Young et al., 1994). However, heparin binding to only two plasma proteins, antithrombin and fibronectin, interferes with heparin-induced platelet activation (Salzman et al., 1980; Chong and Ismail, 1989) or with binding of heparin to platelets (Horne and Chao, 1990).

III. NONIDIOSYNCRATIC HEPARIN-INDUCED PLATELET ACTIVATION

The functional consequence of heparin binding to platelets is subtle cell stimulation. Antibody-independent activation of platelets by heparin in vitro has been reported from many laboratories. However, the results of these studies have varied, presumably because of differences in experimental conditions. In plasma, for example, heparin alone causes slight platelet aggregation, whereas platelets suspended in laboratory buffers are reported to aggregate either briskly or not at all in response to heparin (Eika, 1972; Salzman et al., 1980; Chong and Ismail, 1989; Westwick et al., 1986). In citrate-anticoagulated plasma, heparin also potentiates platelet activation by agonists, such as ADP and collagen (Holmer et al., 1980; Chen and Sylvén, 1992), and this effect is more pronounced in patients with acute illness, arterial disease, and anorexia nervosa (Mikhailidis et al., 1985; Reininger et al., 1996; Burgess and Chong, 1997).

The platelet proaggregatory effect of heparin does not appear to be an artifact of low ionized calcium concentration in the presence of citrate anticoagulant: Chen and colleagues (1992) observed that heparin enhanced collagen-induced platelet aggregation in a dose-dependent fashion even in whole blood anticoagulated with hirudin (i.e., physiological calcium concentrations). On the other hand, the responsiveness of washed platelets to agonists, when resuspended in buffers containing physiological calcium, has been reported to be both increased and decreased by heparin (Saba et al., 1984; Westwick et al., 1986). Although the data are not always consistent, this much seems clear: direct heparin-induced platelet aggregation requires metabolic energy and is mediated by fibrinogen; therefore, it depends on platelet fibrinogen receptors (platelet glycoprotein IIb/IIIa complexes) and divalent cations (Chong and Ismail, 1989). There is also evidence that heparin can antagonize platelet inhibition by prostacyclin (Saba et al., 1979; Eldor and Weksler, 1979; Fortini et al., 1985; Berglund and Wallentin, 1991).

The properties of heparin that influence its platelet binding also influence its stimulatory effects on platelets: heparin of a high molecular weight is more active than low molecular weight heparin, and heparin with low affinity for antithrombin and fibronectin is more active (because it is more available) than heparin with high affinity for these plasma proteins (Salzman et al., 1980; Holmer et al., 1980; Westwick et al., 1986; Chong and Ismail, 1989; Brace and Fareed, 1990).

The latter observation implies that the anticoagulant (antithrombin-dependent) activities of heparin are distinct from its platelet stimulatory effects. Furthermore, nonheparin polysaccharides can mimic the proaggregatory effects of heparin on platelets if they are sufficiently large and charged (Tiffany and Penner, 1981). In contrast, heparan sulfate (the predominant anticoagulant glycosaminoglycan found in danaparoid) has negligible platelet-activating properties, as it has a relatively low degree of sulfation, despite sharing a carbohydrate backbone similar to heparin (Burgess and Chong, 1997; Lindahl and Kjellén, 1991).

IV. PLATELET-RELATED PROHEMORRHAGIC EFFECTS OF HEPARIN

Paradoxically, despite the in vitro evidence that heparin stimulates platelets, there is evidence that heparin causes bleeding partly because of its effects on platelet function (Hirsh, 1984; John et al., 1993). Heparin, for example, causes prolongation of the skin-bleeding time unrelated to any effects on platelet counts (Hjort et al., 1960; Heiden et al., 1977; Kelton, 1986; Ljungberg et al., 1988). Also, the structural characteristics of heparin associated with platelet stimulation in vitro (e.g., increased heparin size and sulfation; decreased affinity for antithrombin) are associated with enhanced bleeding in animal models (Hjort et al., 1960; Carter et al., 1982; Ockelford et al., 1982; Fernandez et al., 1986; Borowska et al., 1988; Van Ryn-McKenna et al., 1989).

The apparent inhibition of platelet function in vivo may be related to two specific actions of heparin: inhibition of thrombin-induced platelet activation, and reduction of von Willebrand factor (vWF)-dependent platelet function. Thrombin is a ''strong'' platelet activator (i.e., it stimulates platelet secretion without intermediate platelet aggregation; Ware and Coller, 1995). However, in the presence of antithrombin, heparin essentially eliminates stimulation of platelets by thrombin (Westwick et al., 1986; Cofrancesco et al., 1988). This effect is likely responsible for the marked prolongation of bleeding time seen in patients receiving high doses of heparin during heart surgery (Kestin et al., 1993). Heparin also binds to vWf, preventing binding of vWF to platelets (Sobel et al., 1991, 1992). This reduces vWF-mediated subendothelial adhesion of platelets flowing at high shear rates, perhaps also contributing to heparin-related prolongation of the bleeding time.

V. NONIMMUNE HEPARIN-ASSOCIATED THROMBOCYTOPENIA (NONIMMUNE HAT)

Nonimmune HAT describes the common clinical situation in which a patient develops a fall in the platelet count within the first few days of receiving heparin.

Often, there are concomitant clinical factors to explain the thrombocytopenia (e.g., hemodilution, bacteremia, or disseminated intravascular coagulation; DIC). In some patients, however, it is possible that a direct proaggregatory effect of the heparin is responsible for the platelet count fall (Salzman et al., 1980). The designation *associated* helps to convey the uncertain role of heparin in causing thrombocytopenia in an individual patient, and the term *nonimmune* distinguishes this syndrome from (immune-mediated) HIT (Warkentin et al., 1998).

Nonimmune HAT is typically mild, transient, and clinically inconsequential (Chong, 1988; Gollub and Ulin, 1962; Johnson et al., 1984; Warkentin and Kelton, 1994). There is debate whether this represents a real in vivo phenomenon, or whether the apparent thrombocytopenia is instead related to ex vivo platelet aggregation (Davey and Lander, 1968). Indeed, some investigators were unable to show this event at all (Heinrich et al., 1988). Sometimes, however, apparent nonimmune HAT is a dramatic clinical syndrome that can be confused with HIT (Chong et al., 1982; see Chap. 12).

Balduini et al. (1993) observed that an early fall in platelet count was more frequent and of greater magnitude in patients receiving heparin following streptokinase therapy for acute myocardial infarction, compared with control patients who received streptokinase alone. The heparin-treated patients also showed greater ex vivo spontaneous platelet aggregation, suggesting that heparin may have had a direct proaggregatory effect.

VI. HEPARIN–PLATELET INTERACTIONS IN THE PATHOGENESIS OF HIT

Heparin also binds to several proteins that are secreted from stimulated platelets. One of these, platelet factor 4 (PF4), binds heparin with unusually high affinity (Capitanio et al., 1985; Loscalzo et al., 1985; Horne, 1993). Unlike antithrombin or fibronectin, however, PF4 does not prevent heparin from binding to platelets. In fact, it appears that heparin can bind to platelets in complexes with PF4 (Horne and Hutchison, 1998).

Heparin-bound PF4 has been identified as the primary target of the antibodies characteristic of HIT (Amiral et al., 1992; Visentin et al., 1994; Kelton et al., 1994). Because platelets have specific-binding sites for PF4, this protein was originally assumed to mediate the attachment of HIT immune complexes to the platelet surface (Kelton et al., 1994). However, it was recently demonstrated that heparin, rather than PF4, serves this purpose; that is, the binding to platelets of heparin–PF4 complexes occurs at heparin-binding sites, rather than PF4-binding sites (Greinacher et al., 1993; Horne and Hutchison, 1998). Thus, nonimmune heparin binding to platelets is fundamental to the pathogenesis of HIT in at least two ways. First, nonidiosyncratic heparin-induced platelet activation leads to release of PF4 from alpha-granules, permitting formation of the immunogenic PF4–heparin complexes; and second, localization of the PF4–heparin complexes to the platelet surface occurs at heparin-binding sites, thereby facilitating interaction of HIT antibodies with the platelet Fc receptors.

Because immune complexes that comprise heparin, PF4, and IgG from HIT patients bind to platelets at heparin-binding sites, they must compete with free heparin for binding to the platelet surface (Horne and Alkins, 1996; Horne and Hutchison, 1998). When free heparin is in molar excess, heparin–PF4–IgG complexes are displaced from the platelet surface (Fig. 2). When PF4 is in excess, there is no free heparin, and binding of the complexes is the only option.

These stoichiometric considerations may explain why some patients develop HIT IgG antibodies (HIT–IgG) without developing thrombocytopenia, and why HIT is more common in certain clinical settings than in others, such as following surgery (Amiral et al., 1995, 1996; Kappers-Klunne et al., 1997; Bauer

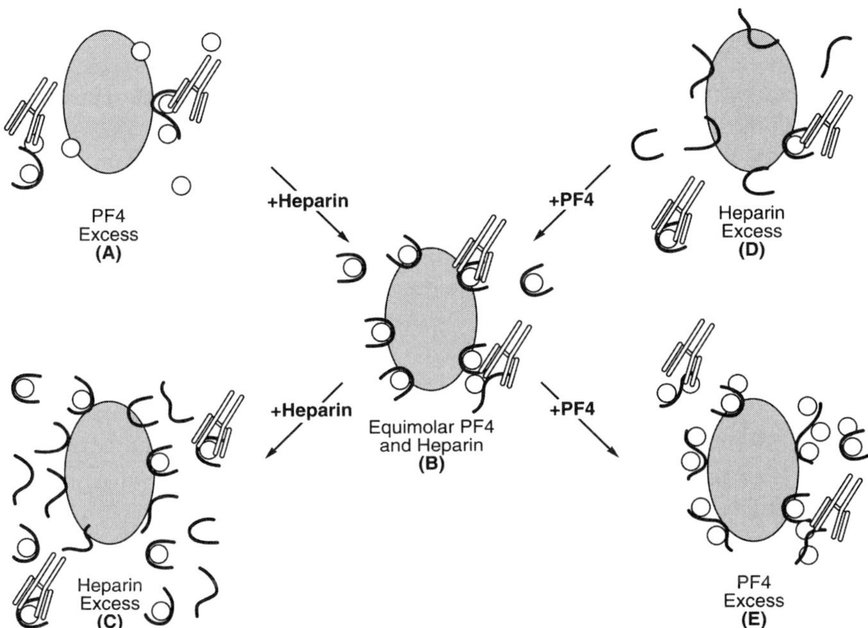

Figure 2 Cartoon illustrating the importance of the molar ratio of heparin to PF4 in determining binding of HIT immune complexes to platelets. Maximal binding of HIT–IgG occurs when heparin and PF4 are present in equimolar concentrations. Note that IgG Fc interactions with platelet Fc receptors are not shown in this figure. (From Horne and Hutchison, 1998.)

et al., 1997; Visentin et al., 1996; Boshkov et al., 1993; Warkentin et al., 1995). When a patient is given heparin, the plasma concentration of PF4 rises because PF4 is displaced from the endothelial surface, where it is normally bound to heparan sulfate (Dawes et al., 1982; Rao et al., 1983; O'Brien et al., 1985). PF4 neoantigens (or cryptic antigens) are formed, leading to the HIT immune response (Chong and Newman, 1997). However, complexes of heparin, PF4, and IgG are harmless unless they become bound to platelets, and this cannot happen as long as there is sufficient free heparin to compete effectively for the limited number of platelet-binding sites (Horne and Hutchison, 1998). Therefore, as long as heparin remains in molar excess over PF4, heparin–PF4–IgG binding to platelets is minimized, and platelet activation and thrombocytopenia do not develop.

In most clinical settings, free heparin is in considerable molar excess over PF4. For example, therapeutic concentrations of heparin (0.2–0.4 U/mL) correspond to about 100–200 nmol/L of heparin. When heparin is given to normal individuals, plasma concentrations of PF4 from endothelial reservoirs reach only about 8 nM (Dawes et al., 1982). For PF4 concentrations to approach 100–200 nmol/L, marked activation of circulating platelets is necessary. Complete activation of platelets in a concentration of 250×10^9/L will generate a plasma PF4 concentration of about 200 nM (Horne, 1993). Therefore, a molar excess of PF4 over therapeutic concentrations of heparin would be highly unlikely outside extreme clinical circumstances. On the other hand, prophylactic doses of heparin (e.g., 5000 U every 8–12 h by subcutaneous injection) administered in a setting associated with some platelet activation (e.g., postoperative orthopedic patients) might well produce molar ratios of heparin and PF4 that would favor platelet binding of heparin–PF4 complexes, and—if an immune response had occurred—platelet binding of heparin–PF4–IgG complexes. Indeed, such scenarios are the ones in which HIT is reported most frequently (Warkentin et al., 1995; Ganzer et al., 1997).

VII. IMPLICATIONS OF NONIMMUNE HEPARIN BINDING TO PLATELETS FOR THE PREVENTION OR TREATMENT OF HIT

Heparin's molecular size influences its platelet-binding affinity and capacity and its stimulating effect on platelets. Similarly, heparin's affinity and capacity for PF4 are related to its size: large heparin molecules have higher affinity for PF4 and can bind several PF4 molecules, whereas smaller heparin molecules have less affinity for PF4 and can bind fewer PF4 molecules (Lane et al., 1984; Bock et al., 1980; Marshall et al., 1984). Therefore, it should be no surprise that low molecular weight heparins are associated with a lower frequency of HIT than standard heparin (Warkentin et al., 1995), and that in some instances low molecular weight heparin has been given to patients with HIT without adverse consequences (Slocum et al., 1996). Smaller heparins complex less efficiently with PF4, thereby reducing immunogenicity, and bind less avidly to platelets, thereby reducing immune complex binding to the cells. Indeed, the very smallest heparin, the antithrombin-binding pentasaccharide (M_r 1714), theoretically is an ideal anticoagulant agent for patients with HIT (see Chap. 8). The pentasaccharide neither stimulates platelets nor binds to PF4 (Walenga et al., 1997; Elalamy et al., 1995).

Similarly, the safety and efficacy of treating HIT patients with danaparoid, a so-called heparinoid, can be explained by the fact that its major component (approximately 84% heparin sulfate) does not bind to platelets (Magnani, 1993; Horne, 1988). On the other hand, danaparoid sometimes cross-reacts with HIT antibodies in laboratory tests for HIT. This is perhaps mediated by a minor component of danaparoid (about 12% dermatan sulfate), which does have weak affinity for both platelets and PF4 (Barber et al., 1972; Horne, 1988).

REFERENCES

Amiral J, Bridey F, Dreyfus M, Vissac AM, Fressinaud E, Wolf M, Meyer D. Platelet factor 4 complexed to heparin is the target for antibodies generated in heparin-induced thrombocytopenia [letter]. Thromb Haemost 68:95–96, 1992.

Amiral J, Bridey F, Wolf M, Boyer-Neumann C, Fressinaud E, Vissac AM, Peynaud-Debayle E, Dreyfus M, Meyer D. Antibodies to macromolecular platelet factor 4–heparin complexes in heparin-induced thrombocytopenia: a study of 44 cases. Thromb Haemost 73:21–28, 1995.

Amiral J, Peynaud-Debayle E, Wolf M, Bridey F, Vissac AM, Meyer D. Generation of antibodies to heparin–PF4 complexes without thrombocytopenia in patients treated with unfractionated or low-molecular-weight heparin. Am J Hematol 52:90–95, 1996.

Balduini CL, Noris P, Bertolino G, Previtali M. Heparin modifies platelet count and function in patients who have undergone thrombolytic therapy for acute myocardial infarction [letter]. Thromb Haemost 69:522–523, 1993.

Barber AF, Kaser-Glanzmann R, Jakabova M, Luscher EF. Characterization of a chondroitin 4-sulfate proteoglycan carrier for heparin neutralizing activity (platelet factor 4) released from human blood platelets. Biochim Biophys Acta 286:312–329, 1972.

Bauer TL, Arepally G, Konkle BA, Mestichelli B, Shapiro SS, Cines DB, Poncz M, McNulty S, Amiral J, Hauck WW, Edie RN, Mannion JD. Prevalence of heparin-associated antibodies without thrombosis in patients undergoing cardiopulmonary bypass surgery. Circulation 95:1242–1246, 1997.

Berglund U, Wallentin L. Influence on platelet function by heparin in men with unstable coronary artery disease. Thromb Haemost 66:648–651, 1991.

Bock PE, Luscombe M, Marshall SE, Pepper DS, Holbrook JJ. The multiple complexes formed by the interaction of platelet factor 4 with heparin. Biochem J 191:769–776, 1980.

Borowska A, Lauri D, Maggi A, Dejana E, De Gaetano G, Donati MB, Pangrazzi J. Impairment of primary haemostasis by low molecular weight heparins in rats. Br J Haematol 68:339–344, 1988.

Boshkov LK, Warkentin TE, Hayward CPM, Andrew M, Kelton JG. Heparin-induced thrombocytopenia and thrombosis: clinical and laboratory studies. Br J Haematol 84:322–328, 1993.

Brace LD, Fareed J. Heparin-induced platelet aggregation. II. Dose/response relationships for two low molecular weight heparin fractions (CY 216 and CY 222). Thromb Res 59:1–14, 1990.

Burgess JK, Chong BH. The platelet proaggregating and potentiating effects of unfractionated heparin, low molecular weight heparin and heparinoid in intensive care patients and healthy controls. Eur J Haematol 58:279–285, 1997.

Capitanio AM, Niewiarowski S, Rucinski B, Tuszynski GP, Cierniewski CS, Hershock D, Kornecki E. Interaction of platelet factor 4 with human platelets. Biochim Biophys Acta 839:161–173, 1985.

Carter CJ, Kelton JG, Hirsh J, Cerskus A, Santos AV, Gent M. The relationship between the hemorrhagic and antithrombotic properties of low molecular weight heparin in rabbits. Blood 59:1239–1245, 1982.

Casu B, Petitou M, Provasoli M, Sinaÿ P. Conformational flexibility: a new concept for explaining binding and biological properties of iduronic acid-containing glycosaminoglycans. Trends Biochem Sci 13:221–225, 1988.

Chen J, Sylvén C. Heparin potentiation of collagen-induced platelet aggregation is related to the GPIIb/GPIIIa receptor and not to the GPIb receptor, as tested by whole blood aggregometry. Thromb Res 66:111–120, 1992.

Chen J, Karlberg KE, Sylvén C. Heparin enhances platelet aggregation irrespective of anticoagulation with citrate or with hirudin. Thromb Res 67:253–262, 1992.

Chong BH. Heparin-induced thrombocytopenia. Blood Rev 2:108–114, 1988.

Chong BH, Ismail F. The mechanism of heparin-induced platelet aggregation. Eur J Haematol 43:245–251, 1989.

Chong BH, Newman PM. The antigenic epitope in heparin-induced thrombocytopenia resides solely on platelet factor 4 [abstr]. Blood 90(suppl 1):461a, 1997.

Chong BH, Pitney WR, Castaldi PA. Heparin-induced thrombocytopenia: association of thrombotic complications with heparin-dependent IgG antibody that induces thromboxane synthesis and platelet aggregation. Lancet 2:1246–1249, 1982.

Cofrancesco E, Colombi M, Manfreda M, Pogliani EM. Effect of heparin and related glycosaminoglycans (GAGs) on thrombin-induced platelet aggregation and release. Haematologica 73:471–475, 1988.

Davey MG, Lander H. Effect of injected heparin on platelet levels in man. J Clin Pathol 21:55–59, 1968.

Dawes J, Pumphrey CW, McLaren KM, Prowse CV, Pepper DS. The in vivo release of human platelet factor 4 by heparin. Thromb Res 27:65–76, 1982.

Eika C. The platelet aggregating effect of eight commercial heparins. Scand J Haematol 9:480–482, 1972.

Elalamy I, Lecrubier C, Potevin F, Abdelouahed M, Bara L, Marie JP, Samama MM. Absence of in vitro cross-reaction of pentasaccharide with the plasma heparin-dependent factor of twenty-five patients with heparin-associated thrombocytopenia [letter]. Thromb Haemost 74:1384–1385, 1995.

Eldor A, Weksler BB. Heparin and dextran sulfate antagonize PGI_2 inhibition of platelet aggregation. Thromb Res 16:617–628, 1979.

Fernandez F, N'guyen P, Van Ryn J, Ofosu FA, Hirsh J, Buchanan MR. Hemorrhagic doses of heparin and other glycosaminoglycans induce a platelet defect. Thromb Res 43:491–495, 1986.

Fortini A, Modesti PA, Abbate R, Gensini GF, Neri Serneri GG. Heparin does not interfere with prostacyclin and prostaglandin D_2 binding to platelets. Thromb Res 40:319–328, 1985.

Ganzer D, Gutezeit A, Mayer G, Greinacher A, Eichler P. Thromboemboliepropylaxe als Auslöser thrombembolischer Komplikationen. Eine Untersuchung zur Inzidenz der Heparin-induzierten Thrombozytopenie (HIT) Typ II. Z Orthop 135:543–549, 1997.

Gollub S, Ulin AW. Heparin-induced thrombocytopenia in man. J Lab Clin Med 59:430–435, 1962.

Greinacher A. Antigen generation in heparin-associated thrombocytopenia: the nonimmunologic type and the immunologic type are closely linked in their pathogenesis. Semin Thromb Hemost 21:106–116, 1995.

Greinacher A, Michels I, Liebenhoff U, Presek P, Mueller-Eckhardt C. Heparin-associated thrombocytopenia: immune complexes are attached to the platelet membrane by the negative charge of highly sulphated oligosaccharides. Br J Haematol 84:711–716, 1993.

Heiden D, Mielke CH Jr, Rodvien R. Impairment by heparin of primary haemostasis and platelet [^{14}C]5-hydroxytryptamine release. Br J Haematol 36:427–436, 1977.

Heinrich D, Görg T, Schulz M. Effects of unfractionated and fractionated heparin on platelet function. Haemostasis 18(suppl 3):48–54, 1988.

Hirsh J. Heparin-induced bleeding. Nouv Rev Fr Hematol 26:261–266, 1984.

Hjort PF, Borchgrevink CF, Iversen OH, Stormorken H. The effect of heparin on the bleeding time. Thromb Diath Haemorrh 4:389–399, 1960.

Holmer E, Lindahl U, Bäckström G, Thunberg L, Sandberg H, Söderström G, Andersson L-O. Anticoagulant activities and effects on platelets of a heparin fragment with high affinity for antithrombin. Thromb Res 18:861–869, 1980.

Horne MK III. Heparin binding to normal and abnormal platelets. Thromb Res 51:135–144, 1988.

Horne MK III. Heparin binds normally to platelets digested with *Streptomyces griseus* protease. Thromb Res 61:155–158, 1991.

Horne MK III. The effect of secreted heparin-binding proteins on heparin binding to platelets. Thromb Res 70:91–98, 1993.

Horne MK III, Alkins BR. Platelet binding of IgG from patients with heparin-induced thrombocytopenia. J Lab Clin Med 127:435–442, 1996.

Horne MK III, Chao ES. Heparin binding to resting and activated platelets. Blood 74: 238–243, 1989.

Horne MK III, Chao ES. The effect of molecular weight on heparin binding to platelets. Br J Haematol 74:306–312, 1990.

Horne MK III, Hutchison KJ. Simultaneous binding of heparin and platelet factor-4 to platelets: further insights into the mechanism of heparin-induced thrombocytopenia. Am J Hematol 58:24–30, 1998.

John LCH, Rees GM, Kovacs IB. Inhibition of platelet function by heparin. An etiologic factor in postbypass hemorrhage. Thorac Cardiovasc Surg 105:816–822, 1993.

Johnson RA, Lazarus KH, Henry DH. Heparin-induced thrombocytopenia: a prospective study. Am J Hematol 17:349–353, 1984.

Kappers-Klunne MC, Boon DMS, Hop WCJ, Michiels JJ, Stibbe J, van der Zwaan C, Koudstaal PJ, van Vliet HHDM. Heparin-induced thrombocytopenia and thrombosis: a prospective analysis of the incidence in patients with heart and cerebrovascular diseases. Br J Haematol 96:442–446, 1997.

Kelton JG. Heparin-induced thrombocytopenia. Haemostasis 16:173–186, 1986.

Kelton JG, Smith JW, Warkentin TE, Hayward CPM, Denomme GA, Horsewood P. Immunoglobin G from patients with heparin-induced thrombocytopenia binds to a complex of heparin and platelet factor 4. Blood 83:3232–3239, 1994.

Kestin AS, Valeri CR, Khuri SF, Loscalzo J, Ellis PA, MacGregor H, Birjiniuk V, Ouimet H, Pasche B, Nelson MJ, Benoit SE, Rodino LJ, Barnard MR, Michelson AD. The platelet function defect of cardiopulmonary bypass. Blood 82:107–117, 1993.

Lanc DA, Denton J, Flynn AM, Thunberg L, Lindahl U. Anticoagulant activities of heparin oligosaccharides and their neutralization by platelet factor 4. Biochem J 218: 725–732, 1984.

Lindahl U, Kjellén L. Heparin or heparan sulfate—what is the difference? Thromb Haemost 66:44–48, 1991.

Ljungberg B, Beving H, Egberg N, Johnsson H, Vesterqvist O. Immediate effects of heparin and LMW heparin on some platelet and endothelial derived factors. Thromb Res 51:209–217, 1988.

Loscalzo J, Melnick B, Handin RI. The interaction of platelet factor four and glycosaminoglycans. Arch Biochem Biophys 240:446–455, 1985.

Magnani HN. Heparin-induced thrombocytopenia (HIT): an overview of 230 patients treated with Orgaran (Org 10172). Thromb Haemost 70:554–561, 1993.

Marshall SE, Luscombe M, Pepper DS, Holbrook JJ. The interaction of platelet factor 4 with heparins of different chain length. Biochim Biophys Acta 797:34–39, 1984.

Mikhailidis DP, Barradas MA, Jeremy JY, Gracey L, Wakeling A, Dandona P. Heparin-induced platelet aggregation in anorexia nervosa and in severe peripheral vascular disease. Eur J Clin Invest 15:313–319, 1985.

O'Brien JR, Etherington MD, Pashley MA. The heparin-mobilisable pool of platelet factor 4: a comparison of intravenous and subcutaneous heparin and Kabi heparin fragment 2165. Thromb Haemost 54:735–738, 1985.

Ockelford PA, Carter CJ, Cerskus A, Smith CA, Hirsh J. Comparison of the in vivo hemorrhagic and antithrombotic effects of a low antithrombin-III affinity heparin fraction. Thromb Res 27:679–690, 1982.

Rao AK, Niewiarowski S, James P, Holt JC, Harris M, Elfenbein B, Bastl C. Effect of heparin on the in vivo release and clearance of human platelet factor 4. Blood 61: 1208–1214, 1983.

Reininger CB, Greinacher A, Graf J, Lasser R, Steckmeier B, Schweiberer L. Platelets

of patients with peripheral arterial disease are hypersensitive to heparin. Thromb Res 81:641–649, 1996.
Saba HI, Saba SR, Blackburn CA, Hartmann RC, Mason RG. Heparin neutralization of PGI_2: effects upon platelets. Science 205:499–501, 1979.
Saba HI, Saba SR, Morelli GA. Effect of heparin on platelet aggregation. Am J Hematol 17:295–306, 1984.
Salzman EW, Rosenberg RD, Smith MH, Lindon JN, Favreau L. Effect of heparin and heparin fractions on platelet aggregation. J Clin Invest 65:64–73, 1980.
Sappington SW. The use of heparin in blood transfusions. JAMA 113:22–25, 1939.
Slocum MM, Adams JG Jr, Teel R, Spadone DP, Silver D. Use of enoxaparin in patients with heparin-induced thrombocytopenia syndrome. J Vasc Surg 23:839–843, 1996.
Sobel M, Adelman B. Characterization of platelet binding of heparins and other glycosaminoglycans. Thromb Res 50:815–826, 1988.
Sobel M, McNeill PM, Carlson PL, Kermode JC, Adelman B, Conroy R, Marques D. Heparin inhibition of von Willebrand factor-dependent platelet function in vitro and in vivo. J Clin Invest 87:1787–1793, 1991.
Sobel M, Soler DF, Kermode JC, Harris RB. Localization and characterization of a heparin binding domain peptide of human von Willebrand factor. J Biol Chem 267:8857–8862, 1992.
Tiffany ML, Penner JA. Heparin and other sulfated polyanions: their interaction with the blood platelet. Ann NY Acad Sci 370:662–667, 1981.
Van Ryn-McKenna J, Ofosu FA, Hirsh J, Buchanan MR. Antithrombotic and bleeding effects of glycosaminoglycans with different degrees of sulphation. Br J Haematol 71:265–269, 1989.
Visentin GP, Ford SE, Scott JP, Aster RH. Antibodies from patients with heparin-induced thrombocytopenia/thrombosis are specific for platelet factor 4 complexed with heparin or bound to endothelial cells. J Clin Invest 93:81–88, 1994.
Visentin GP, Malik M, Cyganiak KA, Aster RH. Patients treated with unfractionated heparin during open heart surgery are at high risk to form antibodies reactive with heparin:platelet factor 4 complexes. J Lab Clin Med 128:376–383, 1996.
Walenga JM, Jeske WP, Bara L, Samama MM, Fareed J. Biochemical and pharmacologic rationale for the development of a synthetic heparin pentasaccharide. Thromb Res 86:1–36, 1997.
Ware AJ, Coller BS. Platelet morphology, biochemistry, and function. In: Beutler E, Lichtman MA, Coller BS, Kipps TJ, eds. Williams Hematology. 5th ed. New York: McGraw-Hill, 1995, pp 1161–1201.
Warkentin TE, Kelton JG. Interaction of heparin with platelets, including heparin-induced thrombocytopenia. In: Bounameaux H, ed. Low-Molecular-Weight Heparins in Prophylaxis and Therapy of Thromboembolic Diseases. New York: Marcel Dekker, 1994, pp 75–127.
Warkentin TE, Levine MN, Hirsh J, Horsewood P, Roberts RS, Gent M, Kelton JG. Heparin-induced thrombocytopenia in patients treated with low-molecular-weight heparin or unfractionated heparin. N Engl J Med 332:1330–1335, 1995.
Warkentin TE, Chong BH, Greinacher A. Heparin-induced thrombocytopenia: towards consensus. Thromb Haemost 79:1–7, 1998.
Westwick J, Scully MF, Poll C, Kakkar VV. Comparison of the effects of low molecular

weight heparin and unfractionated heparin on activation of human platelets in vitro. Thromb Res 42:435–447, 1986.

Young E, Wells P, Holloway S, Weitz J, Hirsh J. Ex-vivo and in-vitro evidence that low molecular weight heparins exhibit less binding to plasma proteins than unfractionated heparin. Thromb Haemost 71:300–304, 1994.

6

Heparin-Dependent Antigens in Heparin-Induced Thrombocytopenia

Jean Amiral
HYPHEN BioMed, Andresy, France

Dominique Meyer
INSERM U-143, Hôpital de Bicêtre, Bicêtre, France

I. INTRODUCTION

Recently, platelet factor 4 (PF4) complexed to heparin (PF4–H) was identified as the major target antigen for heparin-dependent antibodies involved in the pathogenesis of immune heparin-induced thrombocytopenia (HIT) (Amiral et al., 1992, 1995; Greinacher et al., 1994, 1995; Kelton et al., 1994; Visentin et al., 1994; Gruel et al., 1993). Occasionally, other antigens can be involved, such as interleukin-8 (IL-8) or neutrophil-activating peptide-2 (NAP-2), two CXC chemokines of the PF4 superfamily (Amiral et al., 1996a). There is now increasing evidence that the risk of HIT depends on the type of heparin used, its sulfation grade, the therapy duration, and the patient's clinical context (Kelton, 1992; Warkentin and Kelton, 1996; see Chap. 4). However, many questions remain unresolved: How are antibodies generated? Why are they observed in only a subgroup of patients receiving heparin? How do they become pathogenic in only a few of the latter? Indeed, antibodies to PF4–H develop surprisingly often in many heparin-treated patients, especially in the context of platelet activation (e.g., heart surgery using cardiopulmonary bypass) (Amiral et al., 1996b; Visentin et al., 1996).

Clinical complications of HIT are especially associated with high-titer PF4–H antibodies of the IgG isotype, usually in patients with comorbid disease who are receiving unfractionated heparin (UFH). The frequency of HIT is lower with the use of low molecular weight heparin (LMWH) (Warkentin et al., 1995). However, recent studies suggest this complication can also develop in the absence of IgG isotypes (Amiral et al., 1996c). In up to 20% of patients with HIT, only IgA or IgM isotypes are present, usually in high concentrations.

In this chapter, the current understanding of PF4–H antibody generation and its contribution to the complications of HIT will be discussed. Formation of the PF4–H antigen complexes and their binding to blood and endothelial cells, thus targeting the immune response onto these cells (Cines et al., 1987; Horne et al., 1998; Visentin et al., 1994; Visentin and Aster, 1995), will be analyzed. Finally, the possibility that HIT can be caused in the absence of detectable antibodies to PF4–H will be discussed, including the hypothesis that preexisting antibodies to other chemokines could become pathogenic during heparin treatment.

II. ANTIGENICITY OF PF4 IN THE PRESENCE OF HEPARIN

Antibodies to self-antigens, including certain autologous plasma proteins, can develop as result of immune dysfunction, resulting in chronic autoimmune disease. Sometimes, however, formation of complexes between an autologous protein and a foreign substance leads to new antigens, potentially even on the self-protein. These can be described as *cryptic autoantigens*, or *neoantigens*. The immune stimulation resulting from such an altered self-epitope quickly abates when the inducing foreign substance is no longer present. Such a model appears relevant to explain some of the clinical complications observed in HIT (see Chap. 3). In HIT, PF4 constitutes the self-antigen, with one or more cryptic autoepitopes formed when complexes are formed under optimal conditions with the foreign substance, heparin (discussed subsequently). Thus, the antibodies to PF4–H complexes effectively behave as autoantibodies in the presence of heparin (Shoenfeld, 1997).

PF4 is a positively charged tetrameric glycoprotein member of the CXC chemokine family (Brandt and Flad, 1992). The tetramer forms by sequential noncovalent association of PF4 monomers: two dimers are formed that self-associate into the fundamental tetrameric structure. As found within platelet α-granules, PF4 is released into blood only after platelet activation, such as seen with trauma, surgery, atherosclerosis (Dunlop et al., 1987), diabetes, cardiopulmonary bypass, inflammation, cancer, infections, and so on. In vivo, PF4 has many different biological functions, including immunoregulation, inhibition of megakaryocytopoiesis and angiogenesis, and mediation of cell response. When released from platelets, PF4 is in a complex of eight tetramers linked to a chondroitin-containing proteoglycan dimer: the entire complex has a molecular weight (MW) of 350 kDa. The PF4 complexes can also bind to endothelial cell proteoglycans (hcparan sulfate). Heparin, when present, having a greater affinity for PF4, displaces PF4 from the endothelial cell glycosaminoglycans, thereby forming PF4–H complexes that are released into the circulation.

The interaction between heparin and PF4 has been intensively studied (Bock et al., 1980; Cowan et al., 1986; Maccarana et al., 1993; Stuckey et al., 1992). In the presence of a stoichiometric concentration of heparin and PF4 (which corresponds to 27 international units [IU] of heparin per milligram of PF4), multimolecular PF4–H complexes (Greinacher et al., 1994; Amiral et al., 1995) are generated. With stoichiometric concentrations, heparin wraps around the PF4 molecule, altering its structure and rendering it antigenic. Figure 1 shows the different complexes that can be formed between heparin and PF4, depending on the respective concentrations of both substances. Only multimolecular complexes are believed to be antigenic in heparin-treated patients. Thus, the immunogenicity of complexes is strictly dependent on the respective concentrations of heparin and PF4. If we consider the usual therapeutic range for heparin (0.1–1 IU/mL), the amount of PF4 required for the generation of multimolecular PF4–H complexes is from 3 to 40 μg/mL. In patients undergoing cardiopulmonary bypass who receive higher heparin concentrations (up to 3 IU/mL), the corresponding higher PF4 concentrations required for the formation of the immunogenic PF4–H complexes may result from intense platelet activation, resulting from exposure of blood to the extracorporeal circuit. In general, the existence of favorable conditions allowing the formation of multimolecular PF4–H complexes

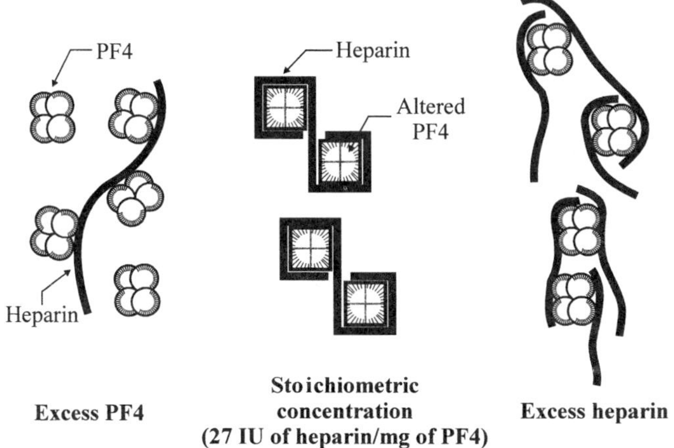

Figure 1 Formation of heparin and PF4 complexes at different concentrations of heparin and PF4: In the presence of stoichiometric concentrations of both substances, multimolecular complexes are formed. Heparin then wraps around the PF4 tetramer, altering its structure and rendering it antigenic.

may depend as much on the underlying disease that is promoting platelet activation as on the dose of heparin given (see Chap. 4).

The intensity of the heparin-dependent immune response thus depends on the presence and, presumably, persistence of the multimolecular PF4–H complexes. In particular, high concentrations of PF4–H complexes may be important in triggering an immune response. However, heparin concentrations vary considerably in treated patients, and the concentrations allowing PF4–H complex formation may occur frequently. But, if low PF4 concentrations are present, formation of immunogenic complexes can occur only at corresponding very low levels of heparin (e.g., 0.027 IU/mL of heparin for 100 ng/mL of PF4, which is the approximate PF4 concentration in normal subjects receiving heparin). The chances of developing a significant immune response in this setting would be low. The potentially important role of individual responsiveness to a given PF4 antigenic stimulus is unknown.

Although antibodies to PF4–H complexes are present in most patients who develop HIT, they are absent in some patients with apparent HIT, including patients with positive activation assays for HIT antibodies. Antibodies to IL-8 or to NAP-2 have been observed in some of these patients (Amiral, 1996a), but in others, no specific heparin-dependent antibodies have been identified. As discussed later, antibodies to IL-8 or to NAP-2 are generated by mechanisms different from those involved in PF4–H antibody formation, and may be true autoantibodies (Bendtzen et al., 1995).

III. PATHOGENICITY OF HEPARIN-DEPENDENT ANTIBODIES

Anti-PF4–H antibodies of the IgG isotype are present in at least 80% of patients with clinical HIT. In the remaining cases, only IgA, IgM, or both, isotypes, in high concentrations, are observed. These intriguing observations require explanation for how these antibodies trigger thrombocytopenia, with or without thrombosis.

Antibodies to PF4–H are believed to become pathogenic when they interact with platelets or other blood and endothelial cells. This can occur only if the PF4–H complexes bind to the cell surfaces, predominantly through their heparin-binding sites (Horne et al., 1996, 1998; Van Rijn et al., 1987), but possibly also through PF4-binding sites (Capitanio et al., 1985; Rybak et al., 1989). Although the HIT antibodies recognize PF4–H complexes in the fluid phase (Newman et al., 1998), it is uncertain whether this typically occurs in vivo before interaction of PF4–H–IgG complexes with the platelet surface, or whether HIT antibodies only bind after PF4–H complexes are attached to the platelet surface.

Regardless, the clinical state of patients—determining the extent of platelet and endothelial cell activation—seems to be a key factor for determining whether clinical HIT results (Boshkov et al., 1993; Reininger et al., 1996). This contribution occurs in several ways: activated platelets generate high PF4 concentrations that can complex with heparin, and activated cells also expose a higher density of heparin-binding sites (Horne and Chao, 1989). Furthermore, these platelets may be more readily activated by heparin-dependent antibodies. This situation occurs in patients with acute or chronic blood activation associated with cardiopulmonary bypass, atherosclerosis, inflammation, infections, cancer, diabetes, orthopedic surgery, among others.

Another factor determining HIT antibody formation is the type of heparin used for heparin binding to PF4 which depends on its oligosaccharide composition, polysaccharide length, and grade of sulfation (Greinacher et al., 1995; Lindahl et al., 1994). Formation of PF4–H complexes requires a heparin molecule with at least 12–14 oligosaccharide units and a high sulfation grade (more than three sulfate groups per disaccharide) (Amiral et al., 1995). Furthermore, binding of heparin to blood and endothelial cells also increases with heparin molecule length and sulfation grade (Horne and Chao, 1990; Harenberg et al., 1994; Sobel and Adelman, 1988). Heparin structure thus has a dual effect in HIT: it is required to form PF4–H complexes, and also to target these complexes onto cells. These factors could explain the higher frequency of PF4–H antibody development and of HIT in patients receiving UFH, compared with LMWH. With UFH, PF4–H complexes are more easily formed and require a lower heparin concentration than with LMWH. For the latter drug, only the subset of molecules containing at least 12–14 oligosaccharide units (MW $>$ 3600 Da) can generate immunoreactive PF4–H complexes. Thus, because LMWH has a lower propensity to form PF4–H complexes, and binds less readily to platelets and endothelial cells, LMWH therapy may be less likely to result in thrombocytopenia even in the presence of pathogenic HIT antibodies.

PF4–H-reactive antibodies targeted to platelets induce platelet activation, resulting in thrombocytopenia and, oftentimes, thrombosis. Occasionally, heparin-induced thrombosis occurs in the absence of thrombocytopenia (Hach-Wunderle et al., 1994; Bux-Gewehr et al., 1996). Platelet activation by the IgG isotype antibodies is mediated by interaction with the platelet FcγRIIA receptors (Kelton et al., 1994; Denomme et al., 1997). Some studies suggest an important role for FcγRIIA polymorphism (Brandt et al., 1995; Burgess et al., 1995). However, the role of the FcγRIIA receptor polymorphism is controversial (Arepally et al., 1997; Bachelot-Loza et al., 1998, Denomme et al., 1997; Suh et al., 1997; see Chap. 9).

Platelet activation might also occur through other mechanisms, such as direct antibody binding to exposed cell antigens (Rubinstein et al., 1995), a phenomenon that is dependent on the antigen electric charge (Schattner et al., 1993). Heparin is highly electronegative. Evidence for direct activation through antigen binding is supported by the positive platelet aggregation produced by some patient plasma samples containing only antibodies of the IgM or IgA isotypes. Furthermore, in vivo, platelets are in their blood and endothelial environment. Formation of heparin-containing immune complexes on cell surfaces can initiate blood and endothelial cell interactions, and this can enhance the activating effect. Cell–cell interactions may occur and be amplified through release products that chemoattract and activate cells, or through transcellular metabolism (Marcus et al., 1995; Nash et al., 1994). Platelet products (e.g., PF4) and platelet-derived microparticles (Warkentin et al., 1994) can induce activation of leukocytes (Aziz

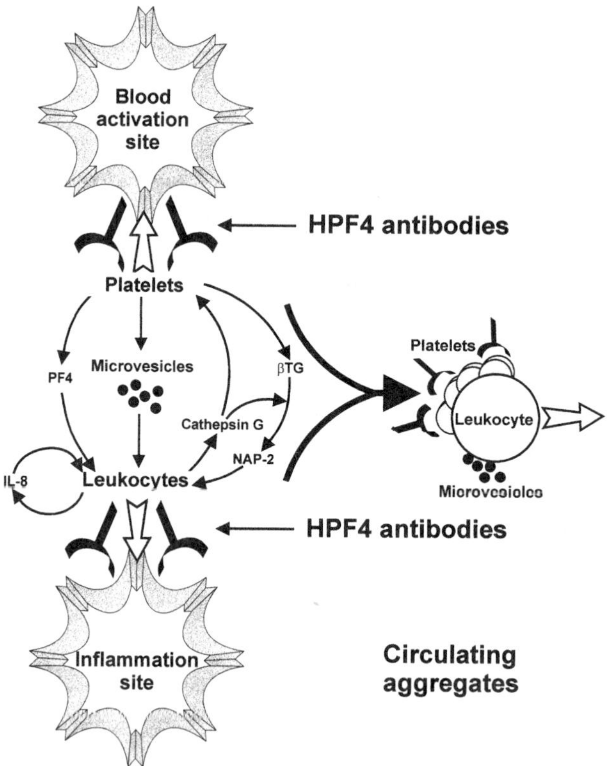

Figure 2 Occurrence of cell–cell interactions at the neighborhood of blood activation or inflammation sites: Presence of heparin-dependent antibodies increases the amount of cells available at these sites, amplifies cell–cell interactions and cellular activation, and can lead to blood clotting or release of circulating cell aggregates. HPF4, heparin–platelet factor 4; IL-8, interleukin-8; NAP-2, neutrophil-activating peptide 2; βTG, β-thromboglobulin

et al., 1995; Jy et al., 1995; Petersen et al., 1996). Leukocyte-release products, such as cathepsin G, can directly activate platelets and cleave β-thromboglobulin to the active chemokine NAP-2, thus establishing an amplification loop. Platelet–leukocyte aggregates can form in vivo contributing to vascular occlusion, especially in limb vessels (Fig. 2).

Various characteristics of PF4–H antibodies are another key factor for induction of HIT. Platelet activation induced by PF4–H antibodies is usually weak and is only pathogenic when amplified. This is demonstrated by the variable lag phase observed in platelet aggregation studies with different plasmas or sera from HIT patients. Antibody concentration is an important factor for determining the extent of platelet activation. Antibody affinity is also very important: the higher the affinity, the lower the concentration of antibodies required for activating platelets. When IgM or IgA isotypes are present, affinity for PF4–H complexes is usually lower than that of IgG isotypes and, consequently, high concentrations are necessary for pathogenicity. Lastly, HIT antibodies do not all bind to the same epitope on PF4–H complexes, and this specificity could be an important factor in their action (Horsewood et al., 1996; Pouplard et al., 1997; Suh et al., 1998). Anti-PF4–H antibodies are not equivalent, and those with the strongest affinity are most pathogenic. Recent data show that primary platelet activation in HIT involves ADP receptors (Polgar et al., 1998), and that platelet aggregation involves GPIIb/IIIa (Hérault et al., 1997; Jeske et al., 1997). These findings further emphasize the importance of platelet activation amplification loops for producing the clinical manifestations of HIT.

IV. PREEXISTING ANTICHEMOKINE ANTIBODIES

Preexisting antibodies to chemokines, such as IL-8 or NAP-2, or possibly to PF4 itself, may be present in some patients even before heparin therapy (Bendtzen et al., 1995; Sylvester et al., 1992). These antibodies may occur naturally and have a regulatory role in inflammation (Reitamo et al., 1993). In some disease states, they are present at high concentrations. Antibodies to IL-8 are most common (Reitamo et al., 1993). However, in some patients, true autoantibodies to PF4 alone can also be observed. In the absence of heparin, these antibodies do not demonstrate clear pathogenicity. During heparin therapy, PF4 and other chemokines are released into the circulation from their storage pools. Heparin localizes these chemokines to blood and endothelial cells. Thus, naturally occurring heparin-dependent antibodies could then be targeted to these cells, initiating immune injury. The amount of chemokine–heparin complexes bound to blood and endothelial cells depends on different factors: the amount of releasable chemokines (i.e., the patient's clinical state); the type and dose of heparin used; and the presence of activated cells with an increased capacity to bind heparin-like antibodies against PF4–H complexes. As with antibodies against PF4–H complexes, these natural antichemokine antibodies could initiate cell activation and cell–cell interactions, as well as generate circulating cell aggregates that could lead to vessel occlusion.

V. CONCLUSIONS

The conditions that permit formation of the molecular PF4–H target antigen for HIT antibodies involve the properties of the heparin used, dose and duration of therapy, and the clinical context of the treated patient. Immunoreactive complexes between PF4 and heparin are formed only under certain conditions. Their formation in high concentrations is facilitated if underlying disease favors platelet activation and release. Similar conditions enhance the pathogenicity of the HIT-generated antibodies. These considerations help unravel the apparent random generation of HIT antibodies in heparin-treated patients, as well as the seemingly random occurrence of thrombotic events.

REFERENCES

Amiral J, Bridey F, Dreyfus M, Vissac AM, Fressinaud E, Wolf M, Meyer D. Platelet factor 4 complexed to heparin is the target for antibodies generated in heparin induced thrombocytopenia [letter]. Thromb Haemost 68:95–96, 1992.

Amiral J, Bridey F, Wolf M, Boyer-Neumann C, Fressinaud E, Vissac AM, Peynaud-Debayle E, Dreyfus M, Meyer D. Antibodies to macromolecular platelet factor 4 heparin complexes in heparin-induced thrombocytopenia: a study of 44 cases. Thromb Haemost 73:21–28, 1995.

Amiral J, Marfaing-Koka A, Wolf M, Alessi MC, Tardy B, Boyer-Neumann C, Vissac AM, Fressinaud E, Poncz M, Meyer D. Presence of auto-antibodies to interleukin-8 or neutrophil-activating peptide-2 in patients with heparin-associated-thrombocytopenia. Blood 88:410–416, 1996a.

Amiral J, Peynaud-Debayle E, Wolf M, Bridey F, Vissac AM, Meyer D. Generation of antibodies to heparin–PF4 complexes without thrombocytopenia in patients treated with unfractionated or low molecular weight heparin. Am J Hematol 52:90–95, 1996b.

Amiral J, wolf M, Fischer AM, Boyer-Neumann C, Vissac AM, Meyer D. Pathogenicity of IgA and/or IgM antibodies to heparin–PF4 complexes in patients with heparin-induced thrombocytopenia. Br J Haematol 92:954–959, 1996c.

Arepally G, McKenzie SE, Jiang X-M, Poncz M, Cines DB. FcγRIIA H/R^{131} polymorphism, subclass-specific IgG anti-heparin/platelet factor 4 antibodies and clinical course in patients with heparin-induced thrombocytopenia and thrombosis. Blood 89:370–375, 1997.

Aziz KA, Cawley JC, Zuzel M. Platelets prime PMN via released PF4: mechanism of priming and synergy with GM–CSF. Br J Haematol 91:846–853, 1995.

Bachelot-Loza C, Saffroy R, Lasne D, Chatellier G, Aiach M, Rendu F. Importance of the FcγRIIA-Arg/His-131 polymorphism in heparin-induced thrombocytopenia diagnosis. Thromb Haemost 79:523–528, 1998.

Bendtzen K, Hansen MB, Ross C, Poulsen LK, Svenson M. Cytokines and autoantibodies to cytokines. Stem Cells 13:206–222, 1995.

Bock PE, Luscombe M, Marshall SE, Pepper DS, Holbrook JJ. The multiple complexes formed by the interaction of platelet factor 4 with heparin. Biochem J 191:769–776, 1980.

Boshkov LK, Warkentin TE, Hayward CPM, Andrew M, Kelton JG. Heparin-induced thrombocytopenia and thrombosis: clinical and laboratory studies. Br J Haematol 84:322–328, 1993.

Brandt E, Flad HD. Structure and function of platelet-derived cytokines of the β-thromboglobulin/interleukin 8 family. Platelets 3:295–305, 1992.

Brandt J, Isenhart CE, Osborne JM, Ahmed A, Anderson CL. On the role of platelet FcγRIIa phenotype in heparin-induced thrombocytopenia. Thromb Haemost 74: 1564–1572, 1995.

Burgess JK, Lindeman R, Chesterman CN, Chong BH. Single amino acid mutation of Fcγ receptor is associated with the development of heparin-induced thrombocytopenia. Br J Haematol 91:761–766, 1995.

Bux-Gewehr I, Helmling E, Sefert UT. HAT type II and platelets within a normal range. Kardiologia 85:656–660, 1996.

Capitanio AM, Niewiarowski S, Rucinski B, Tuszynski GP, Cierniewski CS, Hershock D, Kornecki E. Interaction of platelet factor 4 with human platelets. Biochim Biophys Acta 839:161–173, 1985.

Cines DB, Tomaski A, Tannenbaum S. Immune endothelial-cell injury in heparin-associated thrombocytopenia. N Engl J Med 316:581–589, 1987.

Cowan SW, Bakshi EN, Machin KJ, Isaacs NW. Binding of heparin to human platelet factor 4. Biochem J 234:485–488, 1986.

Denomme GA, Warkentin TE, Horsewood P, Sheppard JI, Warner MN, Kelton JG. Activation of platelets by sera containing IgG1 heparin-dependent antibodies: an explanation for the predominance of the FcγRIIa ''low responder'' (his_{131}) gene in patients with heparin-induced thrombocytopenia. J Lab Clin Med 130:278–284, 1997.

Dunlop MG, Prowse CV, Dawes J. Heparin-induced platelet factor 4 release in patients with atherosclerotic peripheral vascular disease. Thromb Res 46:409–410, 1987.

Greinacher A, Pötzsch B, Amiral J, Dummel V, Eichner A, Mueller-Eckhardt C. Heparin-associated thrombocytopenia: isolation of the antibody and characterization of a multimolecular PF4–heparin complex as the major antigen. Thromb Haemost 71: 247–251, 1994.

Greinacher A. Antigen generation in heparin-associated thrombocytopenia: the nonimmunologic type and the immunologic type are closely linked in their pathogenesis. Semin Thromb Hemost 21:106–116, 1995.

Greinacher A, Alban S, Dummel V, Franz G, Mueller-Eckhardt C. Characterization of the structural requirements for a carbohydrate based anticoagulant with a reduced risk of inducing the immunological type of heparin-associated thrombocytopenia. Thromb Haemost 74:886–892, 1995.

Gruel Y, Boizard-Boval B, Wautier JL. Further evidence that alpha-granule components such as platelet factor 4 are involved in platelet–IgG–heparin interactions during heparin-associated thrombocytopenia. Thromb Haemost 70:374–375, 1993.

Hach-Wunderle V, Kainer K, Krug B, Müller-Berghaus G, Pötzsch B. Heparin-associated thrombosis despite normal platelet counts. Lancet 344:469–470, 1994.

Harenberg J, Malsch R, Piazolo L, Heene DL. Binding of heparin to human leukocytes. Haemostaseologie 14:16–24, 1994.

Hérault J.P, Lalé A, Savi P, Pflieger AM, Herbert JM. In vitro inhibition of heparin-induced platelet aggregation in plasma from patients with HIT by SR 121566, a newly developed Gp IIb/IIIa antagonist. Blood Coagul Fibrinolysis 8:206–207, 1997.

Horne MK III, Alkins BR. Platelets binding of IgG from patients with heparin-induced thrombocytopenia. J Lab Clin Med 127:435–442, 1996.

Horne MK III, Chao ES. Heparin binding to resting and activated platelets. Blood 74: 238–243, 1989.

Horne MK III, Chao ES. The effect of molecular weight on heparin binding to platelets. Br J Haematol 74:306–312, 1990.

Horne MK III, Hutchison KJ. Simultaneous binding of heparin and platelet factor-4 to platelets: further insights into the mechanism of heparin-induced thrombocytopenia. Am J Hematol 58:24–30, 1998.

Horsewood P, Warkentin TE, Hayward CPM, Kelton JG. The epitope specificity of heparin-induced thrombocytopenia. Br J Haematol 95:161–167, 1996.

Jeske WP, Walenga JM, Szatkowski E, Ero M, Herbert JM, Haas S, Bakhos M. Effect of glycoprotein IIb-IIIa antagonists on the HIT serum induced activation of platelets. Thromb Res 88:271–281, 1997.

Jy W, Mao WW, Horstman LL, Tao J, Ahn YS. Platelet microparticles bind, activate and aggregate neutrophils in vitro. Blood Cells Mol Dis 21:217–231, 1995.

Kelton JG, Smith JW, Warkentin TE, Hayward CPM, Denomme GA, Horsewood P. Immunoglobulin G from patients with heparin-induced thrombocytopenia binds to a complex of heparin and platelet factor 4. Blood 83:3232–3239, 1994.

Kelton J. Pathophysiology of heparin-induced thrombocytopenia [letter]. Br J Haematol 82:778–784, 1992.

Lindahl U, Lidholt K, Spillmann D, Kjellen L. More to ''heparin'' than anticoagulant. Throm Res 75:1–32, 1994.

Maccarana M, Lindahl U. Mode of interaction between platelet factor 4 and heparin. Glycobiology 3:271–277, 1993.

Marcus AJ, Safier LB, Broekman MJ, Islam N, Fliessbach JH, Hajjar KA, Kaminski WE, Jendraschak E, Silverstein RL, von Schacky C. Thrombosis and inflammation as multicellular processes: significance of cell–cell interactions. Thromb Haemost 74: 213–217, 1995.

Nash GB. Adhesion between neutrophils and platelets: a modulator of thrombotic and inflammatory events? Thromb Res 74:S3–S11, 1994.

Petersen F, Lidwig A, Flad HD, Brandt E. TNF-α renders human neutrophils responsive to platelet factor 4. J Immunol 156:1954–1962, 1996.

Polgar J, Eichler P, Greinacher A, Clemetson KJ. Adenosine diphosphate (ADP) and ADP receptor play a major role in platelet activation/aggregation induced by sera from heparin-induced thrombocytopenia patients. Blood 91:549–554, 1998.

Pouplard C, Amiral J, Borg JY, Vissac AM, Delahousse B, Gruel Y. Differences in specificity of heparin-dependent antibodies developed under low-molecular-weight-heparin therapy and higher cross-reactivity with Orgaran. Br J Haematol 99:273–280, 1997.

Reininger CB, Greinacher A, Graf J, Lasser R, Steckmeier B, Schweiberer L. Platelets of patients with peripheral arterial disease are hypersensitive to heparin. Thromb Res 81:641–649, 1996.

Reitamo S, Remitz A, Varga J, Ceska M, Effenberger F, Jimenez S, Uitto J. Demonstration of interleukin 8 and autoantibodies to interleukin 8 in the serum of patients with sytemic sclerosis and related disorders. Arch Dermatol 129:189–193, 1993.

Rubinstein E, Boucheix C, Worthington RE, Carroll RC. Anti-platelet antibody interactions with Fcγ receptor. Semin Thromb Haemost 21:10–22, 1995.

Rybak ME, Gimbrone MA, Davies PF, Handin RI. Interaction of platelet factor four with cultured vascular endothelial cells. Blood 73:1534–1539, 1989.

Schattner M, Lazzari M, Trevani AS, Malchiodi E, Kempfer AC, Isturiz MA, Geffner JR. Activation of human platelets by immune complexes prepared with cationized human IgG. Blood 82:3045–3051, 1993.

Shoenfeld Y. Heparin-induced thrombocytopenia as an autoimmune disease: idiotypic evidence for the role of anti-heparin–PF4 autoantibodies. Isr J Med Sci 33:243–245, 1997.

Sobel M, Adelman B. Characterization of platelet binding of heparins and other glycosaminoglycans. Thromb Res 50:815–826, 1988.

Stuckey JA, St Charles R, Edwards B. A model of the platelet factor 4 complex with heparin. Proteins 14:277–287, 1992.

Suh JS, Malik MI, Aster RH, Visentin GP. Characterization of the humoral immune response in heparin-induced thrombocytopenia. Am J Hematol 54:196–201, 1997.

Suh JS, Aster RH, Visentin GP. Antibodies from patients with heparin-induced thrombocytopenia/thrombosis recognize different epitopes on heparin: platelet factor 4. Blood 91:916–922, 1998.

Sylvester L, Yoshimura T, Sticherling M, Schröder JM, Ceska M, Peichi P, Leonard EJ. Neutrophil attractant protein-1–immunoglobulin G immune complexes and free anti-NAP-1 antibody in normal human serum. J Clin Invest 90:471–481, 1992.

Van Rijn JLML, Trillou M, Mardiguian J, Tobelem G, Caen J. Selective binding of heparins to human endothelial cells. Implications for pharmacokinetics. Thromb Res 45: 211–222, 1987.

Visentin GP, Aster RH. Heparin induced thrombocytopenia and thrombosis. Curr Opin Hematol 2:351–357, 1995.

Visentin GP, Ford SE, Scott JP, Aster RH. Antibodies from patients with heparin-induced thrombocytopenia/thrombosis are specific for platelet factor 4 complexed with heparin or bound to endothelial cells. J Clin Invest 93:81–88, 1994.

Visentin GP, Malik M, Cyganiak KA, Aster RH. Patients with unfractionated heparin during open heart surgery are at high risk to form antibodies reactive with heparin: platelet factor 4 complexes. J Lab Clin Med 128:376–383, 1996.

Warkentin TE, Kelton JG. A 14-year study of heparin-induced thrombocytopenia. Am J Med 101:502–507, 1996.

Warkentin TE, Hayward CPM, Boshkov LK, Santos AV, Sheppard JI, Bode AP, Kelton JG. Sera from patients with heparin-induced thrombocytopenia generate platelet-derived microparticles with procoagulant activity: an explanation for the thrombotic complications of heparin-induced thrombocytopenia. Blood 84:3691–3699, 1994.

Warkentin TE, Levine MN, Hirsh J, Horsewood P, Roberts RS, Gent M, Kelton JG. Heparin-induced thrombocytopenia in patients treated with low-molecular-weight heparin or unfractionated heparin. N Engl J Med 332:1330–1335, 1995.

7
Molecular Immunopathogenesis of Heparin-Induced Thrombocytopenia

Gian Paolo Visentin and Steven G. Bacsi
Blood Research Institute, The Blood Center of Southeastern Wisconsin, Inc., Milwaukee, Wisconsin

Richard H. Aster
Medical College of Wisconsin and Blood Research Institute, The Blood Center of Southeastern Wisconsin, Inc., Milwaukee, Wisconsin

I. INTRODUCTION

Thrombocytopenia occurs commonly during heparin therapy, usually as a transient fall in platelet count 1–3 days after initiation of treatment. In most patients, this is of no clinical significance, and platelet levels return to normal within 3 days, with or without discontinuing the heparin administration. In contrast, a relatively small group of patients develop thrombocytopenia, with a characteristic delay that is usually 5–10 days after starting heparin therapy, although some patients recently exposed to heparin develop an abrupt onset of thrombocytopenia. Paradoxically, many of these patients experience venous or arterial thromboembolism (see Chap. 3). To early investigators, this profile of a delay in onset of thrombocytopenia, as well as abrupt recurrence on rechallenge, suggested an immune pathogenesis (see Chap. 1).

Today, there is an emerging consensus that this immune-mediated syndrome, designated heparin-induced thrombocytopenia (HIT), is an important life- and limb-threatening complication of heparin therapy. HIT is more common in patients receiving certain types of heparin, such as unfractionated heparin (UFH) of beef lung versus porcine mucosal origin, or unfractionated versus low molecular weight forms of porcine-derived heparin (see Chap. 4). HIT can be triggered by standard therapeutic-dose heparin, low-dose (prophylactic) treatment (Hrushesky, 1978), low molecular weight heparin (LMWH) (Lecompte, 1991; Tardy, 1991), and even by minute quantities given to ''flush'' intravascular catheters (Heeger and Backstrom, 1986; Ling and Warkentin, 1998). Various aspects of the pathogenesis of this disorder are also summarized in Chapters 6, 8, 9, and 10.

Early investigations showed that IgG antibodies associated with HIT could induce platelet activation in the presence of pharmacological (0.2–1 U/mL) or even lower doses of heparin. By taking advantage of this property, two ''activation'' diagnostic tests were developed for HIT: the platelet aggregation test (PAT) and the serotonin-release assay (SRA; see Chap. 11). Because activation of platelets by IgG from patients with HIT in the presence of heparin could be inhibited by a monoclonal antibody that blocks the platelet FcγRIIA receptor (Kelton et al., 1988), it was assumed that the antibodies react with heparin to form immune complexes which, in turn, activate platelets. However, early studies failed to demonstrate binding of heparin-induced antibodies to platelets in the presence of heparin, in contrast to the behavior of platelet-reactive antibodies induced by other drugs, such as quinidine and quinine. Moreover, the putative heparin–IgG complexes could not be identified in most studies (Green et al., 1978; Warkentin and Kelton, 1991; Greinacher et al., 1992). Thus, it remained unclear how heparin induces platelet activation and thrombocytopenia in patients with HIT.

A new understanding of the pathogenesis of HIT and associated thrombosis emerged when Amiral and co-workers (1992) suggested that antibodies in HIT might be specific for complexes of heparin and platelet factor 4 (PF4), rather than for heparin alone. We (Visentin et al., 1994) and others (Greinacher et al., 1994; Kelton et al., 1994) confirmed these findings. We added the observation that HIT antibodies recognize PF4 bound to heparan sulfate, normally found on the surface of endothelial cells in the form of proteoglycan, and speculated that binding of antibodies to PF4 on endothelial cells might promote endothelial cell damage predisposing to thrombosis (Visentin et al., 1994). These advances enabled the development of hypotheses to explain thrombocytopenia and thrombosis in HIT, but our understanding of the pathogenesis of this disorder is still incomplete.

II. HEPARIN AND PLATELET FACTOR 4

Heparin and heparan sulfate constitute a distinct class of glycosaminoglycans (GAG). GAGs are long, linear polymers composed of repeating disaccharide subunits. Heparin and heparan sulfate belong to a family of polysaccharide species, the chains of which are made up of alternating 1–4-linked and variously sulfated residues of hexuronic (D-glucuronic or L-iduronic) acid and D-glucosamine. The two substances differ in their hexuronic acid composition and pattern of substitution, with heparin having a higher content of sulfates and, consequently, a greater linear charge density. Commercially available heparin preparations are heterogeneous and polydisperse, consisting of polysaccharide fragments ranging in length from 3,000 to 30,000 kDa (10–100 saccharide residues; see Chap. 8).

Heparan sulfate, together with chondroitin sulfate and dermatan sulfate, is widely distributed in all tissues, whereas heparin is found only in lung, ileum, skin, lymph nodes, thymus, and appendix where mast cells are concentrated (Gomes and Dietrich, 1982). Metachromatic granules of mast cells are the major reservoir of heparin (Metcalfe et al., 1979). Heparan sulfate and other GAGs are also found in mast cell granules, but are expressed mainly on the surface of nearly all adherent mammalian cells in the form of proteoglycans, consisting of oligosaccharides covalently linked to a core protein (syndecan) (Höök et al., 1984).

PF4, a heparin-binding protein normally found in platelet α-granules, is secreted when platelets are activated by various stimuli. Human PF4 is a member of a large family of homologous proteins, encoded by genes located on chromosomes 4 and 17, which have been designated "chemokines," and are involved in chemotaxis, coagulation, inflammation, and cell growth (Oppenheim et al., 1991; Rollins, 1997; Luster, 1998). This family has been separated into four branches, designated CX_3C, CXC, CC, and C, based on the relative position of the first two conserved cysteines. PF4 belongs to the CXC family, which includes among others, interleukin-8 (IL-8), interferon-γ-inducible protein (IP-10), platelet basic protein (PBP), and two proteins derived from PBP by proteolytic cleavage: β-thromboglobulin (β-TG) and neutrophil-activating protein-2 (NAP-2). Human PF4 is a symmetrical, tetrameric molecule made up of identical subunits, each containing 70 amino acid residues of known sequence (Poncz et al., 1987), including two disulfide bonds, a single tyrosine, but no tryptophan. The molecule is positively charged at physiological pH (Handin and Cohen, 1976). The crystal structure of human PF4 has been resolved (Zhang et al., 1994). Lysine residues on the exterior faces of α-helices at the COOH-terminus of each monomer are critical for heparin binding (Loscalzo et al., 1985). However, residues located elsewhere on the tetramer are probably also important for this interaction (Maccarana and Lindbahl, 1993; Mayo et al., 1995b).

III. NATURE OF THE EPITOPES RECOGNIZED BY HIT ANTIBODIES

A. The Role of Polyanion

The HIT antibodies fail to recognize PF4 or heparin alone, but bind avidly to the PF4–heparin complex (Visentin et al., 1994). Antibody epitopes, therefore, could be composed of either combinatorial epitopes, consisting partly of heparin and partly of PF4, or conformational epitopes on the PF4 molecule induced by heparin binding. Alternatively, a conformational change elsewhere on the PF4 molecule, created when the complex forms, could be targeted.

Heparin is a linear polyanion, and Maccarana and Lindahl (1993) have suggested that it binds to positively charged PF4 by nonspecific, electrostatic interactions, rather than by specific oligosaccharide sequence recognition. However, Stringer and Gallagher (1997) have described a sequence on heparan sulfate consisting of a 9-kDa fragment, with sulfated domains at each end separated by a central, *N*-acetylated region, that may confer some specificity for PF4 binding. Regardless of whether PF4-heparin interaction is to some extent specific, non-GAG molecules can be substituted for heparin in detecting HIT antibodies. Kelton et al. (1994) found that highly sulfated polysaccharides, including heparan sulfate, pentosan polysulfate, and dextran sulfate, could be used, provided that they contained 1.0–1.5 sulfate groups per saccharide residue. Chondroitin sulfates A, B, and C, containing an average of only 0.5 sulfates per saccharide residue, were inactive. Highly sulfated, but low molecular weight substances, such as glucose-1,3,6-trisulfate, 1,2-cyclohexanediol disulfate, and heparin disaccharide, were likewise inactive. Greinacher and colleagues (1992, 1995) also characterized the structural requirements of polysaccharides active in generating HIT antibody epitopes. They showed that the β1,4-linkage between disaccharides, characteristic of heparin and other GAGs, was not essential, that heparin fractions containing fewer than ten residues were unable to promote platelet serotonin release by HIT antibodies, and that branched glucan sulfates were more effective than linear glucan sulfates of the same molecular weight. Similarly, Amiral and co-workers (1995) found that the extent of polysaccharide sulfation is positively correlated with the ability to interact with PF4 in facilitating the binding of HIT antibodies.

Studies conducted in our laboratory (Visentin et al., 1997a) showed that UFH of bovine and porcine origin, as well as LMWH formed complexes with PF4 that were recognized equally well by a panel of HIT antibodies. In studies with heparin fragments of known size, a length of at least ten saccharide residues was required to form complexes with PF4 that reacted (weakly) with this antibody panel. For optimal antibody recognition, fragments containing at least 12 saccharide residues were required. Also, sulfated GAGs other than heparin (e.g., heparan sulfate) as well as non-GAG sulfated polysaccharides (e.g., fucoidan and dextran sulfate) behaved similarly to heparin in their ability to form antibody-binding complexes with PF4. However, the heparinoid anticoagulant danaparoid (Orgaran), a mixture of nonheparin low molecular weight GAGs having a low degree of sulfation, formed complexes that reacted with only about one-third of patient samples tested (Visentin et al., 1997a). Our findings, together with those of Kelton, Greinacher, and Amiral already cited, indicate that the ability of GAGs and other sulfated polysaccharides to substitute for heparin in promoting platelet activation by HIT antibodies and to form complexes with PF4 to which the antibodies bind, is directly related to the size and degree of sulfation of the polysaccharide.

To determine whether or not a polysaccharide structure is necessary for the formation of HIT antibody epitopes, we evaluated a series of linear, nonsaccharide, polyanionic compounds and, unexpectedly, polyvinyl sulfate, polyvinyl sulfonate, polyvinyl phosphate, polyvinyl phosphonate, and polyanethole sulfonate all react with PF4 to form complexes recognized by HIT-associated antibodies (Visentin et al., 1997a). Thus, neither a saccharide chain nor sulfate side groups is essential for a polyanion to react with PF4 and to create sites for antibody binding, arguing strongly against the possibility that HIT antibodies are specific for ''compound epitopes'' consisting partially of GAG and partially of peptide sequence at sites where the molecules making up the complex come into close contact. This observation, together with the finding that HIT antibodies fail to recognize heparin complexed with protamine (unpublished observation), excludes the possibility that they recognize a configuration of the sulfated saccharide that is stabilized on binding to a small, positively charged, spherical protein.

It appears likely, therefore, that sites for antibody binding are created when linear polyanionic compounds bind to PF4 and alter its three-dimensional configuration. Heparin-induced antibodies associated with HIT bind avidly to complexes formed between PF4 and heparin fragments attached by end-linkage to agarose beads, but fail to recognize PF4 complexed with heparin molecules immobilized by multiple cross-linkages (Suh et al., 1998). Thus, another requirement for the formation of heparin–PF4 complexes for which HIT antibodies are specific is that the saccharide chain making up the heparin molecule must be in a flexible, relatively unconstrained state.

Although heparin–PF4 complexes have not yet yielded to structural analysis, some informative data about the nature of heparin–PF4 interaction and its effect on PF4 structure are available. Both bovine (St. Charles et al., 1989) and human (Zhang et al., 1994) PF4 tetramers have been crystallized and have similar structure. Each PF4 monomer consists of a COOH-terminal amphiphilic α-helix overlying a three-stranded antiparallel β-sheet, a structure typical of CXC chemokine family members (Luster, 1998). Two PF4 monomers associate side by side to produce a six-stranded antiparallel β-sheet, with overlying antiparallel α-helices (AB dimer). Each AB dimer associates with an identical CD dimer through surface interaction between the β-sheets. The elements of PF4 structure are shown schematically in Fig. 1a.

Crystallographic studies have shown that both bovine (St. Charles et al., 1989) and human (Zhang et al., 1994) PF4 contain a ring of positively charged lysine, arginine, and histidine residues that encircle the tetramer along a line perpendicular to the α-helices and are available for interaction with solvent. Modeling studies (Stuckey et al., 1992) support the possibility that a negatively

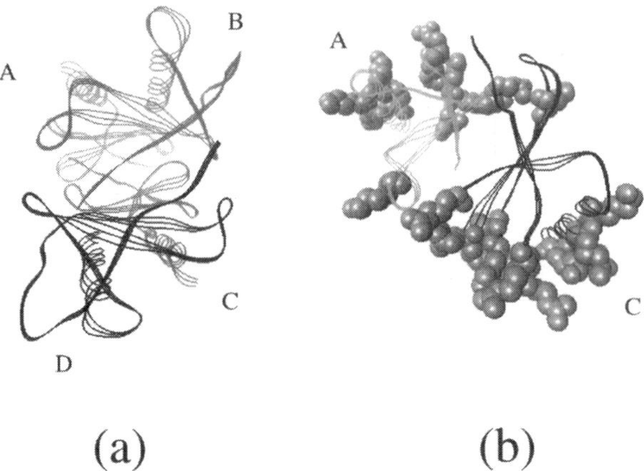

Figure 1 (a) Computer-generated model (WebLab ViewerPro; Molecular Simulation Inc., San Diego, CA) of the human PF4 tetramer, based on the crystallographic coordinates. (b) AC dimer view of human PF4: the amino acid residues crucial for heparin binding are displayed. (From: a, Zhang et al., 1994; b, Loscalzo et al., 1985; Mayo et al., 1995a).

charged heparin molecule, containing 18 saccharide residues (MW ~ 5.4 kDa), interacts with these positively charged residues spanning about half the tetramer. Mayo et al. (1995a,b) created a PF4 mutant (PF4-M2) in which the NH_2-terminal 11 residues were replaced by eight residues from the homologous CXC chemokine interleukin-8, to create a tetramer that binds heparin with the same avidity as native PF4, but is more nearly symmetrical around all three axes, facilitating NMR structural analysis. Their data, contrary to PF4–heparin-binding models that center around COOH-terminal α-helix lysines, indicate that arginines 20, 22, and 49, and to a lesser extent histidine 23, threonine 25, and lysine 46, are also important for heparin binding (Fig. 1b and Fig. 2). On the basis of these findings, it was speculated that heparin does not bind perpendicularly to the α-helices of the AB dimer, as had been suggested (Stuckey et al., 1992), but instead, reacts with the α-helix at an angle, interacting preferentially with PF4 along the AD dimer, where it would encounter arginine and other positively charged residues. In either model, it is plausible that binding of a linear polyanion of sufficient length and linear charge density to positively charged residues on the surface of PF4, could cause the structural rearrangement throughout the entire tetramer necessary for generation of HIT antibody epitopes.

On the basis of these reports and our own observations, it is possible to propose a model of how heparin and other linear polyanions react with PF4 to produce configurational changes in the tetramer and create sites for HIT antibody

```
        1                 10
        E A E E D G D L Q C L C V K T

      20                  30
T S Q V[R]P[R][H]I[T]S L E V I K A G P H

      40                  50
C P T A Q L I A T L[K]N G[R]K I C L D L
  •  •  •                 •               •

      60                  70
Q A P L Y[K K I I K K]L L E S
  •
```

Figure 2 Amino acid composition of human PF4 monomers: Residues crucial for heparin binding [COOH-terminal α-helix residues encompassing lysines 61–62 and 65–66 (Loscalzo et al., 1985), arginines 20, 22, and 49, histidine 23, threonine 25, and lysine 46 (Mayo, 1995b)] are boxed. Filled circles identify the six residues (37,38,39,49,55, and 57) in the 47 COOH-terminal region of PF4 at which human and rat PF4 differ.

binding. We suggest that linear polyanions, such as heparin, that carry appropriately spaced, strong negative charges interact with PF4 by binding to the ring of positive charges extending between the A and D or B and C subunits, or both. The minimum length for a fully active polyanion is about 50 A, equivalent to six disaccharide subunits (12-mer), with each disaccharide measuring about 8.4 A in length (Visentin et al., 1997a). Reconfiguration of the tetramer, resulting from binding of the polyanion, creates the neoepitope(s) for which HIT antibodies are specific.

B. The Role of Protein

Only a few investigators have attempted to map the actual epitopes on heparin–PF4 complexes recognized by HIT antibodies. Horsewood et al. (1996) studied a total of 29 antibodies from patients with HIT that were positive in the PF4–heparin enzyme-linked immunosorbent assay (ELISA) and in the serotonin release assay (SRA). Five of these antibodies also reacted with reduced–alkylated PF4 in the presence of heparin. The same five antibodies also recognized a peptide containing the 19 COOH-terminal amino acid residues of the PF4 monomer, a region that encompasses a positively charged α-helical domain thought to be critical for heparin binding (Loscalzo et al., 1985). However, neither reduced PF4 nor the COOH-terminal peptide could inhibit binding of HIT antibodies to heparin–PF4 complexes, even at high concentrations. Therefore, the clinical significance of the five antibodies is uncertain.

Amiral and co-workers (1996) studied a subgroup of 15 patients thought to have HIT whose antibodies were positive in a platelet aggregation test, but negative in heparin–PF4 ELISA. Nine of these patients had antibodies that recognized NAP-2 or IL-8, or both, two members of the CXC chemokine family that are homologous with PF4. These findings are of interest because five of the nine patients had thrombotic episodes. However, reactions of these antibodies against NAP-2 or IL-8 in their normal configurations (not immobilized on plastic) were not described, and their relation to antibodies that recognize heparin–PF4 complexes is uncertain.

Ziporen et al. (1998) studied the binding of antibodies from 50 HIT patients to different constructs of PF4, which contained a single amino acid substitution, and chimeric proteins, which contained various portions of human PF4 and NAP-2. Mutation to alanine of three (K62, K65, K66) of the four lysine residues in the COOH-terminal α-helix, had only minimal effect on the binding of HIT antibodies, and the K61 $\rightarrow$ A mutation reduced antibody binding by only about 50%, suggesting that the COOH-terminal lysines of PF4 do not constitute the major antigenic site for HIT antibodies. NH_2-terminal PF4–NAP-2 chimeras exhibited only slightly reduced antibody binding. In contrast, the PF4–NAP-2 chimera, in which the portion of PF4 lying between the third and fourth cysteine residue (amino acids 37–47) was substituted by the corresponding NAP-2 sequence, was almost totally nonreactive.

With a different approach, we found that, although human PF4 has 74% protein sequence identity to bovine and rat PF4, neither bovine nor rat PF4 complexed to heparin are recognized by HIT antibodies (Visentin et al., 1997b). Yet, rat PF4 differs from its human counterpart at only 6 of its 47 COOH-terminal amino acids (Doit et al., 1987; Poncz et al., 1987; see Fig. 2). To characterize the binding sites for HIT antibodies on PF4–heparin, we constructed seven PF4 mutants in which the human sequence (reactive) was converted to the corresponding residues of rat PF4 (nonreactive) and determined the effect of each change on HIT antibody binding to the construct complexed with heparin. The PF4 constructs tested were comparable with wild-type PF4 in their avidity for heparin. Each of 15 antibodies from HIT patients recognized PF4–heparin complexes containing PF4 constructs bearing mutations: E4 $\rightarrow$ S, L11 $\rightarrow$ V, and T16 $\rightarrow$ S at the NH_2-terminus, or A57 $\rightarrow$ V at the COOH-terminus just as well as wild-type human PF4-heparin complexes. In contrast, complexes containing other COOH-terminal mutants: P37 $\rightarrow$ A/T38 $\rightarrow$ V/A39 $\rightarrow$ P, R49 $\rightarrow$ S, and L55 $\rightarrow$ R exhibited varying degrees of reduced binding. The HIT antibodies tested recognized PF4 mutated at positions 49 and 55 only at a higher ratio of heparin to PF4 (0.8 U/mL vs. 0.5 U/mL). None of the 15 antibodies recognized peptides comprising the 26 or 15 COOH-terminal amino acid residues of the PF4 monomer, or reduced–alkylated human PF4 either in presence or absence of heparin (Fig. 3).

These results, together with the observations by Ziporen and associates (1998), point to the region of PF4 between the third and fourth cysteine residues as the major antigenic site for HIT antibodies' binding. Our observations with

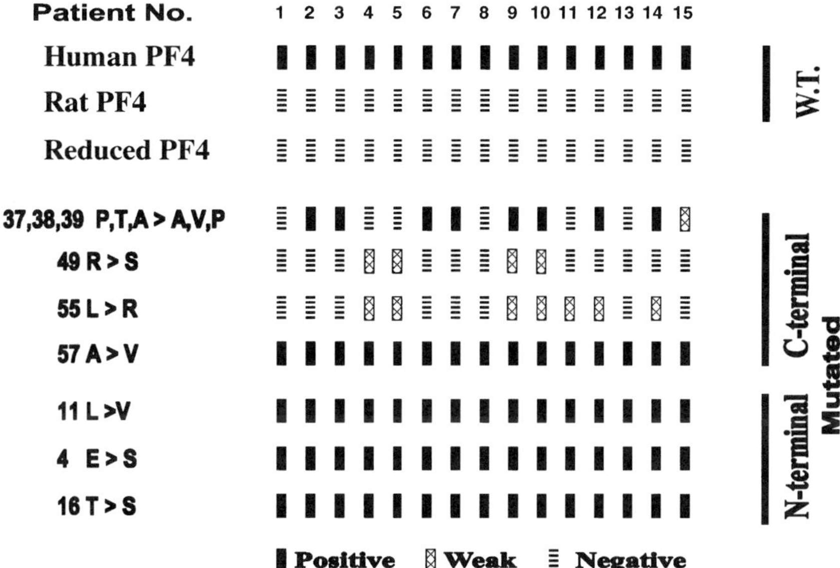

Figure 3 Summary of the reactions (obtained in PF4–heparin enzyme-linked immunosorbent assay; ELISA) of 15 HIT antibodies vs. complexes made up of PF4 mutants and heparin. Negative results were confirmed using a wide range of heparin concentrations (0.01–2 U/mL) vs. a fixed concentration (10 μg/mL) of PF4 construct.

biotin-labeled affinity-purified HIT antibodies in a competitive inhibition assay (Suh et al., 1998), indicate that at least three dominant HIT antibody recognition sites can be distinguished and further support the idea that HIT antibodies recognize conformation-dependent neoepitopes formed on PF4 when it binds to heparin.

IV. THE CELLULAR IMMUNE RESPONSE

The finding that HIT antibodies can be of the IgM, IgG, or IgA isotype (Visentin et al., 1994; Greinacher et al., 1994; Kelton et al., 1994; Amiral et al., 1995, 1996b; Arepally et al., 1997; Suh et al., 1997) indicates that class switching, likely requiring helper T cells, takes place in patients mounting a humoral immune response to heparin–PF4. Although HIT is a drug-induced disorder, parallels for the role of T cells in HIT may be drawn from studies of autoimmune conditions, such as systemic lupus erythematosus, systemic sclerosis, and insulin autoimmune syndrome (Ito et al., 1993; Crow et al., 1994; Kuwana et al., 1995b).

In both lupus and scleroderma, T-helper cells mediate antigen-specific autoantibody production by B cells (Adams et al., 1991; Mohan et al., 1993; Kuwana et al., 1995a).

We have used T-cell receptor (TCR) spectratyping (Maslanka et al., 1995), also called immunoscope (Cochet et al., 1992; Pannetier et al., 1993), and clonotyping (Maslanka et al., 1996) to characterize the T-cell response to PF4–heparin complexes in HIT. The TCRs of more than 95% of peripheral blood T cells are composed of two highly variable α- and β-chain glycoproteins, which function together in a complex with five other invariant molecules (CD3 complex) on the surface of the cell. The genes encoding the TCR β-chain subunit undergo sequential rearrangements analogous to that of the immunoglobulin superfamily of genes, during which D and J segments first, and then V segments, are combined to form various VDJ sequences (LaRoque and Robinson, 1996). Diversity is further increased by the random removal and insertion of nucleotides between the V, D, and J segments. The resulting VDJ sequence encodes the so-called third complementarity region or CDR3 loop, the primary region involved in peptide recognition by the TCR (LaRoque and Robinson, 1996). Through allelic exclusion, only a single β-chain is expressed on the surface of a T cell, thus the β-chain CDR3 sequence provides a clonal marker for T-cell lineages and has been used to assess T-cell repertoires. TCR spectratyping is a polymerase chain reaction (PCR)-based technique that provides a readout of TCR β-chain diversity in a given T-cell population. TCR clonotyping is a refinement of spectratyping whereby oligonucleotide probes specific to a given CDR3 loop region from a particular TCR β-chain (thus a ''clonotype'') are used to detect the presence or absence of the clonotype in a given T-cell population.

Culture of peripheral blood mononuclear cells (PBMC) from patients experiencing HIT incubated with heparin–PF4 complexes, but not heparin or PF4 alone, leads to selective expansion of T-cell subsets (De Palma et al., 1995; Bacsi et al., 1999). On in vitro culturing of PBMC from two HIT patients, the PF4–heparin complexes preferentially stimulated T cells expressing TCR with β-chains of the V 5.1 family, with a shared core CDR3 region amino acid motif (TGPG) (Bacsi et al., 1999). In a study of a third HIT patient, we found heparin–PF4-specific expansion of several βV 17 TCR clonotypes with yet another shared core CDR3 region amino acid motif (TSG) (Bacsi et al., 1997).

It is presently unclear why patients with HIT mount a brisk humoral immune response to an autologous protein (PF4). PF4 is undoubtedly processed, under normal circumstances, by antigen-presenting cells (APC) without triggering immunity. One possible explanation for the induction of a response to PF4 after injection of heparin is that heparin may perturb the processing of PF4 by APC in a way such that peptides not ordinarily produced (cryptic peptides) are generated and presented to T cells in the context of class II MHC molecules. Studies in murine systems provide examples of ''autoimmune'' states triggered by exogenous agents that perturb protein processing (Hess et al., 1991; Griem et al., 1996), but this phenomenon is not well characterized in the context of human disease. Our studies support a model in which pharmacological doses of heparin cause aberrant processing of PF4 by APCs, leading to the presentation of peptides not ordinarily seen by the immune system. This hypothesis can be tested directly if T-cell clones can be developed from mononuclear cells responding to heparin–PF4 cultures.

It appears that multiple factors influence the formation of antibodies specific for heparin–PF4 complexes in patients receiving heparin. Currently, there is no evidence to support genetic predisposition as a basis for antibody formation in patients receiving heparin. Unlike the situation in alloimmune thrombocytopenia (de Waal et al., 1986; Mueller-Eckhardt et al., 1989), no connection between HIT and human leukocyte antigens (HLA) has been found (Greinacher and Mueller-Eckhardt, 1993). IgM antibodies specific for heparin–PF4 complexes are a common finding in HIT (Visentin et al., 1994, 1997), indicating a primary immune response, and it could be speculated that patients who received UFH previously may be at greater risk to produce heparin–PF4-specific antibodies and develop HIT, if rechallenged with heparin. However, Cadroy et al. (1994) described a patient with a history of HIT who mounted a brisk IgM response when challenged again with UFH 3 years later. A recent report by Warkentin and Kelton (1998) suggests that there is no anamnestic immune response in HIT (i.e., patients either have ''typical'' HIT [onset at days 5–10] or ''rapid'' HIT, the latter apparently caused by residual circulating HIT antibodies, rather than a secondary immune response). Furthermore, HIT did not necessarily recur in patients who were exposed to heparin a second time.

V. IMPLICATIONS

The identification of mutations of human PF4 that lead to loss of HIT antibody binding will not necessarily localize the epitopes at which antibodies attach because the actual binding site(s) could be elsewhere in the PF4 tetramer. Moreover, HIT antibodies appear to recognize multiple sites on PF4-heparin (Suh et al., 1998). Because the PF4 molecule is a nearly symmetrical tetramer (Ibel et al., 1986), the HIT epitope could be expressed four times on each heparin–PF4 heterodimer, creating the potential for even a single antibody clone to react with four sites on a PF4 tetramer complexed with heparin. Studies from our group (Visentin et al., 1994, 1996) and others (Amiral et al., 1995; Arepally et al., 1995) have shown that, although antibodies reactive with heparin–PF4 complexes are nearly always present in patients with HIT, not all patients who form such antibodies experience thrombosis, or even thrombocytopenia. Factors that could predispose antibody formers to develop the HIT syndrome include the formation of unusually potent (high-titer) antibodies (Suh et al., 1997) and the presence of underlying conditions, congenital or acquired, that predispose to thrombosis. It can be speculated that antibodies recognizing certain sites on heparin–PF4 form immune complexes that are particularly effective in activating platelets. The same antibodies might be more likely to promote vessel injury when they bind to PF4 complexed with GAG on endothelial cells. Alternatively, patients who make antibodies that recognize multiple sites on heparin–PF4 may be more likely to produce pathogenic immune complexes, leading to more severe symptomatology.

ACKNOWLEDGMENTS

Supported in part by Grants HL-13629 and HL-44612 from the National Heart, Lung, and Blood Institute.

REFERENCES

Adams S, Leblanc P, Datta SK. Junctional region sequences of T-cell receptor beta-chain genes expressed by pathogenic anti-DNA autoantibody-inducing helper T cells from lupus mice: possible selection by cationic autoantigens. Proc Natl Acad Sci USA 88:11271–11275, 1991.

Amiral J, Bridey F, Dreyfus M, Vissac AM, Fressinaud E, Wolf M, Meyer D. Platelet factor 4 complexed to heparin is the target for antibodies generated in heparin-induced thrombocytopenia [letter]. Thromb Haemost 68:95–96, 1992.

Amiral J, Bridey F, Wolf M. Antibodies to macromolecular platelet factor-4 heparin complexes in heparin-induced thrombocytopenia: a study of 44 cases. Thromb Haemost 73:21–28, 1995.

Amiral J, Marfaing-Koka A, Wolf M, Alessi MC, Tardy B, Boyer-Neumann C, Vissac AM, Fressinaud E, Poncz M, Meyer D. Presence of autoantibodies to interleukin-8 or neutrophil-activating peptide-2 in patients with heparin-associated thrombocytopenia. Blood 88:410–416, 1996a.

Amiral J, Wolf M, Fischer AM, Boyer-Neumann C, Vissac AM, Meyer D. Pathogenicity of IgA and/or IgM antibodies to heparin–PF4 complexes in patients with heparin-induced thrombocytopenia. Br J Haematol 92:954–959, 1996b.

Arepally G, Reynolds C, Tomaski A, Amiral J, Jawad A, Poncz M, Cines DB. Comparison of PF4–heparin ELISA assay with the ^{14}C-serotonin release assay in the diagnosis of heparin-induced thrombocytopenia. Am J Clin Pathol 104:648–654, 1995.

Arepally G, McKenzie SE, Jiang XM, Poncz M, Cines DB. FcγRIIA H/R^{131} polymorphism, subclass-specific IgG anti-heparin/platelet factor 4 antibodies and clinical course in patients with heparin-induced thrombocytopenia and thrombosis. Blood 89:370–375, 1997.

Bacsi S, De Palma R, Visentin GP, Gorski J, Aster RH. Complexes of heparin and platelet factor 4 specifically stimulate T cells from patients with heparin-induced thrombocytopenia/thrombosis. Blood 94:208–215, 1999.

Bacsi S, Geoffrey R, Gorksi J, Aster R. Antigen-specific expansion of T cell clonotypes in heparin-induced thrombocytopenia/thrombosis (HITT) patient cultured T cells [abstr]. Blood 90(suppl):403a, 1997.

Cadroy Y, Amiral J, Raynaud H, Brunel P, Mazaleyrat A, Sauer M, Sie P. Evolution of antibodies anti-PF4/heparin in a patient with a history of heparin-induced thrombocytopenia reexposed to heparin [letter]. Thromb Haemost 71:247–251, 1994.

Cochet M, Pannetier C, Regnault A, Darche S, Leclerc C, Kourilsky P. Molecular detection and in vivo analysis of the specific T cell response to a protein antigen. Eur J Immunol 22:2639–2647, 1992.

Crow MK, DelGiudice-Asch G, Zehetbauer JB, Lawson JL, Brot N, Weissbach H, Elkon KB. Autoantigen-specific T cell proliferation induced by the ribosomal P2 protein in patients with systemic lupus erythematosus. J Clin Invest 94:345–352, 1994.

De Palma R, Gorski J, Aster RH, Visentin GP. The immune response in heparin-induced thrombocytopenia/thrombosis (HITP): preferential use of the Vβ11 family of the T cell receptor (TCR) repertoire [abstr]. Blood 86(suppl):537a, 1995.

de Waal LP, van Dalen CM, Engelfriet CP, von dem Borne AEGK. Alloimmunization against the platelet specific Zw^a antigen, resulting in neonatal alloimmune thrombocytopenia or posttransfusion purpura, is associated with the supertypic DRw52 antigen including DR3 and DRw6. Hum Immunol 17:45–53, 1986.

Doi T, Greenberg SM, Rosenberg RD. Structure of the rat platelet factor 4 gene: a marker for megakaryocyte differentiation. Mol Cell Biol 7:898–904, 1987.

Gomes PB, Dietrich CP. Distribution of heparin and other sulfated glycosaminoglycans in vertebrates. Comp Biochem Physiol 73B:857–863, 1982.

Green D, Harris K, Reynolds N, Roberts M, Patterson R. Heparin immune thrombocytopenia: evidence for heparin–platelet complex as the antigenic determinate. J Lab Clin Med 91:167–175, 1978.

Greinacher A, Mueller-Eckhardt C. Heparin-associated thrombocytopenia: no association of immune response with HLA. Vox Sang 65:151–153, 1993.

Greinacher A, Michels I, Mueller-Eckhardt C. Heparin-associated thrombocytopenia: the antibody is not heparin specific. Thromb Haemost 67:545–549, 1992.

Greinacher A, Pötzsch B, Amiral J, Dummel V, Eichner A, Mueller-Eckhardt C. Heparin-associated thrombocytopenia: isolation of the antibody and characterization of a multimolecular PF4–heparin complex as the major antigen. Thromb Haemostas 71: 247–251, 1994.

Greinacher A, Alban S, Dummel V, Franz G, Mueller-Eckhardt C. Characterization of the structural requirements for a carbohydrate-based anticoagulant with a reduced risk of inducing the immunological type of heparin-associated thrombocytopenia. Thromb Haemost 74:886–892, 1995.

Griem P, Panthel K, Kalbacher H, Gleichmann E. Alteration of a model antigen by Au(III) leads to T cell sensitization to cryptic peptides. Eur J Immunol 26:279–287, 1996.

Handin RI, Cohen HJ. Purification and binding properties of human platelet factor four. J Biol Chem 251:4273–4282, 1976.

Heeger PS, Backstrom JT. Heparin flushes and thrombocytopenia. Ann Intern Med 105: 143, 1986.

Hess EV. Drug-related lupus [review]. Curr Opin Rheumatol 3:809–814, 1991.

Horsewood P, Warkentin TE, Hayward CPM, Kelton JG. The epitope specificity of heparin-induced thrombocytopenia. Br J Haematol 95:161–167, 1996.

Höök M, Kjellén L, Johansson S, Robinson J. Cell-surface glycosaminoglycans. Annu Rev Biochem 53:847–869, 1984.

Hrushesky WJ. Subcutaneous heparin-induced thrombocytopenia. Arch Intern Med 138: 1489–1491, 1978.

Ibel K, Polland GA, Baldwin JP, Pepper DS, Luscombe M, Holbrook JJ. Low-resolution structure of the complex of human platelet factor 4 with heparin determined by small-angle neutron scattering. Biochim Biophys Acta 870:58–63, 1986.

Ito Y, Nieda M, Uchigata Y, Nishimura M, Tokunaga K, Kuwata S, Obata F, Tadokoro K, Hirata Y, Omori Y, Juji T. Recognition of human insulin in the context of HLA-DRB1*0406 products by T cells of insulin autoimmune syndrome patients and healthy donors. J Immunol 151:5770–5776, 1993.

Kelton JG, Sheridan D, Santos A, Smith J, Steeves K, Smith C, Brown C, Murphy WG. Heparin-induced thrombocytopenia: laboratory studies. Blood 72:925–930, 1988.

Kelton JG, Smith JW, Warkentin TE, Hayward CPM, Denomme GA, Horsewood P. Immunoglobulin G from patients with heparin-induced thrombocytopenia binds to a complex of heparin and platelet factor 4. Blood 83:3232–3239, 1994.

Kelton JG, Warkentin TE. Heparin-induced thrombocytopenia. Diagnosis, natural history, and treatment options [review]. Postgrad Med 103:169–171, 175–178, 1998.

Kuwana M, Medsger TA Jr, Wright TM. T cell proliferative response induced by DNA topoisomerase I in patients with systemic sclerosis and healthy donors. J Clin Invest 96:586–596, 1995a.

Kuwana M, Medsger TA Jr, Wright TM. T and B cell collaboration is essential for the autoantibody response to DNA topoisomerase I in systemic sclerosis. J Immunol 155:2703–2714, 1995b.

LaRoque R, Robinson MA. Diversity in the human T cell receptor beta chain [review]. Hum Immunol 48:3–11, 1996.

Lecompte T. Thrombocytopenia associated with low-molecular-weight heparin [letter]. Lancet 338:1217, 1991.

Ling E, Warkentin TE. Intraoperative heparin flushes and subsequent acute heparin-induced thrombocytopenia. Anesthesiology 89:1567–1569, 1998.

Loscalzo J, Melnick B, Handin RI. The interaction of platelet factor 4 and glycosaminoglycans. Arch Biochem Biophys 240:446–455, 1985.

Luster AD. Chemokines—chemotactic cytokines that mediate inflammation [review]. N Engl J Med 338:436–445, 1998.

Maccarana M, Linbahl U. Mode of interaction between platelet factor 4 and heparin. Glycobiology 3:271–277, 1993.

Máslanka K, Piatek T, Gorski J, Yassai M, Gorski J. Molecular analysis of T cell repertoires. Spectratypes generated by multiplex polymerase chain reaction and evaluated by radioactivity or fluorescence. Hum Immunol 44:28–34, 1995.

Maslanka K, Yassai M, Gorski J. Molecular identification of T cells that respond in a primary bulk culture to a peptide derived from a platelet glycoprotein implicated in neonatal alloimmune thrombocytopenia. J Clin Invest 98:1802–1808, 1996.

Mayo KH, Roongta V, Ilyina E, Milius R, Barker S, Quinlan C, La Rosa G, Daly TJ. NMR solution structure of the 32-kDa platelet factor 4 ELR-motif N-terminal chimera: a symmetric tetramer. Biochemistry 34:11399–11409, 1995a.

Mayo KH, Ilyina E, Roongta V, Dundas M, Joseph J, Lai CK, Maione T, Daly TJ. Heparin binding to platelet factor-4. An NMR and site-directed mutagenesis study: arginine residues are crucial for binding. Biochem J. 312:357–365, 1995b.

Metcalfe DD, Lewis RA, Silbert JE, Rosenberg RD, Wasserman SI, Austen KF. Isolation and characterization of heparin from human lung. J Clin Invest 64:1537–1543, 1979.

Mohan C, Adams S, Stanik V, Datta SK. Nucleosome: a major immunogen for pathogenic autoantibody-inducing T cells of lupus. J Exp Med 177:1367–1381, 1993.

Mueller-Eckhardt C, Kiefel V, Kroll H, Mueller-Eckhardt G. HLA-DRw6, a new immune response marker for immunization against the platelet alloantigen Br^a. Vox Sang 57:90–91, 1989.

Oppenheim JJ, Zachariae COC, Mukaida N, Matsushima K. Properties of the novel proinflammatory supergene "intercrine" cytokine family. Annu Rev Immunol 9:617–648, 1991.

Pannetier C, Cochet M, Darche S, Casrouge A, Zöller M, Kourilsky P. The sizes of the CDR3 hypervariable regions of the murine T-cell receptor β chains vary as a function of the recombined germ-line segments. Proc Natl Acad Sci USA 90:4319–4323, 1993.

Poncz M, Surrey S, LaRocco P, Weiss MJ, Rappaport EF, Conway TM, Schwartz E. Cloning and characterization of platelet factor 4 cDNA derived from a human erythroleukemic cell line. Blood 69:219–223, 1987.

Rollins BJ. Chemokines [review]. Blood 90:909–928, 1997.

St. Charles R, Walz DA, Edwards BFP. The three-dimensional structure of bovine platelet factor 4 at 3.0-A resolution. J Biol Chem 264:2092–2099, 1989.

Stringer SE, Gallagher JT. Specific binding of the chemokine platelet factor 4 to heparan sulfate. J Biol Chem 272:20508–20514, 1997.

Stuckey JA, St. Charles R, Edwards DFP. A model of the platelet factor 4 complex with heparin. Proteins 14:277–287, 1992.

Suh JS, Malik MI, Aster RH, Visentin GP. Characterization of the humoral immune response in heparin-induced thrombocytopenia. Am J Hematol 54:196–201, 1997.

Suh JS, Aster RH, Visentin GP. Antibodies from patients with heparin-induced thrombocytopenia/thrombosis recognize different epitopes on heparin:platelet factor 4 complexes. Blood 91:916–922, 1998.

Tardy B. Thrombocytopenia associated with low-molecular-weight heparin [letter]. Lancet 338:1217, 1991.

Visentin GP, Ford SE, Scott PJ, Aster RH. Antibodies from patients with heparin-induced thrombocytopenia/thrombosis are specific for platelet factor 4 complexed with heparin or bound to endothelial cells. J Clin Invest 93:81–88, 1994.

Visentin GP, Malik M, Cyganiak KA, Aster RH. Patients treated with unfractionated heparin during open heart surgery are at high risk to form antibodies reactive with heparin:platelet factor 4 complexes. J Lab Clin Med 128:376–383, 1996.

Visentin GP, Moghaddam M, Aster RH. Antibodies associated with heparin-induced thrombocytopenia/thrombosis (HITP) recognize sites on platelet factor 4 (PF4) induced by the binding of linear polyanionic compounds [abstr]. Thromb Haemost 77(suppl):362, 1997a.

Visentin GP, Aster RH, Geoffrey RA. Identification of critical amino acids in human platelet factor 4 (PF4)-heparin complex required for antibody recognition in heparin-induced thrombocytopenia/thrombosis (HITP) [abstr]. Thromb Haemost 77(suppl):362, 1997b.

Warkentin TE, Kelton JG. Heparin-induced thrombocytopenia. Prog Hemost Thromb 10: 1–34, 1991.

Warkentin TE, Kelton JG. Timing of heparin-induced thrombocytopenia (HIT) in relation to previous heparin use: absence of an anamnestic immune response, and implications for repeat heparin use in patients with a history of HIT [abstr]. Blood 92(suppl):182a, 1998.

Zhang X, Chen L, Bancroft DP, Lai CK, Maione TE. Crystal structure of recombinant human platelet factor 4. Biochemistry 33:8361–8366, 1994.

Ziporen L, Li ZQ, Park KS, Sabnekar P, Liu WY, Arepally G, Shoenfeld Y, Kieber-Emmons T, Cines DB, Poncz M. Defining an antigenic epitope on platelet factor 4 associated with heparin-induced thrombocytopenia. Blood 92:3250–3259, 1998.

8

Role of Sulfated Polysaccharides in the Pathogenesis of Heparin-Induced Thrombocytopenia

Susanne Alban
University of Regensburg, Regensburg, Germany

Andreas Greinacher
Ernst-Moritz-Arndt University, Greifswald, Germany

I. INTRODUCTION

Unfractionated heparin (UFH) and low molecular weight heparin (LMWH) are the anticoagulants of choice when parenteral anticoagulation with a short half-life is required. Both can be given subcutaneously or intravenously, and both are effective in a variety of clinical settings (Hirsh et al., 1998). UFH in particular has several limitations. These include its poor bioavailability after subcutaneous injection, as well as the marked variability in the anticoagulant response to UFH treatment in patients with acute thromboembolism (Hirsh, 1991; Young et al., 1992). Another problem is the risk of inducing heparin-induced thrombocytopenia (HIT). These limitations are closely linked (Greinacher, 1995): the underlying cause is the high density of negative charges of the heparin molecule, leading to nonspecific binding of heparin to plasma proteins other than antithrombin (AT). This results in inhibition of the anticoagulant effects of heparin, as well as changes in the conformational structure of the proteins following binding to heparin, with the potential for exposure of neoepitopes, or cryptic epitopes, toward which an immune response can be induced.

In this chapter, the mechanism and structural requirements for complex formation between sulfated carbohydrates, especially heparin, and proteins, such as platelet factor 4 (PF4), are reviewed. The pathophysiological consequences of these interactions in causing HIT are summarized. From these considerations, the prospects for development of carbohydrate-based heparin alternatives that would not cause immune thrombocytopenia are discussed.

II. INTERACTIONS OF PF4 WITH SULFATED CARBOHYDRATES

A. Structure of PF4

Heparin activity is neutralized by platelet factor 4 (PF4), a protein released from the α-granules of activated platelets (Sear and Poller, 1973; Klener and Kubisz, 1978; Niewiarowski, 1976; Luscher and Kaser-Glanzman, 1975; Walsh, 1976) that attaches to the endothelial surface by binding to glycosaminoglycans (GAGs) (Novotny et al., 1993). PF4 is a compact homotetrameric globular protein with a subunit molecular weight (MW) of 7780 Da (70 amino acid residues per subunit) (Kaplan and Niewiarowski, 1985; Mayo et al., 1995) containing 6.0% arginine, 3.2% histidine, and 12.3% lysine basic amino acids (Moore et al., 1975). The NH_2-terminal residues form antiparallel β-sheet–like structures that induce non-covalent associations between dimers and also contribute to the cohesion of the tetrameric unit. Furthermore, electrostatic interactions of multiply charged amino acid side chains and hydrogen-bonding interactions at the AB/CD dimer interface serve to stabilize the tetrameric structure. The COOH-terminal α-helices, which contain four lysine residues each of which are thought to be intimately involved in binding heparin, are arranged as antiparallel pairs on the surface of each extended β-sheet (St. Charles et al., 1989). These lysine residues are predominantly on one side, resulting in a ring of strong, positive charge that runs perpendicularly across the helices (Stuckey et al., 1992; Zhang et al., 1994; see Fig. 1 in Chap. 7).

B. Structure of Heparin

Heparin is a polydisperse mixture of GAGs with MWs ranging from 5 to 40 kDa, with an average MW of 13 kDa (Linhardt and Toida, 1997). It is composed of alternating D-glucosamine residues linked 1 → 4 to either L-iduronic acid or D-glucuronic acid (Casu, 1985). The principal repeating unit in heparin is the trisulfated disaccharide [→ 4)-*O*-α-L-iduronic acid-2-sulfate (1 → 4)-*O*-α-D-glucosamine-2, 6-disulfate (1 →] (Fig. 1), which represents 75–90% of the heparin chain (Linhardt et al., 1992). The remaining 10–25% disaccharide units differ in their degree and positions of sulfation (Linhardt et al., 1988). Besides, there are disaccharides consisting of unsulfated glucuronic acid and/or *N*-acetylglucosamine. With a SO_3^-/COO^- ratio of 2.0–2.5, heparin is the GAG with the highest charge density. By binding to domains containing positively charged amino acids, especially arginine and lysine, it interacts with many proteins, resulting in mani-

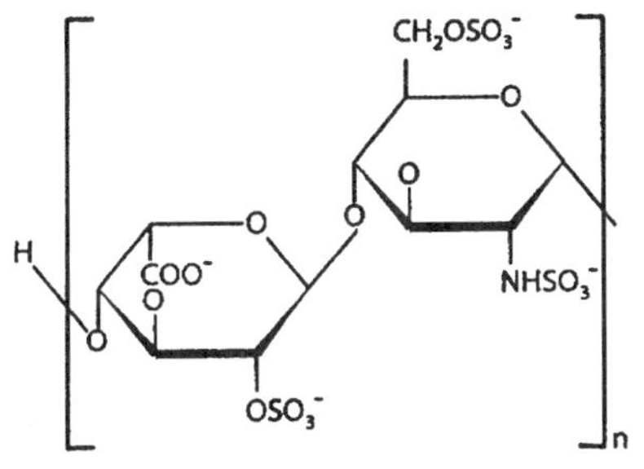

[4)-α-L-Ido*p*A-(1→4)-α-D-Glc*p*N2S,6S-(1→]

Figure 1 Main disaccharide unit of heparin composed of 75–90% heparin.

fold biological activities. The most prominent example is a well-defined pentasaccharide sequence with a central α-D-glucosamine-2,3,6-trisulfate unit, which binds specifically to AT (Choay, 1989). About 30% of the heparin chains contain this pentasaccharide (Fig. 2), which is called high-affinity heparin in contrast to the low-affinity heparin without this AT-binding site (Casu, 1990). AT is a natural serine protease inhibitor that controls blood coagulation by forming equimolar covalent complexes with certain coagulation enzymes. The anticoagulant action of heparin is based mainly on accelerating the slow rate of factor Xa (FXa) and thrombin (FIIa) inhibition by AT (Björk et al., 1989). Whereas the heparin pentasaccharide is sufficient for FXa inhibition, thrombin inhibition requires a mini-

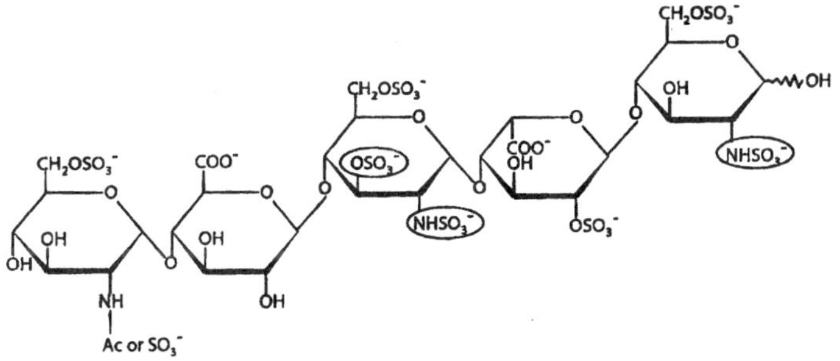

[4)-α-D-Glc*p*N2S/Ac,6S-(1→4)-β-D-Glc*p*A-(1→4)-α-D-Glc*p*N2S,3S,6S-(1→4)-α-L-Ido*p*A2S-(1→4)-α-D-Glc*p*N2S,6S-(1→]

Figure 2 Pentasaccharide sequence of the antithrombin (AT)-binding site of heparin: Sulfate groups essential for the AT-binding are encircled.

mum heparin chain length of 18 monosaccharides (5400 Da) to permit simultaneous binding of heparin to both AT and thrombin.

C. PF4-Sulfated Polysaccharide Complexes

Platelet factor 4 has the highest affinity to heparin among proteins stored within the platelet α-granules. Large heparin molecules (> 30 monosaccharides) bind to PF4 by ionic interactions with all four lysine residues on the helix of each monomer, wrapped around the tetramer along the ring of positive charges (Stuckey et al., 1992). At low concentrations (0.1–1.0 IU/mL) of shorter heparin chains, and high concentrations of PF4, the binding capacity of a PF4 tetramer for heparin is not saturated by one heparin molecule, thus permitting simultaneous binding to more than one heparin chain. If a heparin molecule is longer than 16 monosaccharides, it is able to bind to, and thereby bridge, two PF4 tetramers. Thus, at certain concentrations of heparin and PF4, formation of large, multimolecular PF4–heparin complexes occurs that can become dissociated in the presence of high heparin concentrations (Bock et al., 1980; Greinacher et al., 1995, 1994c; see Fig. 2 in Chap. 5 and Fig. 1 in Chap. 6).

Only heparin molecules containing 16 or more monosaccharides completely bind to immobilized PF4, resulting in total neutralization of their antifactor Xa (anti-Xa) and antithrombin (anti-IIa) activities, whereas progressively smaller oligosaccharides (without anti-IIa activity) become increasingly resistant to neutralization of their anti-Xa activity by PF4 (Denton et al., 1983; Lane et al., 1984). Because of their reduced sensitivity to inactivation by PF4, LMWHs are more active than UFH in platelet-rich plasma (Beguin et al., 1989), despite their lower activity in platelet-poor plasma (Samama et al., 1994). However, in contrast with their anti-Xa activity, the anti-IIa activity of LMWHs, which is mediated by molecules with a MW of more than 5400 Da, can be completely neutralized by higher PF4 concentrations (Padilla et al., 1992; Bendetowicz et al., 1994).

Formation of the PF4–heparin complex is independent of the AT-binding site, because heparin of either low or high affinity to AT binds to PF4 with a similar apparent K_d (Loscalzo et al., 1985). The interaction appears to be mediated by electrostatic interactions, as shown by studies of heparin oligosaccharides with different charge densities (Maccarana and Lindahl, 1993). Therefore, the complexes are dissociable. Indeed, heparin can be displaced from PF4 by sulfated polysaccharides, such as other GAGs (Handin and Cohen, 1976), dextran sulfate (Loscalzo et al., 1985), or xylan sulfate (Campbell et al., 1987). The molar ratios required for complex formation increase in the order: UFH < LMWH < heparan sulfate < dermatan sulfate < chondroitin-6-sulfate < chondroitin-4-sulfate (Handin and Cohen, 1976). Besides the degree of sulfation (DS), other structural parameters, such as the type of the uronic acid and the location of the sulfate groups

Table 1 Main Disaccharide Units of Mammalian Glycosaminoglycans, Arranged by Increasing Affinity to PF4

Glycosaminoglycan	Main disaccharide unit	DS[a]
Hyaluronic acid	[4)-β-D-GlcpA-(1 → 3)-β-D-GlcpNAc-(1 →]	0
Keratan sulfate	[3)-β-D-Gal-(1 → 4)-β-D-GlcpNAc6S-(1 →]	< 1.0
Chondroitin sulfate A	[4)-β-D-GlcpA-(1 → 3)-β-D-GalpNAc4S-(1 →]	< 1.0
Chondroitin sulfate C	[4)-β-D-GlcpA-(1 → 3)-β-D-GalpNAc6S-(1 →]	< 1.0
Dermatan sulfate = ChS B	[4)-α-L-IdopA-(1 → 3)-β-D-GalpNAc4S-(1 →]	1.0
Heparan sulfate	[4)-β-D-GlcpA-(1 → 4)-α-D-GlcpNAc6S-(1 →]	1.0–1.5
Low molecular weight heparin[b]	[4)-α-L-IdopA2S-(1 → 4)-α-D-GlcpN2S,6S-(1 →]	2.0–2.5
Unfractionated heparin	[4)-α-L-IdopA2S-(1 → 4)-α-D-GlcpN2S,6S-(1 →]	2.0–2.5

[a] DS, degree of sulfation (sulfate groups per disaccharide unit).
[b] Produced by degradation of unfractionated heparin.

on the amino sugar in the case of GAGs, influence the affinity of a polysaccharide to PF4 (Table 1).

D. Interactions of PF4 with Sulfated Polysaccharides In Vivo

Intravenous injection of heparin causes an increase in plasma PF4 level, whereas subcutaneous injection does not (O'Brien et al., 1985). The maximum amount of PF4 released corresponds to only about 5% of total platelet PF4 (Dawes et al., 1982). Some GAGs that have no significant effects on platelets are still able to increase plasma PF4 levels (Cella et al., 1986). Thus, endothelial-bound, rather than platelet-stored, PF4 seems to be the predominant source of the PF4 released by heparin. Most likely, heparin and other high-sulfated polysaccharides are able to displace PF4 from endothelial heparan sulfate in relation to their affinity for PF4 (O'Brien et al., 1985).

III. PF4–HEPARIN COMPLEXES AS THE MAJOR ANTIGEN RECOGNIZED BY HIT ANTIBODIES

A. Formation of Immune Complexes by HIT Antibodies

Two types of platelet count reduction associated with heparin treatment must be distinguished (Greinacher, 1995; Warkentin et al., 1995, 1998). Mild thrombocytopenia that occurs within the first 4 days of heparin treatment is most common, usually with high doses of heparin, or under certain clinical circumstances (e.g., following thrombolytic therapy or during the perioperative period). Known as nonimmune heparin-associated thrombocytopenia, the platelet count fall is typically unaccompanied by clinically adverse events, and the platelet count recovers despite continued use of heparin. In contrast, HIT occurs between the 5th and 20th days after starting heparin therapy. HIT is often associated with thromboembolic complications.

Whereas nonimmune heparin-associated thrombocytopenia may be caused by direct platelet-activating effects of heparin (see Chap. 5), HIT results from an immune mechanism (Amiral et al., 1992). However, both thrombocytopenic syndromes are closely linked in their pathogenesis (Greinacher, 1995), as the strong anionic character of heparin plays a pathogenic role for each. Heparin adheres to both endothelial-bound and platelet-bound PF4, with a further PF4 increase resulting from the platelet-activating effects of heparin. Heparin binding to PF4 exposes one or more neoepitopes, or cryptic autoantigens, on PF4. Some patients develop antibodies, predominantly IgG, but also IgM or IgA isotypes (Amiral, 1997) against the multimolecular PF4–heparin complexes, which thus represent the major antigen of HIT (Visentin et al., 1994; Greinacher et al., 1994c). Most HIT antibodies recognize a noncontiguous conformational epitope on the PF4 molecule that is produced when four to eight PF4 molecules are bound together by heparin (Horsewood et al., 1996). The antibodies recognize two, and probably three, distinct sites on the PF4–heparin complexes (Suh et al., 1998). Furthermore, the heparin molecules must be in a flexible, relatively unconstrained state to react with PF4 in such a way that they create sites for HIT antibody binding.

In a few cases, PF4 alone can be recognized by the HIT antibodies (Greinacher et al., 1994c). Here, endogenous GAGs may take the role of heparin, but the clinical effect of these antibodies is unknown. In some patients with acute myocardial infarction, HIT antibodies were apparently detected at baseline, even though the patients had never previously been exposed to heparin (Suzuki et al., 1997). This might be due to platelet activation connected with release of PF4 binding to endogenous GAGs. Antibodies with cross-reactivity to PF4–heparin complexes may have been generated against such endogenous GAG–PF4 complexes, even before the first heparin treatment.

B. Effects of HIT Antibody-Containing Immune Complexes

Heparin-induced thrombocytopenia antibodies bind to PF4–heparin complexes by their $F(ab')_2$ domains (Horne and Alkins, 1996), with the predominant immunoglobulin isotype being IgG (Amiral et al., 1996b). Thus, divalent IgG binding to multimolecular PF4–heparin complexes leads to the formation of large immune complexes containing HIT–IgG on the platelet surface. The interaction of the HIT–IgG Fc with the platelet FcγIIa receptors leads to cross-linking of these receptors and, consequently, platelet activation (Kelton et al, 1988, 1994; Chong et al., 1989a; see Chap. 9). The HIT antibody-mediated platelet activation can be inhibited by a monoclonal antibody specific for the FcγIIa receptor, by high concentrations of Fc fragments derived from normal IgG, and by excess heparin saturating all binding sites on PF4, and thus preventing the formation of multimolecular complexes (Greinacher et al., 1994b; Visentin et al., 1994).

Besides these effects on platelets, polyclonal HIT antibodies bind to endothelial cells (Cines et al., 1987; Visentin et al., 1994). The most convincing evidence demonstrating that these antibodies are the same ones that cause platelet activation was provided by classic adsorption–elution experiments (Greinacher et al., 1994c). Purified IgG obtained from sera of HIT patients gave positive reactions in both activation (serotonin release) and antigen (anti-PF4–heparin) assays. This IgG fraction was then adsorbed using cultured endothelial cells and, after extensive washing, the cells were eluted. The eluate again tested positive in both activation and antigen assays. Thus, these experiments showed that the antibodies recognize the same epitope on platelets, endothelial cells, and PF4–heparin complexes coated onto a microtiter plate. It appears most likely that the epitope on endothelial cells comprises surface GAGs (Cines et al., 1987; Greinacher et al., 1994c; Visentin et al., 1994). Endothelial cell activation by HIT antibodies can be inhibited by excess heparin, but not by anti-FcγIIa receptor monoclonal antibodies.

In addition to platelet and endothelial cell activation, there is concomitant activation of coagulation, as shown by marked elevations in thrombin–AT complex levels (Warkentin et al., 1997; Warkentin, 1998). The simultaneous activation of platelets, endothelium, and coagulation factors could explain the development of thrombocytopenia combined with thrombosis or disseminated intravascular coagulation in patients with HIT.

C. Importance of HIT Antibodies in Clinical HIT

The HIT antibodies occur commonly in heparin-treated patients. However, as many patients develop neither thrombocytopenia nor thrombosis (Amiral et al., 1996a; Kappers-Klunne et al., 1997; Arepally et al., 1997; Bauer et al., 1997), it is evident that pathogenicity requires additional factors. Two possible factors are high titers of HIT antibodies (Suh et al., 1997), as well as optimal (equimolar) concentrations of heparin and PF4 in the blood circulation, such that formation of the macromolecular PF4–heparin antigen complexes is permitted (Horne and Alkins, 1996). Thus, during low-dose heparin prophylaxis in a setting of minimal platelet activation, clinical HIT may occur less often than in a patient receiving high heparin doses together with activated platelets (Fondu, 1995). In accordance with this working hypothesis, HIT antibodies are most frequently induced by UFH in patients following cardiopulmonary bypass surgery (~50%), followed by patients undergoing major orthopedic surgery (~15%), and least frequently in medical patients (~3%) (see Chap. 4).

Further factors favoring the development of clinical HIT are prethrombotic or inflammatory situations (e.g., open heart surgery) (Visentin et al., 1996), greater susceptibility of the platelets to activation by HIT antibodies (Salem and van der Weyden, 1983), perhaps mediated by differences in PF4 binding to platelets (Capitanio et al., 1985), and increased expression of FcγIIa receptors (Chong et al., 1993). Also, polymorphism of the FcγIIa receptor at position Arg–His^{131} seems to be associated with a predisposition to HIT (Carlsson et al., 1998). Consequently, although HIT antibodies play an important role in the pathogenesis of clinical HIT, they are not the only factor responsible for the clinical manifestation of HIT. Thus, although monitoring for HIT antibodies should identify patients at risk for HIT (Elalamy et al., 1996), it remains uncertain whether this would lead to improved clinical outcomes versus simply monitoring the platelet count to make an early diagnosis of HIT.

IV. CROSS-REACTIVITY OF HIT ANTIBODIES WITH OTHER SULFATED CARBOHYDRATES

A. Interactions with Low Molecular Weight Heparins

Generation of the HIT antigen depends not only on the concentration, but also on the chain length of heparin. LMWH preparations (Table 2) have reduced affinity for platelets, endothelial cells, and plasma proteins, such as PF4 (Horne, 1993; O'Brien et al., 1985; Turpie, 1996). Accordingly, LMWH is less likely to form multimolecular complexes with PF4 (Greinacher et al., 1993); hence, they may induce an immune response less often than UFH. This is corroborated by a prospective study in which patients receiving LMWH after hip replacement surgery had a lower frequency of HIT antibody formation than patients receiving UFH (Warkentin et al., 1995).

Despite its lower immunogenicity, LMWH exhibits nearly 100% in vitro cross-reactivity to HIT antibodies using sensitive assays (Greinacher et al., 1994a,b; Amiral et al., 1996b; Amiral, 1997; Warkentin et al., 1995). The small variations found with different LMWH preparations are probably based on their individual structural parameters, such as DS and MW (Fareed et al., 1988). Homogeneous heparin fragments containing 20, 18, 16, 14, and 12 carbohydrate residues form multimolecular complexes recognized by the antibodies; fragments containing 10 residues induce antigen formation only weakly; fragments containing 8 and 6 residues are less (Amiral et al., 1995; Greinacher et al., 1995) or nonreactive (Visentin et al., 1997). Small heparin molecules may bind to PF4 (Bock et al., 1980; Denton et al., 1983; Greinacher et al., 1995), but only large molecules are able to bridge four to eight PF4 molecules, thus producing the noncontiguous conformational epitopes recognized by most HIT antibodies (Horsewood et al., 1996).

Table 2 Characteristics of Commercial LMWHs and the Heparinoid Danaparoid

INN (WHO)	Trade names	Company	Code number	Preparation method	Mean MW (kDa)	Anti-Xa U/mg LMWH[a]	Anti-Xa/anti-IIa ratio[b]
Ardeparin sodium	Normiflo	Hepar/Wyeth-Ayerst	RD11885	Peroxidative degradation	3.8	100	2.1
Certoparin sodium	Mono-Embolex NM Sandoparin	Novartis Pharma	—	Isoamylnitrite degradation	6.0	94	2.0 (2.0–2.2)[c]
Dalteparin sodium	Fragmin(e)	Pharmacia & Upjohn/Kissei	Kabi 2165	Nitrous acid degradation	5.0	142	2.7
Enoxaparin sodium	Clexane, Lovenox	Rhône-Poulenc Rorer	PK10169	Benzylation and alkaline β-elimination	4.5	100	3.7 (3.3–5.3)[d]
Nadroparin calcium	Fraxiparin(e), Seleparin	Sanofi Winthrop	CY216	Ethanol precipitation/nitrous acid degradation	4.3	95	3.6 (2.5–4.0)[d]
Parnaparin sodium	Fluxum	Opocrin	OP 2123	Peroxidative degradation and ethanol extraction	3.5–5.0	83	3.5
Reviparin sodium	Clivarin(e), Divitine	Knoll	—	Nitrous acid degradation	3.9	105	3.5 (3.0–5.0)[c]
Tinzaparin sodium	Logiparin, Innohep	Novo/LEO/Dupont/Braun	LHN-1	Enzymatic (heparinase) β-elimination	4.5	87	1.9
Danaparoid sodium	Orgaran	Organon	Org 10172	Degradation of a porcine intestine GAG mixture	6.0	20	> 22

[a] According to the First International Standard.
[b] Ratio of the specific anti-Xa to the anti-II activity (ratio = 1 for unfractionated heparin).
[c] According to the manufacturer.
[d] European pharmacopeia 1997.
INN, International Nonproprietary Name; WHO, World Health Organization.

B. Interactions with Other Sulfated Carbohydrates

The formation of platelet-activating immune complexes is not limited to heparin (Greinacher et al., 1992, 1993). Various other sulfated polysaccharides bind PF4 to form antigen complexes recognized by HIT antibodies. This cross-reaction depends on their structure, especially on their DS and MW (Amiral et al., 1995; Greinacher et al., 1992, 1995; Kelton et al., 1994). In vitro assays demonstrate that pentosan polysulfate, dextran sulfate, as well as a highly sulfated chondroitin sulfate can substitute for heparin. In contrast, neither dextran, dermatan sulfate, de-*N*-sulfated heparin, nor the AT-binding pentasaccharide, react in these assays. Accordingly, pentosan polysulfate and highly sulfated chondroitin sulfate have induced thrombocytopenia and thrombosis in vivo (Greinacher et al., 1993; Tardy et al., 1994). The corresponding antibodies can be detected by conventional PF4–heparin enzyme-linked immunosorbent assay (PF4–H ELISA), demonstrating the cross-reactivity with heparin (Gironell et al., 1996).

C. Relation Between the Anticoagulant Activity of β-1,3-Glucan Sulfates and Their Cross-Reaction with HIT-Associated Antibodies

To establish the structural requirements for the anticoagulant activity of sulfated carbohydrates, as well as for the development of platelet-activating immune complexes in the presence of HIT antibodies, we synthesized structurally well-defined sulfated polysaccharides (Greinacher et al., 1995). The resulting β-1,3-glucan sulfates (GluS) varied in their DS, MW, sulfation pattern, and their chemically introduced glycosidic side chains (Fig. 3). Although these heparinoids differ structurally from heparin, they exhibit structure-dependent anticoagulant as well as antithrombotic activities (Alban et al., 1995; Franz and Alban, 1995). They also induce platelet activation in the presence of HIT antibodies (Greinacher et al., 1995). Therefore, neither uronic acids, amino groups, nor the α-1,4- or β-1,4-glycosidic linkages found in heparin are essential for these biological properties.

An increase in the DS results in improved anticoagulant activity and, after binding to PF4, an increased formation of HIT antibody-binding sites. The MW is a second important structural parameter for anticoagulant potency of a sulfated polysaccharide, as well as its capacity to cause platelet activation in the presence of HIT antibodies. Fractions with hydrodynamic volumes between 38 and 60 kDa showed the most prominent effects (Alban and Franz, 1994a; Greinacher et al., 1995) (the hydrodynamic volumes were determined by gel permeation chromatography using neutral pullulans as MW standards; because these have lower hydrodynamic volumes owing to the missing sulfate groups, the measured hydrodynamic volumes are higher than the real MW; e.g., UFH had a mean hydrodynamic volume of 30 kDa). Therefore, this MW range seems to represent

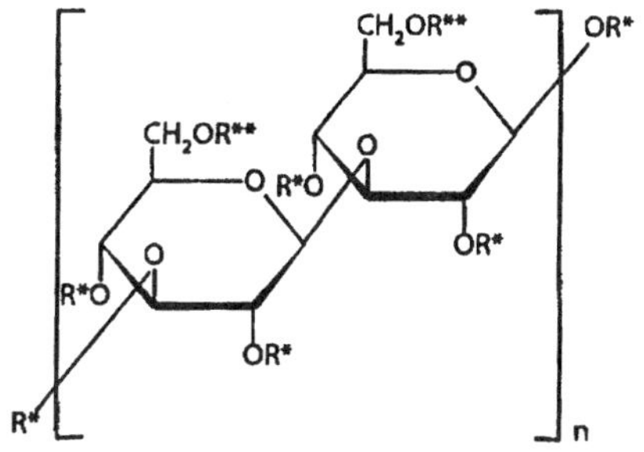

R* = H or SO_3^-
R** = SO_3^- or H or glycosidic side chain

Figure 3 Repeating unit of β-1,3-glucan sulfates: The primary OH-group in position 6 is preferentially sulfated. Glycosidic-branched β-1,3-glucan sulfates are substituted by a glucose, rhamnose, or arabinose unit, respectively, in position 6.

the optimal chain length both for the interaction with proteins involved in the coagulation cascade as well as with PF4 to form HIT antigens. Beyond the optimal chain length, higher concentrations are required to form multimolecular PF4–GluS complexes (Greinacher et al., 1995).

Compared with linear GluS having similar DS and MW, glycosidic-branched products generally exhibit higher anticoagulant activity than the respective linear derivatives (Alban, 1993, 1997). Glycosidic substitution changes the three-dimensional structure of the polysaccharide chain, enhancing its flexibility and improving the interaction with proteins (Kindness et al., 1980). As the side chains are more accessible to sulfation, they represent clusters of negative charges (Alban and Franz, 1994b), facilitating binding to PF4, which results in an increased cross-reactivity with HIT antibodies.

V. IMPLICATIONS FOR THE DEVELOPMENT OF CARBOHYDRATE-BASED HEPARIN ALTERNATIVES

A. Structural Requirements of Carbohydrate-Based Heparin Alternatives

A carbohydrate-based antithrombotic drug with a reduced risk to generate the HIT antigen should meet the following criteria (Greinacher et al., 1995):

1. The molecule should not be branched to reduce its flexibility and to minimize charge clusters.

2. Its DS should be lower than 1.0, if its chain length exceeds ten monosaccharides.
3. Its MW should be lower than 2.4 kDa (about seven monosaccharides), if its DS is higher than 1.0.
4. If the MW is higher than 2.4 kDa and the DS higher than 1.0, then at least the therapeutic concentration must be lower than that exhibiting cross-reactivity with HIT antibodies.

B. Danaparoid

Danaparoid sodium (Orgaran) is the alternative anticoagulant most often used to treat patients with HIT (see Chap. 14). This heparinoid consists of a depolymerized mixture of GAGs extracted from porcine intestinal mucosa, with a mean MW of 6 kDa. Its components are approximately 80% low molecular weight heparan sulfate, 10% dermatan sulfate, 5% chondroitin sulfate, and a small proportion of heparan sulfate (4%) with high affinity for AT (Meuleman, 1992). Apart from the minor AT-binding heparan sulfate component, the constituents of danaparoid have a DS between 0.5–0.7, as well as a low MW. Thus, the two important requirements to form multimolecular complexes with PF4 are not met. This is consistent with the low cross-reactivity rate of danaparoid (about 10%) (Wilde and Markham, 1997; see Chaps. 11 and 14). As danaparoid even inhibits platelet activation by HIT antibodies in the presence of heparin (Chong et al., 1989b), it is possible that the GAG mixture binds to PF4 without producing the antigen. Consequently, less PF4 is available for the small amount of higher-sulfated heparan sulfate molecules responsible for AT binding and, presumably, PF4 binding resulting in cross-reactivity with HIT antibodies (Greinacher et al., 1992).

C. Pentasaccharide

Within the scope of developing new carbohydrate-based antithrombotics applicable to HIT patients, a synthetic pentasaccharide (ORG 31540; MW = 1727 Da; DS = 1.6; 864 anti-Xa U/mg) corresponding to the AT-binding site of heparin is currently under clinical investigation (Van Amsterdam et al., 1995; Heráult et al., 1997; Lormeau et al., 1997; Petitou et al., 1997) (Fig. 4). As expected, owing to the structure–activity relations previously discussed, this pentasaccharide did not cross-react with HIT antibodies in any concentration tested, either in the PF4–H-ELSIA or in the serotonin release assay (Amiral et al., 1997; Greinacher et al., 1995).

However, in our laboratory, a higher-sulfated pentasaccharide, ORG 32701 (MW = 1991 Da; DS = 2.0) exhibiting higher anticoagulant activity (1150 anti-Xa U/mg) (Herbert et al., 1996) (Fig. 5) induced platelet activation in the pres-

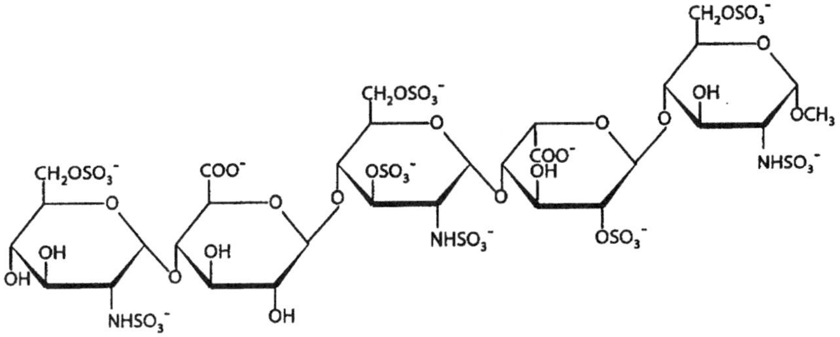

Figure 4 Chemical structure of the synthetically produced pentasaccharide, ORG 31540 (MW = 1727 kDa; DS = 1.6; 864 anti-Xa U/mg), with eight sulfate groups corresponding to the natural antithrombin-binding site.

ence of HIT antibodies. This proves the DS plays a critical parameter in HIT antigen formation. The influence of the MW is reflected by the concentrations required for platelet activation, which are about 1000-fold higher for this pentasaccharide derivative, compared with heparin.

D. Conclusions

From experiments with well-defined GluS, the various structural requirements for a sulfated carbohydrate to form the HIT antigen have become clear. Given

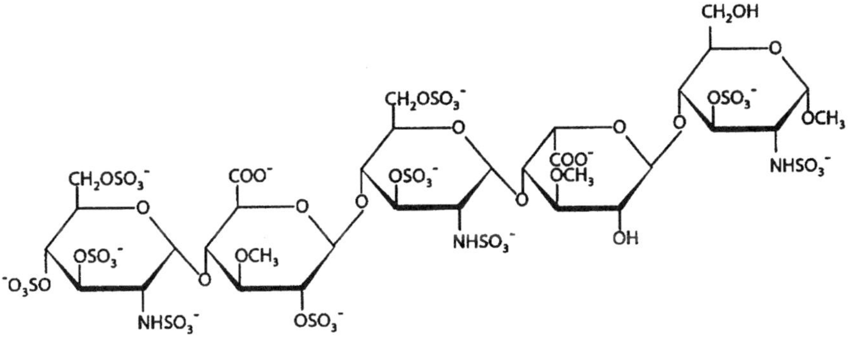

Figure 5 Chemical structure of the synthetically produced pentasaccharide, ORG 32701 (MW = 1991 kDa; DS = 2; 1150 anti-Xa U/mg), with a higher degree of sulfation (ten sulfate groups) than the natural antithrombin-binding site.

this detailed knowledge, at least three carbohydrate-based anticoagulant options can be proposed that should have a negligible risk for inducing HIT antibodies:

1. Mixtures of GAGs consisting predominantly of low-sulfated carbohydrates with correspondingly limited capacity to form antigenic complexes with PF4: A prototype of such an anticoagulant is danaparoid.
2. Oligosaccharides with antithrombotic activity similar to the AT-binding pentasaccharide: One such agent (the pentasaccharide ORG 31540) is currently under clinical investigation.
3. GAGs with highly sulfated, but short, regions that are connected by nonsulfated ''spacers'': Hereby, the thrombin-binding site and the AT-specific pentasaccharide can be expressed in a single molecule without reaching the critical grade of sulfation for HIT antigen formation (Petitou et al., 1999).

The increasing use of LMWH already seems to have reduced the incidence of HIT. We propose that the problem of HIT can be avoided completely by using anticoagulants meeting the foregoing outlined criteria in our treatment arsenal.

ACKNOWLEDGMENTS

Part of this work was supported by Bayerischer Habilitations-Förderpreis 1996/ Hans Zehetmair-Preis (S.A.) and Deutsche Forschungsgemeinschaft, DFG Gr 1096/2-1 and Gr 1096/2-2 (A.G.).

REFERENCES

Alban S. Synthese und physiologische Testung neuartiger Heparinoide. Ph.D dissertation, University of Regensburg, Germany, 1993.

Alban S. Carbohydrates with anticoagulant and antithrombotic properties. In: Witczak ZJ, Nieforth KA, eds. Carbohydrates in Drug Design. New York: Marcel Dekker, 1997: 209–276.

Alban S, Franz G. Anticoagulant activity of curdlan sulfates in dependence on their molecular weight. Pure Appl Chem 66:2403–2406, 1994a.

Alban S, Franz G. Gas liquid chromatography–mass spectrometry analysis of anticoagulant active curdlan sulfates. Semin Thromb Hemost 20:152–158, 1994b.

Alban S, Jeske W, Welzel D, Franz G, Fareed J. Anticoagulant and antithrombotic actions of a semisynthetic β-1,3-glucan sulfate. Thromb Res 78:201–210, 1995.

Amiral J. Le facteur 4 plaquettaire, cible des anticorps anti-héparine: application au diagnostic biologique de la thrombopénie induite par l'éparine (TIH). Ann Med Intern 148:142–149, 1997.

Amiral J, Bridey F, Dreyfus M, Vissac AM, Fressinaud E, Wolf M, Meyer D. Platelet factor 4 complexed to heparin is the target for antibodies generated in heparin-induced thrombocytopenia [letter]. Thromb Haemost 68:95–96, 1992.

Amiral J, Bridey F, Wolf M, Boyer-Neumann C, Fressinaud E, Vissac AM, Peynaud-Debayle E, Dreyfus M, Meyer D. Antibodies to macromolecular platelet factor 4-heparin complexes in heparin-induced thrombocytopenia: a study of 44 cases. Thromb Haemost 73:21–28, 1995.

Amiral J, Peynaud-Debayle E, Wolf M, Bridey F, Vissac AM, Meyer D. Generation of antibodies to heparin–PF4 complexes without thrombocytopenia in patients treated with unfractionated or low-molecular-weight heparin. Am J Hematol 52:90–95, 1996a.

Amiral J, Wolf M, Fischer A, Boyer-Neumann C, Vissac A, Meyer D. Pathogenicity of IgA and/or IgM antibodies to heparin–PF4 complexes in patients with heparin-induced thrombocytopenia. Br J Haematol 92:954–959, 1996b.

Amiral J, Lormeau JC, Marfaing-Koka A, Vissac AM, Wolf M, Boyer-Neumann C, Tardy B, Herbert JM, Meyer D. Absence of cross-reactivity of SR90107A/ORG31540 pentasaccharide with antibodies to heparin–PF4 complexes developed in heparin-induced thrombocytopenia. Blood Coagul Fibrinolysis 8:114–117, 1997.

Arepally G, McKenzie SE, Jiang XM, Poncz M, Cines DB. FcγRIIA H/R^{131} polymorphism, subclass-specific IgG anti-heparin/platelet factor 4 antibodies and clinical course in patients with heparin-induced thrombocytopenia and thrombosis. Blood 89:370–375, 1997.

Beguin S, Mardiguian J, Lindhout T, Hemker HC. The mode of action of low molecular weight heparin preparation (PK10169) and two of its major components on thrombin generation in plasma. Thromb Haemost 61:30–34, 1989.

Bendetowicz AV, Kai H, Knebel R, Caplain H, Hemker HC, Lindhout T, Beguin S. The effect of subcutaneous injection of unfractionated and low molecular weight heparin on thrombin generation in platelet rich plasma a study in human volunteers. Thromb Haemost 72:705–712, 1994.

Björk I, Olson ST, Shore JD. Molecular mechanisms of the accelerating effect of heparin on the reactions between antithrombin and clotting proteinases. In: Lane DA, Lindahl U, eds. Heparin, Chemical and Biological Properties, Clinical Applications. London: Edward Arnold, 1989, pp 229–255.

Bock PE, Luscombe M, Marshall SE, Pepper DS, Holbrook JJ. The multiple complexes formed by the interaction of platelet factor 4 with heparin. Biochem J. 191:769–776, 1980.

Campbell A, Nesheim ME, Doctor VM. Mechanism of potentiation of antithrombin III [AT-III] inhibition by sulfated xylans. Thromb Res 47:341–352, 1987

Capitanio AM, Niewiarowski S, Rucinski B, Tuszynski GP, Cierniewski CS, Hershock D, Kornecki E. Interaction of platelet factor 4 with human platelets. Biochim Biophys Acta 839:161–173, 1985.

Carlsson LE, Santoso S, Baurichter G, Kroll H, Papenberg S, Eichler P, Westerdaal NAC, Kiefel V, van de Winkel JGJ, Greinacher A. Heparin-induced thrombocytopenia: new insights into the impact of the FcγRIIa-R-H131 polymorphism. Blood 92: 1526–1531, 1998.

Casu B. Structure and biological activity of heparin. Adv Carbohydr Chem Biochem 43: 51–134, 1985.

Casu B. Heparin structure. Haemostasis 20(suppl 1):62–73, 1990.

Cella G, Scattolo N, Luzzatto G, Stevanato F, Vio C, Girolami ASO. Effects on platelets and on the clotting system of four glycosaminoglycans extracted from hog mucosa and one extracted from aortic intima of the calf. J Med 17:331–346, 1986.

Choay J. Structure and activity of heparin and its fragments: an overview. Semin Thromb Hemost 15:359–364, 1989.

Chong BH, Fawaz I, Chestermann CN, Berndt MC. Heparin-induced thrombocytopenia: mechanism of interaction of the heparin-dependent antibody with platelets. Br J Haematol 73:235–240, 1989a.

Chong BH, Ismail F, Cade J, Gallus AS, Gordon S, Chesterman CN. Heparin-induced thrombocytopenia: studies with a new molecular weight heparinoid, Org 10172. Blood 73:1592–1596, 1989b.

Chong BH, Pilgrim RL, Cooley MA, Chesterman CN. Increased expression of platelet IgG Fc receptors in immune heparin-induced thrombocytopenia. Blood 81:988–993, 1993.

Cines DB, Tomaski A, Tannenbaum S. Immune endothelial-cell injury in heparin-associated thrombocytopenia. N Engl J Med 316:581–589, 1987.

Dawes J, Pumphrey CW, McLaren KM, Prowse CV, Pepper DS. The in vivo release of human platelet factor 4 by heparin. Thromb Res 27:65–76, 1982.

Denton J, Lane DA, Thunberg L, Slater AM, Lindahl U. Binding of platelet factor 4 to heparin oligosaccharides. Biochem J 209:455–460, 1983.

Elalamy I, Potevin F, Lecrubier C, Bara L, Marie JP, Samama MM. A fatal low-molecular-weight heparin-associated thrombocytopenia after hip surgery: possible usefulness of PF4–heparin ELISA test. Blood Coagul Fibrinolysis 7:665–671, 1996.

Fareed J, Walenga JM, Hoppensteadt D, Haun X, Racanelli A. Comparative study on the in vitro and in vivo activities of seven low-molecular-weight heparins. Haemostasis 18(suppl 3):3–15, 1988.

Fondu P. Heparin-associated thrombocytopenia: an update. Acta Clin Belg 50:343–357, 1995.

Franz G, Alban S. Structure–activity relationship of antithrombotic polysaccharide derivatives. Int J Biol Macromol 17:311–314, 1995.

Gironell A, Altes A, Arboix A, Fontcuberta J, Munoz Z, Marti-Vilalta JL. Pentosan polysulfate-induced thrombocytopenia: a case diagnosed with an ELISA test used for heparin-induced thrombocytopenia. Ann Hematol 73:51–62, 1996.

Greinacher A. Antigen generation in heparin-associated thrombocytopenia: the nonimmunologic type and the immunologic type are closely linked in their pathogenesis. Semin Thromb Hemost 21:106–116, 1995.

Greinacher A, Michels I, Mueller-Eckhardt C. Heparin-associated thrombocytopenia: the antibody is not heparin specific. Thromb Haemost 67:545–549, 1992.

Greinacher A, Michels I, Liebenhoff U, Presek P, Mueller-Eckhardt C. Heparin-associated thrombocytopenia: immune complexes are attached to the platelet membrane by the negative charge of highly sulphated oligosaccharides. Br J Haematol 84:711–716, 1993.

Greinacher A, Feigl M, Mueller-Eckhardt C. Crossreactivity studies between sera of patients with heparin-associated thrombocytopenia and a new low molecular weight heparin, reviparin. Thromb Haemost 72:644–645, 1994a.

Greinacher A, Amiral J, Dummel V, Vissac AM, Kiefel V, Mueller-Eckhardt C. Laboratory diagnosis of heparin-associated thrombocytopenia, comparison of platelet aggregation test, heparin-induced platelet activation (HIPA) test, and PF4/heparin ELISA. Transfusion 34:381–385, 1994b.

Greinacher A, Pötzsch B, Amiral J, Dummel V, Eichner A, Mueller-Eckhardt C. Heparin-associated thrombocytopenia: isolation of the antibody and characterization of a multimolecular PF4–heparin complex as the major antigen. Thromb Haemost 71: 247–251, 1994c.

Greinacher A, Alban S, Dummel V, Franz G, Mueller-Eckhardt C. Characterization of the structural requirements for a carbohydrate based anticoagulant with a reduced risk of inducing the immunological type of heparin-associated thrombocytopenia. Thromb Haemost 74:886–892, 1995.

Handin RI, Cohen HJ. Purification and binding properties of human platelet factor four. J Biol Chem 251:4273–4282, 1976.

Heráult JP, Donat F, Barzu T, Crepon B, Bernat A, Lormeau JC, Herbert JM. Pharmacokinetic study of three synthetic AT-binding pentasaccharides in various animal species—extrapolation to humans. Blood Coagul Fibrinolysis 8:161–167, 1997.

Herbert JM, Heráult JP, Bernat A, van Amsterdam RG, Vogel GM, Lormeau JC, Petitou M, Meuleman DG. Biochemical and pharmacological properties of SANORG 32701. Comparison with the ''synthetic pentasaccharide'' (SR 90107/ORG 31540) and standard heparin. Circ Res 79:590–600, 1996.

Hirsh J. Heparin. N Engl J Med 324:1565–1574, 1991.

Hirsh J, Warkentin TE, Raschke R, Granger C, Ohman EM, Dalen J. Heparin and low molecular weight heparin. Mechanisms of action, pharmacokinetics, dosing considerations, monitoring, efficacy and safety. Chest 114:489S–510S, 1998.

Horne MK III. The effect of secreted heparin-binding proteins on heparin binding to platelets. Thromb Res 70:91–98, 1993.

Horne MK III, Alkins BR. Platelet binding of IgG from patients with heparin-induced thrombocytopenia. J Lab Clin Med 127:435–442, 1996.

Horsewood P, Warkentin TE, Hayward CP, Kelton JG. The epitope specificity of heparin-induced thrombocytopenia. Br J Haematol 95:161–167, 1996.

Kaplan KL, Niewiarowski S. Nomenclature of secreted platelet proteins—report of the Working Party on Secreted Platelet Proteins of the Subcommittee on Platelets. Thromb Haemost 53:282–284, 1985.

Kappers-Klunne MC, Boon DM, Hop WC, Michiels JJ, Stibbe J, van der Zwaan C, Koudstaal PJ, van Vliet HH. Heparin-induced thrombocytopenia and thrombosis: a prospective analysis of the incidence in patients with heart and cerebrovascular diseases. Br J Haematol 96:442–446, 1997.

Kelton JG, Sheridan D, Santos A, Smith J, Steeves K, Smith C, Brown C, Murphy WG. Heparin-induced thrombocytopenia: laboratory studies. Blood 72:925–930, 1988.

Kelton JG, Smith JW, Warkentin TE, Hayward CP, Denomme GA, Horsewood P. Immunoglobulin G from patients with heparin-induced thrombocytopenia binds to a complex of heparin and platelet factor 4. Blood 83:3232–3239, 1994.

Kindness G, Long WF, Williamson FB. Anticoagulant effects of sulphated polysaccharides in normal and antithrombin III-deficient plasmas. Br J Pharmacol 69:675–677, 1980.

Klener P, Kubisz PSO. Platelet heparin-neutralizing activity (platelet factor 4). Acta Univ Carol Med (Praha) 24:79–86, 1978.

Lane DA, Denton J, Flynn AM, Thunberg L, Lindahl U. Anticoagulant activities of heparin oligosaccharides and their neutralization by platelet factor 4. Biochem J 218: 725–732, 1984.

Linhardt RJ, Toida T. Heparin oligosaccharides: new analogues development and applications. In: Witczak ZJ, Nieforth KA, eds. Carbohydrates in Drug Design. New York: Marcel Dekker, 1997, pp 277–341.

Linhardt RJ, Rice KM, Kim YS, Lohse DL, Wang HM, Loganathan D. Mapping and quantification of the major oligosaccharide components of heparin. Biochem J 254: 781–787, 1988.

Linhardt RJ, Ampofo SA, Fareed J, Hoppensteadt D, Mulliken JB, Folkman J. Isolation and characterization of human heparin. Biochemistry 31:12441–12445, 1992.

Lormeau JC, Herault JP, Gaich C, Barzu T, van Dinther TG, Visser A, Herbert JM. Determination of the anti-factor Xa activity of the synthetic pentasaccharide SR 90107A/ ORG 31540 and of two structural analogues. Thromb Res 85:67–75, 1997.

Loscalzo J, Melnick B, Handin RI. The interaction of platelet factor four and glycosaminoglycans. Arch Biochem Biophys 240:446–455, 1985.

Luscher EF, Kaser-Glanzman R. Platelet heparin-neutralizing factor (platelet factor 4). Thromb Diath Haemorrh 33:66–72, 1975.

Maccarana M, Lindahl U. Mode of interaction between platelet factor 4 and heparin. Glycobiology 3:271–277, 1993.

Mayo KH, Roongta V, Ilyina E, Milius R, Barker S, Quinlan C, La Rosa G, Daly TJ. NMR solution structure of the 32-kDa platelet factor 4 ELR-motif N-terminal chimera: a symmetric tetramer. Biochemistry 34:11399–11409, 1995.

Meuleman DG. Orgaran (Org 10172): its pharmacological profile in experimental models. Haemostasis 22:58–65, 1992.

Moore S, Pepper DS, Cash JD. Platelet antiheparin activity. The isolation and characterisation of platelet factor 4 released from thrombin-aggregated washed human platelets and its dissociation into subunits and the isolation of membrane-bound antiheparin activity. Biochim Biophys Acta 379:370–384, 1975.

Niewiarowski S. Report of the Working Party on Platelets. Platelet factor 4 (PF4), platelet protein with heparin neutralizing activity. Thromb Haemost 36:273–276, 1976.

Novotny WF, Maffi T, Mehta RL, Milner PG. Identification of novel heparin-releasable proteins, as well as the cytokines midkine and pleiotrophin, in human postheparin plasma. Arterioscler Thromb 13:1798–1805, 1993.

O'Brien JR, Etherington MD, Pashley MA. The heparin-mobilisable pool of platelet factor 4: a comparison of intravenous and subcutaneous heparin and Kabi heparin fragment 2165. Thromb Haemost 54:735–738, 1985.

Padilla A, Gray E, Pepper DS, Barrowcliffe TW. Inhibition of thrombin generation by heparin and low molecular weight (LMW) heparins in the absence and presence of platelet factor 4 (PF4). Br J Haematol 82:406–413, 1992.

Petitou M, Duchaussoy P, Jaurand G, Gourvenec F, Lederman I, Strassel JM, Barzu T, Crepon B, Herault JP, Lormeau JC, Bernat A, Herbert JM. Synthesis and pharmacological properties of a close analogue of an antithrombotic pentasaccharide (SR 90107A/ORG 31540). J Med Chem 40:1600–1607, 1997.

Petitou M. Herault JP, Bernat A, Driguez PA, Duchaussoy P, Lormeau JC, Herbert JM. Synthesis of thrombin-inhibiting heparin mimetics without side effects. Nature 398: 417–422, 1999.

St. Charles R, Walz DA, Edwards BF. The three-dimensional structure of bovine platelet factor 4 at 3.0-A resolution. J Biol Chem 264:2092–2099, 1989.

Salem HH, van der Weyden MB. Heparin-induced thrombocytopenia. Variable platelet-rich plasma reactivity to heparin-dependent platelet aggregating factor. Pathology 15:297–299, 1983.

Samama MM, Bara L, Gerotziafas GT. Mechanisms for the antithrombotic activity in man of low molecular weight heparins (LMWHs). Haemostasis 24:105–117, 1994.

Sear CH, Poller L. Antiheparin activity of human serum and platelet factor 4. Thromb Diath Haemorrh 30:93–105, 1973.

Stuckey JA, St. Charles R, Edwards BF. A model of the platelet factor 4 complex with heparin. Proteins 14:277–287, 1992.

Suh JS, Malik MI, Aster RH, Visentin GP. Characterization of the humoral immune response in heparin-induced thrombocytopenia. Am J Hematol 54:196–201, 1997.

Suh JS, Aster RH, Visentin GP. Antibodies from patients with heparin-induced thrombocytopenia/thrombosis recognize different epitopes on heparin: platelet factor 4, Blood 91:916–922, 1998.

Suzuki S, Koide M, Sakamoto S, Yamamoto S, Matsuo M, Fujii E, Matsuo T. Early onset of immunological heparin-induced thrombocytopenia in acute myocardial infarction. Blood Coagul Fibrinolysis 8:13–15, 1997.

Tardy PB, Tardy B, Grelac F, Reynaud J, Mismetti P, Bertrand JC, Guyotat D. Pentosan polysulfate-induced thrombocytopenia and thrombosis. Am J Hematol 88:803–808, 1994.

Turpie AGG. New therapeutic opportunities for heparins: what does low molecular weight heparin offer? J Thromb Thrombolysis 3:145–149, 1996.

Van Amsterdam RG, Vogel GM, Visser A, Kop WJ, Buiting MT, Meuleman DG. Synthetic analogues of the antithrombin III-binding pentasaccharide sequence of heparin. Prediction of in vivo residence times. Arterioscler Thromb Vasc Biol 15:495–503, 1995.

Visentin GP, Ford SE, Scott JP, Aster RH. Antibodies from patients with heparin-induced thrombocytopenia/thrombosis are specific for platelet factor 4 complexed with heparin or bound to endothelial cells. J Clin Invest 93:81–88, 1994.

Visentin GP, Malik M, Cyganiak KA, Aster RH. Patients treated with unfractionated heparin during open heart surgery are at high risk to form antibodies reactive with heparin: platelet factor 4 complexes. J Lab Clin Med 128:376–383, 1996.

Visentin GP, Moghaddam M, Aster RH. Antibodies associated with heparin-induced thrombocytopenia/thrombosis (HITP) recognize sites on platelet factor four (PF4) induced by the binding of linear polyanionic compounds [abstr]. Thromb Haemost 78(suppl):PD-1483, 1997.

Walsh PN. Platelets, heparin, and blood coagulation. In: Kakkar VV, Thomas DP, eds. Heparin: Chemistry and Clinical Usage. London: Academic Press, 1976, pp 125–43.

Warkentin TE. Limitations of conventional treatment options for heparin-induced thrombocytopenia. Semin Hematol 35(suppl 5):17–25, 1998.

Warkentin TE. Levine MN, Hirsh J, Horsewood P, Roberts RS, Gent M, Kelton JG. Heparin-induced thrombocytopenia in patients treated with low molecular weight heparin or unfractionated heparin. N Engl J Med 332:1330–1335, 1995.

Warkentin TE, Elavathil LJ, Hayward CPM, Johnston MA, Russett JI, Kelton JG. The pathogenesis of venous limb gangrene associated with heparin-induced thrombocytopenia. Ann Intern Med 127:804–812, 1997.

Warkentin TE, Chong BH, Greinacher A. Heparin-induced thrombocytopenia: towards consensus. Thromb Haemost 79:1–7, 1998.

Wilde MI, Markham A. Danaparoid. A review of its pharmacology and clinical use in the management of heparin-induced thrombocytopenia. Drugs 54:903–924, 1997.

Young E, Prins MH, Levine MN, Hirsh J. Heparin binding to plasma proteins, an important mechanism for heparin resistance. Thromb Haemost 67:639–643, 1992.

Zhang X, Chen L, Bancroft DP, Lai CK, Maione TE. Crystal structure of recombinant human platelet factor 4. Biochemistry 33:8361–8366, 1994.

9
The Platelet Fc Receptor in Heparin-Induced Thrombocytopenia

Gregory A. Denomme
University of Toronto and Mount Sinai Hospital,
Toronto, Ontario, Canada

I. INTRODUCTION

Heparin-induced thrombocytopenia (HIT) is a unique immune-mediated disorder. HIT is common, occurring in as many as 5% of certain patient populations. Affected patients often develop the paradox of thrombosis, but not bleeding, despite having thrombocytopenia. One possible reason for this unique clinical profile is the central role of the platelet Fcγ receptor (FcγR) IIa in mediating platelet activation in HIT. Indirect evidence suggesting a crucial role for platelet activation in the pathogenesis of HIT is the observation that thrombocytopenia caused by HIT antibodies is strongly associated with thrombosis, whereas formation of HIT antibodies without thrombocytopenia is not (Warkentin et al., 1995).

It has been known for several years that HIT results from a predominant IgG immune response to antigenic determinants involving heparin bound to the surface of the platelet membrane (Green et al., 1978). Thus, the pathogenesis of HIT resembles a type II immune reaction, i.e., a cytotoxic antibody response (Roitt et al., 1985). However, typical features of a type II immune response, such as phagocytosis, killer cell activity, or complement-mediated lysis, do not seem to predominate in HIT. Instead, thrombocytopenia results primarily from IgG binding to platelet factor 4–heparin (PF4–H) complexes on the platelet surface. The HIT–IgG within these large multimolecular immune complexes interacts with the platelet FcγRIIa; cross-linking of the receptors causes platelet activation, aggregation, and granule release (Chong et al., 1981). Furthermore, HIT antibodies activate endothelium in vitro by interaction with PF4–heparan sulfate complexes (Cines et al., 1987; Greinacher et al., 1994a; Visentin et al., 1994). However, unlike platelets, human endothelium (with the exception of placental villous endothelial cells) do not express any Fc receptors, either constitutively or in the setting of immune complex diseases (Sedmak et al., 1991). Thus, platelet activation and endothelial activation in HIT probably arise from fundamentally distinct processes.

One of the most important unanswered questions in the pathophysiology of this disorder is an explanation for why only a few patients who develop HIT antibodies become thrombocytopenic. This problem has led investigators to study the role of FcγRIIa in explaining, at least partly, the heterogeneous clinical sequelae among patients with HIT. This chapter will (a) review the structure and function of the platelet FcγRIIa; (b) describe the mechanism of HIT antibody-induced platelet activation by FcγRIIa; and (c) summarize the studies that have attempted to identify a role for the FcγRIIa in modifying clinical manifestations of HIT.

II. PLATELET FcγRIIa STRUCTURE, DISTRIBUTION, AND FUNCTION

The platelet FcγRIIa is a member of a family of structurally related glycoproteins, many of which are expressed on hematopoietic cells (Table 1). Twelve different transcripts have been reported, derived from eight distinct genes and grouped into three different classes: I, II, and III (for review see van de Winkel and Capel, 1993; Rascu et al., 1997; Gessner et al., 1998). Allelic polymorphic variants add yet another level of diversity for FcγRIIa, FcγRIIIa, and FcγRIIIb. The affinity for IgG varies among these isoforms and polymorphic variants. Most notably, the FcγRIIa–His^{131} allele has a significantly higher affinity for human IgG2 than FcγRIIa–Arg^{131} (Warmerdam et al., 1991). Furthermore, FcγRIIIa–Val^{158} and FcγRIIIb–NA1 bind nearly twice as much IgG as FcγRIIIa–Phe^{158} and FcγRIIIb–NA2, respectively (Salmon et al., 1990; Koene et al., 1997). When cross-linked, each isoform participates in biological activities through distinct signal transduction pathways that affect cell functions, including antigen presentation, immune complex clearance, phagocytosis and the oxidative burst, release of various cytokines and intracellular granular mediators, antibody-dependent cellular cytotoxicity (ADCC), and negative down-regulation of antibody production.

Only FcγRIIa is expressed on platelets (Rosenfeld et al., 1985; Kelton et al., 1987). The receptor is a single α-chain, 40-kDa glycoprotein, with an extracellular region consisting of two immunoglobulin-like, disulfide-linked domains responsible for ligand binding, a transmembrane region, and an intracellular domain that incorporates an immunoreceptor tyrosine-based activation motif

Table 1 The Family of Fcγ Receptors: Molecular and Structural Characteristics and Tissue Distribution

	FcγRI (CD64)	FcγRII (CD32)	FcγRIII (CD16)
Genes	IA, IB, IC	IIA, IIB, IIC	IIIA, IIIB
Allelic functional variants[a]	None	IIA: Gln/Lys^{127} IIA: Arg/His^{131}	IIIA: Leu/Arg/His^{48} IIIA: Phe/Val^{158} IIIB:NA1/NA2 IIIB: Ala/Asp^{60} (SH)
RNA transcripts[b]	Ia1 Ib1, Ib2 Ic	IIa1, IIa2 IIb1, IIb2, IIb3 IIc	IIIa IIIb
Glycoprotein expressed[c]	Ia	IIa1, sIIa2 IIb1, sIIb2, IIb3 IIc	IIIa IIIb (GPI linked)
Molecular weight (kDa)	72	40	50–80
Extracellular Ig-like domains	3	2	2
Intracellular tyrosine motif[d]	None	ITAM(IIa, IIc) ITIM (IIb)	None
Noncovalent-associated subunits	γ-chain	None	β-chain, γ-chain, ζ-chain
Affinity constant	$10^8 M^{-1}$	$< 10^7 M^{-1}$	IIIa: $3 \times 10^7 M^{-1}$ IIIb: $< 10^7 M^{-1}$
IgG subclass avidity[e]	$3 = 1 > 4 \ggg 2$	IIa-Arg^{131} $3 > 1 \ggg 2 > 4$ IIa-His^{131} $3 > 1 = 2 > 4$ IIb1 $3 > 1 > 4 \ggg 2$	IIIa-Val^{158} $1 > 3 \ggg 2,4$ IIIa-Val^{158} > IIIa-Phe^{158} for 1 and 3 IIIb-NA1 > IIIb-NA2 for 1 and 3
Hematopoietic cell distribution	CD34 progenitor cells, monocytes, macrophages, dendritic cells	IIA: platelets, endothelial cells, monocytes, macrophages, eosino-/baso-/neutrophils, Langerhans/dendritic cells IIB: B cells, monocytes	IIIa: monocytes, macrophages, NK cells, T cells IIIb: neutrophils

[a] Allelic polymorphisms that show differences in IgG binding; NA1/NA2 variants have multiple amino acid differences (Ory et al., 1989); SH+ individuals (Bux et al. 1997) carry three copies of FcγRIIIB (Koene et al., 1998).

[b] Multiple mRNA transcripts from FcγRIB, IIA, and IIB, are the result of alternative splicing of primary transcripts.

[c] Soluble forms of FcγRIIa and IIb (sIIa, sIIb) are devoid of the hydrophobic transmembrane exon; GPI, glycerol phosphatidyl inositol.

[d] Intracellular signal transduction sequences; ITAM, immunoreceptor tyrosine-based activation motif; ITIM, immunoreceptor tyrosine-based inhibition motif.

[e] Numbers represent the relative order of IgG subclass binding to variants of FcγRIIa (Warmerdam et al., 1990), FcγRIIIa (Koene et al., 1997; Wu et al., 1997), and FcγRIIIb (Salmon et al., 1990; Bredius et al., 1994b).

(ITAM) essential for intracellular signal transduction (Qiu et al., 1990). The gene comprises seven exons. A soluble form of the receptor is produced by alternative splicing of primary RNA transcripts to exclude exon five, containing the transmembrane region (Rappaport et al., 1993). The nucleotide region encoding the ITAM is unique in that the two tyrosine motifs are separated by 12 amino acids, rather than the usual 7 (Brooks et al., 1989).

At the amino acid level, the extracellular domain of FcγRIIa shows 96% homology with FcγRIIb and FcγRIIc (Brooks et al., 1989). A G → A nucleotide polymorphism at nucleotide position 519 of the cDNA (position 512 in Genbank Accession M90724) is responsible for the Arg/His^{131} allelic functional variants (Clark et al., 1989). Surprisingly, a 140-nucleotide stretch of the 5′-region of exon 4 that extends seven nucleotides past the G → A polymorphism is reiterated in intron 3, with the exception of one nucleotide deletion and one nucleotide substitution. Therefore, care must be taken to exclude this particular region of intron 3 when designing flanking and sequence-specific primers or oligonucleotide probes for the G → A^{519} polymorphism, because the intron has an invariant G at the position homologous to the polymorphism (Fig. 1).

An additional polymorphism, an A → G at nucleotide 207 of the cDNA, results in a Gln–Trp^{27} substitution in the mature polypeptide (Warmerdam et al., 1991). However, the Arg–His^{131} position is near or within the binding region for IgG Fc (Hulett et al., 1995), and it is this polymorphism that is associated with the affinity differences for human IgG2 (Warmerdam et al., 1991). More recently, another polymorphism proximal to Arg^{131} that affects IgG2 binding has been

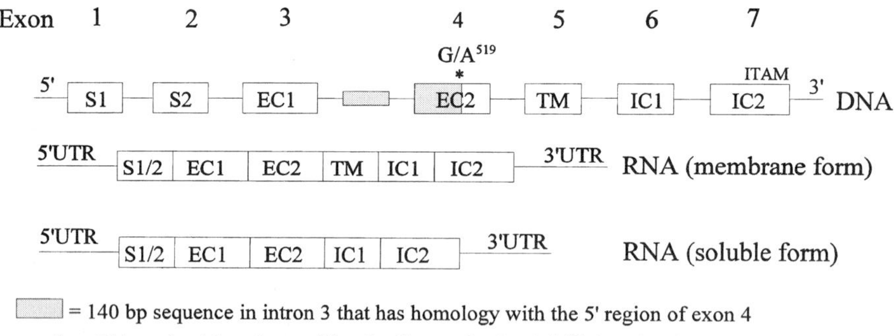

Figure 1 Schematic diagram of the genomic organization and RNA transcripts for the FcγRIIA gene. S, signal sequences; EC, extracellular exons; TM, transmembrane domain; IC, intracellular exons; ITAM, region containing the immunoreceptor tyrosine-based activation motif; UTR, untranslated region.

found in a single healthy individual (Norris et al., 1998): a lysine substitution for glutamine at position 127 demonstrated a significant increase in FcγR-mediated phagocytosis in this homozygous FcγRIIa–Arg^{131} individual.

FcγRIIa has low affinity for IgG ($< 10^7\ M^{-1}$) and interacts only with multivalent antigen–antibody complexes (Warmedam et al., 1991; Parren et al., 1992). The numbers of FcγRIIa receptors expressed on normal resting platelets varies among healthy individuals, but is stable for a given individual (Rosenfeld et al., 1987). Studies using Scatchard analysis report roughly a threefold variation among individuals, with the number of binding sites ranging from 600 to 1500 molecules per platelet when assayed using intact murine monoclonal antibody IV.3 (McCrae et al., 1990), and 1500 to more than 4500 for the monovalent (Fab) preparation of IV.3 (Tomiyama et al., 1992; Brandt et al., 1995). There are no major differences in FcγRIIa number between males and female, among platelets from persons of different ages, or among platelets representing the three possible genotypic classes of the FcγRIIa–Arg/His^{131} allelic variants (Brandt et al., 1995).

III. IMMUNOGLOBULIN G AGONISTS AND PLATELET ACTIVATION

Murine monoclonal antibodies, usually of the IgG1 subclass, against CD9 were among the first studied for their platelet-activating properties. Subsequently, it was determined that monoclonal antibodies to glycoprotein (GP) IIb/IIIa, β_2-microglobulin, GP IV (CD36), and other selected antigens can activate platelets (for review, see Rubinstein et al., 1995). In each instance, platelet activation occurs by a consistent mechanism: first, there is Fab-mediated binding to surface-expressed platelet antigens, then the Fc portion of the antibodies interacts with platelet FcγRIIa. Evidence for FcγRIIa dependency includes the inhibition of platelet activation by a murine monoclonal anti-FcγRIIa antibody (IV.3). However, some platelet GPs (e.g., GP Ib) do not support activation by monoclonal antibodies; others support activation despite their usual sequestered location within platelets (e.g., multimerin); and still other GPs (e.g., GP IIb/IIIa) support activation by only certain monoclonal antibodies (Horsewood et al., 1991). This suggests that specific factors, such as target protein membrane mobility and localization of the target epitope, that permit formation of multimolecular GP antigen–IgG–FcγRIIa complexes, are crucial for platelet activation mediated by FcγRIIa clustering. These murine IgG Fc moieties within the platelet surface immune complexes can interact with either FcγRIIa on the same platelet (intraplatelet activation) or FcγRIIa receptors in close proximity, located on other platelets (interplatelet activation) (Anderson et al., 1991; Horsewood et al., 1991).

Complexed human IgG is also a potent stimulator of platelet activation.

Karas and co-workers (1982) showed that trimeric human IgG and larger immune complexes had significant affinity for platelet FcγRIIa. Presumably, the affinity constants of monomeric and dimeric IgG for FcγRIIa are too low to result in appreciable binding. King et al. (1990) showed that trimeric IgG molecules are necessary for platelet activation. Furthermore, heat-aggregated IgG also is a potent agonist for platelet activation (Warkentin et al., 1994; Warkentin and Sheppard, 1999), as are streptokinase–antistreptokinase antibodies (Lebrazi et al., 1995) and PF4–H-containing immune complexes (Greinacher et al., 1994a). "IgG agonists," such as HIT antibodies, were exceeded only by calcium ionophore in their capacity to produce procoagulant, platelet-derived microparticles (i.e., HIT antibodies can be as potent as physiological platelet agonists under some experimental conditions) (Warkentin and Sheppard, 1999). HIT–IgG also cause the generation of thromboxane A_2 and associated platelet granule release (Chong et al., 1981). Indeed, several different "activation assays" have been developed that detect HIT antibodies by their ability to cause normal platelets to aggregate (Greinacher et al., 1991) and cause granule release (Sheridan et al., 1986), among other activation responses (see Chap. 11).

It appears that ADP is an important autocrine stimulator of platelet activation by HIT–IgG. Chong et al. (1981) demonstrated that ADP release was involved in HIT-dependent platelet aggregation and release. This observation was confirmed by Anderson and Anderson (1990), who showed that FcγRIIa-mediated activation was augmented by ADP. Although ADP potentiates platelet activation by many agonists, Polgàr and co-workers (1998) found that pretreatment of platelets with a potent ADP receptor antagonist completely blocked the activity of HIT sera. This observation indicates that ADP and a functional ADP receptor are crucial to FcγRIIa activation by HIT–IgG, and underscores the importance of certain technical requirements of platelet activation assays (e.g., use of apyrase [an enzyme that proteolyzes ADP] during platelet washing to prevent subsequent refractoriness to ADP-induced platelet activation).

The transduction signal resulting from platelet FcγRIIa clustering is poorly understood. However, the action of phospholipase C, the release of inositol triphosphate, and the mobilization of internal calcium stores appear to be the primary pathways activated by FcγRIIa engagement (Anderson and Anderson, 1990). The clustering of FcγRIIa induces ITAM phosphorylation by unknown tyrosine phosphorylase(s), which then activates tyrosine kinase $p72^{syk}$ through its noncovalent association with the receptor (Chacko et al., 1994). In addition, the phosphoinositol kinase (PI 3-kinase) is associated with the FcγRIIa and tyrosine kinase $p72^{syk}$ (Chacko et al., 1996). Greinacher et al. (1994b) showed that FcγRIIa engagement resulted in the activation of various protein kinases that phosphorylate mainly pleckstrin and myosin light chain. Therefore, FcγRIIa clustering facilitates downstream protein tyrosine phosphorylation by uncertain signaling pathways by protein kinases (e.g., p72^{syk}) with platelet cytoskeletal involvement (shape change) and the generation of IP3 via PI 3-kinase.

IV. FcγRIIa ACTIVATION IN HIT

Although an association between heparin treatment and paradoxical thrombosis was first suspected about 40 years ago (Weismann et al., 1958; Roberts et al., 1964), it was Rhodes and colleagues (1973) who first provided evidence that serum from HIT patients contained a substance, most likely IgG, that aggregated normal platelets in the presence of heparin. This observation was confirmed by Fratantoni et al. (1975), who reported a simple indirect aggregation method for detecting HIT antibodies. In 1986, Sheridan and co-workers (1986) reported a washed platelet activation assay, employing radiolabeled serotonin, as an activation endpoint that was sensitive and specific for detecting clinically significant HIT antibodies. This same group later reported that platelet activation by HIT antibodies was platelet FcγRIIa-dependent, as it could be completely abrogated by a murine monoclonal anti-FcγRIIa antibody, IV.3 (Kelton et al., 1988). Other workers confirmed the central importance of the platelet Fc receptor in mediating platelet activation in HIT (Adelman et al., 1989; Chong et al., 1989a,b). Subsequently, Amiral and colleagues (1992) reported that the major target antigen for HIT was PF4 complexed to heparin, a finding quickly confirmed by other workers (Greinacher et al., 1994a; Kelton et al., 1994; Visentin et al., 1994). HIT–IgG binds to PF4–H complexes on the surface of the platelet, and activation likely occurs by intraplatelet as well as interplatelet interactions between IgG and FcγRIIa (Horsewood et al., 1991).

Monoclonal antibodies against GP Ib can interfere with platelet activation by HIT antibodies, suggesting that FcγRIIa may be closely associated with GP Ib (Adelman et al., 1989). However, the reaction is not GP Ib-dependent, for HIT–IgG-activated platelets from a patient deficient in GP Ib (Bernard-Soulier syndrome) (Chong et al., 1989a).

A. Platelet FcγRIIa Numbers

Variable expression of FcγRIIa numbers among individuals could affect susceptibility to immune complex diseases (Rosenfeld et al., 1987), or even to HIT. The number of platelet surface-expressed FcγRIIa molecules is increased dramatically in patients with HIT, much more than can be explained by normal variability or by changes in platelet size (Chong et al., 1993b). However, increased FcγRIIa expression was also seen after in vitro activation of platelets by HIT antibodies. Thus, elevated FcγRIIa numbers may be a consequence of platelet activation in

HIT, rather than a proximate cause. It remains uncertain whether high baseline (pre-HIT) FcγRIIa numbers represents an important risk factor for HIT.

B. Plasma-Soluble FcγRIIa

Soluble FcγRIIa, which is released from α-granules on platelet activation by thrombin, has been demonstrated in plasma (Gachet et al., 1995). The soluble form of the receptor lacks the amino acids for the transmembrane domain, a result of alternative splicing that removes exon 5 from primary transcripts (Rappaport et al., 1993). However, the relative amount of membrane versus soluble FcγRIIa is fixed (Keller et al., 1993). Gachet and colleagues (1995) reported that approximately 2 ng of soluble FcγRIIa is produced from 10^9 platelets. This value equals 2 ag, or 300 molecules, per platelet compared with roughly ten times as many molecules on the platelet surface. A much larger amount of plasma-soluble FcγRIIa would be needed to inhibit significantly PF4–H immune complexes from binding to platelet FcγRIIa. Therefore, there is likely no effect of soluble FcγRIIa on membrane FcγRIIa-dependent platelet activation, especially considering that immune complexes formed on the platelet surface would sterically hinder soluble receptor interaction. Moreover, plasma levels of soluble FcγRIIa are higher in patients with HIT than in heparin-treated or other nonthrombocytopenic controls, presumably as a marker of in vivo platelet activation in HIT (Saffroy et al., 1997).

C. Plasma IgG Concentrations

Plasma IgG levels appear to influence platelet activation and aggregation by HIT sera. With a platelet-rich plasma (PRP) aggregation test to detect HIT antibodies, Chong et al. (1993a) showed variable platelet sensitivity to aggregation that was stable over time among different platelet donors. One factor that correlated with sensitivity to platelet aggregation was the IgG level of the donor plasma. In addition, Chong and co-workers showed that the addition of purified human IgG to the PRP inhibited platelet aggregation by HIT sera, with complete inhibition at 40 mg/mL. It is possible that the effect of purified IgG is due to the presence of small IgG oligomers, because Karas et al. (1982) demonstrated that monomeric IgG does not bind to the platelet FcγRIIa. Furthermore, Greinacher et al. (1994b) showed that different preparations of intravenous IgG (ivIgG) for therapeutic use varied in their ability to inhibit HIT antibody-induced platelet serotonin release. Only Cohn alcohol-fractionated ivIgG preparations retained the ability to inhibit the reaction at concentrations that can be achieved in vivo (20 mg/mL). Preparations that were treated to reduce IgG oligomers did not inhibit heparin-dependent platelet serotonin release.

Larger IgG immune complexes, such as heat-aggregated IgG, can activate platelets strongly. However, as ivIgG inhibits HIT antibody-induced platelet activation both in vitro and in vivo, this suggests that the oligomers in ivIgG are sufficiently small (i.e., predominantly dimers) that they inhibit, rather than potentiate, platelet activation by the FcγRIIa receptors. Although the use of ivIgG to treat HIT does not appear to be common, it is a rational approach in certain clinical settings (see Chap. 13).

D. FcγRIIa–Arg/His^{131} Polymorphism

There is an arginine–histidine (Arg/His) polymorphism at amino acid 131 of the human FcγRIIa (Clark et al., 1989, Warmerdam et al., 1990). This allelic variation affects the ability of human platelets to be activated by murine monoclonal IgG1 as well as by human IgG2 (Horsewood et al., 1991, Tomiyama et al., 1992, Parren et al., 1992, Bachelot et al., 1995). This prompted Burgess et al. (1995) to suggest that inherited FcγRIIa receptor variants could be a risk factor for developing HIT. In a small cohort of patients, they found an overrepresentation of the FcγRIIa–His^{131} variant. They hypothesized that IgG2 might be an important IgG subclass among HIT–IgG, as this could explain an apparent association between HIT and the FcγRIIa–His^{131} variant.

However, subsequent reports argued against this hypothesis: IgG1 rather than IgG2 was the predominant subclass among HIT–IgG (Arepally et al., 1997; Denomme et al., 1997; Suh et al., 1997). Nevertheless, in support of a biological basis for a possible increased frequency of FcγRIIa–His^{131}, two groups found that HIT antibodies, including those that were predominantly IgG1, preferentially activated washed platelets of the His^{131} variant in vitro (Denomme et al., 1997; Bachelot-Loza et al., 1998). However, Brandt et al. (1995) found the opposite activation profile in platelet aggregation studies using citrated platelet-rich plasma (i.e., the Arg^{131} variant was preferentially activated by HIT plasmas). No consensus has emerged either among the six studies that investigated whether one of the FcγRIIa–Arg/His^{131} phenotypes predominated among patients with HIT: three studies show an overrepresentation of FcγRIIa–His^{131} (Burgess et al., 1995; Brandt et al., 1995; Denomme et al., 1997); two studies found no correlation with either variant (Arepally et al., 1997; Bachelot-Loza et al., 1998); and one study (the largest) showed the reverse correlation (Carlsson et al., 1998). This topic is considered in detail in the following section.

V. FcγRIIa POLYMORPHISMS IN DISEASE

A. Determining the FcγRIIa Polymorphism

The FcγRIIa–Arg/His^{131} polymorphism was first identified on the basis of functional differences effected by anti-CD3 monoclonal antibodies of the murine IgG1 subclass (Tax et al., 1983, 1984). Proliferation assays distinguished ‘‘high’’ and ''low'' responders relative to the effects of these anti-CD3 murine monoclonal antibodies on T-cell–dependent mitogenesis. Subsequently, individuals bearing the FcγRIIa–Arg^{131} phenotype were identified as the ''high responders'' and the functional differences between the two polymorphic variants were later confirmed using other FcγRIIa-dependent assays, such as erythrocyte antigen-rosetting, phagocytosis, and platelet activation (Clark et al., 1989; Warmerdam et al., 1991; Parren et al., 1992; Salmon et al., 1992). Murine monoclonal IgG1 antibodies activate platelets of all three Arg/His^{131} phenotypes, but the homozygous FcγRIIa–Arg^{131} variant requires less murine monoclonal antibody for platelet activation to occur.

The high-affinity binding of human IgG2 to FcγRIIa results when histidine is substituted at amino acid 131 of the mature protein (Warmerdam et al., 1991). FcγRIIa–His^{131} has a greater affinity for human IgG2, but a lower affinity for murine IgG1. Therefore, the terms high and low responder, used historically for the effects of murine monoclonal antibodies on Arg^{131} and His^{131} FcγRIIa phenotypes, respectively, is confusing, as the opposite reaction profile is observed with human IgG2. The high/low responder terminology has been largely replaced in favor of referring simply to the amino acid polymorphism.

The FcγRIIa–Arg/His^{131} variant polymorphism can be determined in three ways: (a) by functional assay, such as T-cell–dependent proliferation or murine monoclonal antibody activation; (b) by specific binding using 41H16, a monoclonal antibody the Fab of which binds exclusively to the FcγRIIa–Arg^{131} variant; and (c) by molecular genotyping. Four DNA-based methods have been developed to genotype for the FcγRIIa–Arg/His^{131} nucleotide substitution (Clark et al., 1991; Osborne et al., 1994; Bachelot et al., 1995; Jiang et al., 1996; Denomme et al., 1997). In one technique, the presence of the FcγRIIa–Arg/His^{131} variant gene is determined using genomic DNA and a sequence-specific primer polymerase chain reaction (PCR) assay. Two PCR reactions are necessary, each containing a common primer paired with a unique primer having different 3′-ends to detect the presence of the G or A variant nucleotide (Clark et al., 1991). This method has been modified using different sequence-specific primers (Flesch et al., 1998) or using a nested sequence-specific PCR (Carlsson et al., 1998). In a second technique, flanking primers are used to amplify a region containing the nucleotide polymorphism, followed by dot-blotting and hybridization with allele-specific, single-stranded oligonucleotide probes (Burgess et al., 1995; Osborne et al., 1994; Denomme et al., 1997). In a third technique, Bachelot and co-workers (1995) developed a denaturing gradient gel electrophoresis assay that distinguishes between the FcγRIIa–Arg/His^{131} variants also using flanking primers that amplify a region containing the polymorphism. Last, restriction endonuclease digestion of PCR-amplified genomic DNA has been developed using one primer immediately proximal to the polymorphic site and containing a mutation such that the polymorphism creates a restriction enzyme site for only one of the alleles (Jiang et al., 1996).

B. Influence of FcγRIIa Polymorphism in Infectious or Autoimmune Disease

A few studies have examined whether expression of the FcγRIIa–Arg/His^{131} polymorphism influences susceptibility to infectious or autoimmune disease. In theory, the weaker binding of human IgG2 to the FcγRIIa–Arg^{131} variant suggests that this gene might be overrepresented among patients with recurrent infections characterized by certain microbes with polysaccharide coats (i.e., involving an IgG2 antibody response), and overrepresented in disease characterized by circulating immune complexes (because phagocytic cells bearing the FcγRIIa–His^{131} variant would clear these complexes more readily). Certainly, a skewed genotypic distribution favoring the FcγRIIa–Arg^{131} variant has been noted in patients with *Haemophilus influenzae* infections (Sanders et al., 1994) and meningococcal septic shock (Bredius et al., 1994a). Furthermore, there is also predominance of FcγRIIa–Arg^{131} in patients with elevated levels of immune complexes and glomerulonephritis complicating systemic lupus erythematosus (Duits et al., 1995; Table 2).

C. FcγRIIa Polymorphism in HIT

It was logical to hypothesize that the platelet FcγRIIa–Arg/His^{131} polymorphism would influence the clinical expression of HIT. First, platelets from normal individuals exhibit considerable variability in their activation by HIT sera (Salem and Van der Weyden, 1983; Pfueller and David, 1986; Warkentin et al., 1992). Second, many patients who form HIT antibodies during heparin treatment do not develop thrombocytopenia (Warkentin et al., 1995; Amiral et al., 1996; Suh et al., 1997). Third, the inciting role of heparin, a sulfated carbohydrate, suggested that there could be an important role for HIT antibodies of IgG2 subclass—that is, the subclass with higher affinity for FcγRIIa–His^{131} that is predominantly formed in response to carbohydrate antigens (Herrmann et al., 1992). (However, HIT epitopes form on the protein PF4 when it undergoes conformation change bound to heparin; see Chaps. 6–8). Consequently, it was speculated that the FcγRIIa variant distribution in HIT would differ significantly from a random control population, and especially differ from patients who did not develop thrombocytopenia during heparin treatment (Denomme et al., 1997; Bachelot-Loza et al., 1998).

The six studies investigating the role of the FcγRIIa–Arg/His^{131} polymorphism have not yielded uniform results (Fig. 2). Three studies showed a predomi-

Table 2 Role of FcγRIIa–Arg/His^{131} Polymorphism in Disease

Disease	Predominant FcγRIIa variant	Comment
Infections by encapsulated bacteria	Arg^{131}	Reduced binding of IgG2 by FcγRIIa–Arg^{131} -MPS cells reduces phagocytosis, conferring susceptibility to infections with bacteria bearing polysaccharide capsules (*Haemophilus*, meningococcus).
Immune complex nephritis (SLE)	Arg^{131}	Reduced clearance of IgG-containing immune complexes by FcγRIIa–Arg^{131} -MPS cells leads to greater glomerular deposition of immune complexes.
HIT with thrombosis	Arg^{131}	Reduced clearance of IgG-containing immune complexes by FcγRIIa–Arg^{131} -MPS cells leads to greater immune complex-dependent activation of platelets and endothelial cells (Carlsson et al., 1998).
HIT with or without thrombosis	His^{131}	Increased activation by HIT–IgG1 and HIT–IgG2 of FcγRIIa–His^{131} platelets, without significant role for MPS cells (Denomme et al., 1997).

Abbreviations: Arg, arginine; FcγRIIa, RcγIIa receptor; His, histidine; MPS, mononuclear phagocytic system (reticuloendothelial system); SLE, systemic lupus erythematosus.

nance of the His^{131} variant in patients with HIT that was significant, compared with control patients. Together with evidence that HIT antibodies preferentially activate platelets in vitro from individuals bearing the FcγRIIa–His^{131} polymorphism (Denomme et al., 1997; Bachelot-Loza et al., 1998), it was suggested that FcγRIIa–His^{131} predominance could reflect a greater potential for these platelets to be activated in vivo by HIT antibodies (see Table 2). Two relatively small studies did not show any significant differences in the Arg/His^{131} phenotypes between HIT patients and controls.

However, the largest of the six studies, involving 389 patients (i.e., more than the 260 HIT patients reported in the previous five studies combined), showed an increase in the frequency of the Arg^{131}, rather than the His^{131}, variant in patients with HIT (Carlsson et al., 1998). Moreover, these workers made the intriguing observation that the increase in Arg^{131} phenotype occurred only in the subset of patients whose HIT was complicated by thrombosis. These investigators proposed that reduced clearance of IgG-containing immune complexes by phagocytic cells bearing FcγRIIa–Arg^{131} leads to greater immune complex-dependent

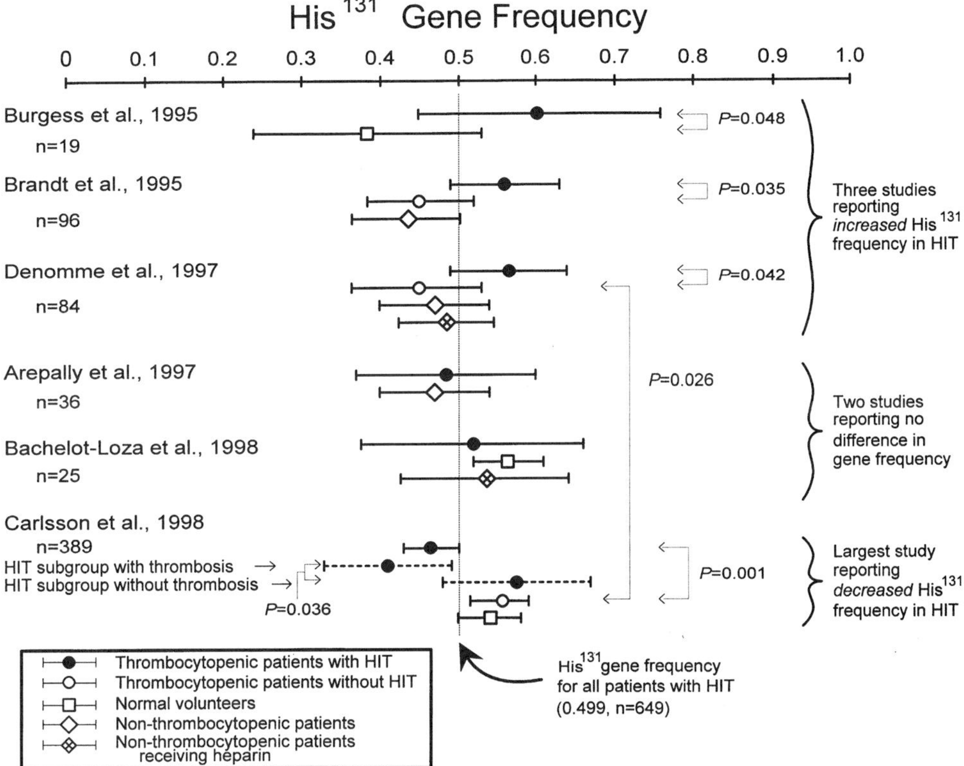

Figure 2 FcγRIIa–His^{131} gene frequencies in six studies of HIT are shown: The first four studies were from North American centers, the last two from Europe. Although the first three studies showed predominance of His^{131} in patients with HIT, the last study showed predominance of Arg^{131} in patients with HIT complicated by thrombosis. A complicating feature is the difference in gene frequencies between certain control populations [e.g., between Denomme et al. (1997) and Carlsson et al. (1998)]. Not shown in the figure is the significant difference between control patients in the studies by Carlsson and Brandt (p = 0.013).

activation of platelets and endothelial cells, thus predisposing to thrombosis (see Table 2). Although Arepally et al. (1997) did not observe a significant increase in the Arg^{131} phenotype among HIT patients with thrombosis, their subset of HIT patients with thrombosis was much smaller than that reported by Carlsson (23 vs. 68 patients).

The explanation for the differences among these various studies is not readily apparent. However, a complicating aspect is noted in Fig. 2: the frequency of the His[131] phenotype is higher in the European controls (Bachelot-Loza et al., 1998; Carlsson et al., 1998), compared with the North American and Australian control populations (Burgess et al., 1995; Brandt et al., 1995; Denomme et al., 1997; Arepally et al., 1997), an observation consistent with population allele frequencies reported by Rascu et al. (1997). Indeed, pairwise χ^2 analysis for the frequency of the His[131] genotype among the various control groups shows that the control population of Carlsson's study differs from that reported by Denomme and Brandt (see Fig. 2). The FcγRIIa–Arg/His[131] polymorphism varies among populations: in whites and African Americans, the gene frequencies have roughly a 50:50 balance (Osborne et al., 1994; Lehrnbecher et al., 1998). In contrast, in the Japanese and Chinese populations, the His[131] gene frequency is approximately 75% (Rascu et al., 1997; Osborne et al., 1994). It is possible that unrecognized differences in population between HIT patients and controls could be important. For example, whereas samples from HIT patients could be referred from a wider geographic area, control patients might have been obtained from a localized area. None of the six studies reported on the Arg/His[131] phenotype distribution among heparin-treated patients who formed HIT antibodies, but who did not develop thrombocytopenia (i.e., the ideal control group for assessing the influence of the FcγRIIa polymorphism).

In summary, the role of the FcγRIIa–Arg/His[131] polymorphism in contributing to the pathogenesis of HIT remains controversial. Regardless of its ultimate resolution, the elucidation of the biological basis for differences in frequency of FcγRIIa phenotype between HIT patients, with or without thrombosis, and control subjects will provide new insights into the pathogenesis of immune-mediated disease.

ACKNOWLEDGMENTS

The author wishes to thank Dr. Lena E. Carlsson for her helpful review of the manuscript. Some of the studies described were supported by a Career Development Fellowship Award of the Canadian Blood Services. The author is a Bayer/Canadian Blood Services/Medical Research Council Scholar.

REFERENCES

Adelman B, Sobel M, Fujimura Y, Ruggeri ZM, Zimmerman TS. Heparin-associated thrombocytopenia: observations on the mechanism of platelet aggregation. J Lab Clin Med 113:204–210, 1989.

Amiral J, Bridey F, Dreyfus M, Vissaco AM, Fressinaud E, Wolf M, Meyer D. Platelet factor 4 complexed to heparin is the target for antibodies generated in heparin-induced thrombocytopenia. Thromb Haemost 68:95–96, 1992.

Amiral J, Peynaud-Debayle E, Wolf M, Bridey F, Vissac A-M, Meyer D. Generation of antibodies to heparin–PF4 complexes without thrombocytopenia in patients treated with unfractionated or low-molecular-weight heparin. Am J Hematol 52:90–95, 1996.

Anderson GP, Anderson CL. Signal transduction by the platelet Fc receptor. Blood 76: 1165–1172, 1990.

Anderson GP, van de Winkel JGJ, Anderson CL. Anti-GPIIb/IIIa (CD41) monoclonal antibody-induced platelet activation requires Fc receptor-dependent cell–cell interaction. Br J Haematol 79:75–83, 1991.

Arepally G, McKenzie SE, Jiang X-M, Poncz M, Cines DB. FcγRIIA H/R^{131} polymorphism, subclass-specific IgG anti-heparin/platelet factor 4 antibodies and clinical course in patients with heparin-induced thrombocytopenia and thrombosis. Blood 89:370–375, 1997.

Bachelot C, Saffroy R, Gandrille S, Aiach M, Rendu F. Role of FcγRIIA gene polymorphism in human platelet activation by monoclonal antibodies. Thromb Haemost 74: 1557–1563, 1995.

Bachelot-Loza C, Saffroy R, Lasne D, Chatellier G, Aiach M, Rendu F. Importance of the FcγRIIa–Arg/His-131 polymorphism in heparin-induced thrombocytopenia diagnosis. Thromb Haemost 79:523–528, 1998.

Brandt JT, Isenhart CE, Osborne JM, Ahmed A, Anderson CL. On the role of platelet FcγRIIa phenotype in heparin-induced thrombocytopenia. Thromb Haemost 74: 1564–1572, 1995.

Bredius RGM, Derkz BHF, Fijen CAP, de Wit TPM, de Haas M, Weening RS, van de Winkel JGJ, Out TA. Fc gamma IIa (CD32) polymorphism in fulminant meningococcal septic shock in children. J Infect Dis 170:848–853, 1994a.

Bredius RGM, Fijen CAP, de Haas M, Kuijper EJ, Weening RS, van de Winkel JGJ, Out TA. Role of neutrophil FcγRIII (CD32) and FcγRIII (CD16) polymorphic forms in phagocytosis of human IgG1- and IgG3-opsonized bacteria and erythrocytes. Immunology 83:624–630, 1994b.

Brooks DG, Qiu WQ, Luster AD, Ravetch JV. Structure and expression of human IgG FcRII (CD32). Functional heterogeneity is encoded by the alternatively spliced products of multiple genes. J Exp Med 170:1369–1385, 1989.

Burgess JK, Lindeman R, Chesterman CN, Chong BH. Single amino acid mutation of Fcγ receptor is associated with the development of heparin-induced thromboctyopenia. Br J Haematol 91:761–766, 1995.

Bux J, Stein EL, Bierling P, Fromont P, Clay ME, Stoncek DF, Santoso S. Characterization of a new alloantigen (SH) on the human neutrophil Fcγ receptor IIIb. Blood 89: 1027–1034, 1997.

Carlsson LE, Santoso S, Baurichter G, Kroll H, Papenberg S, Eichler P, Westerdaal NAC, Kiefel V, van de Winkel JGJ, Greinacher A. Heparin-induced thrombocytopenia: new insights into the impact of the FcγRIIa-R–H131 polymorphism. Blood 92: 1526–1531, 1998.

Chacko GW, Duchemin A-M, Coggeshall KM, Osborne JM, Brandt JT, Anderson CL.

Clustering of the platelet Fcγ receptor induces noncovalent association with the tyrosine kinase p72syk. J Biol Chem 269:32435–32440, 1994.

Chacko GW, Brandt JT, Coggeshall KM, Anderson CL. Phosphoinositide 3-kinase and p72syk noncovalently associate with the low affinity Fcγ receptor on human platelets through an immunoreceptor tyrosine-based activation motif. J Biol Chem 271: 10775–10781, 1996.

Chong BH, Grace CS, Rozenberg MC. Heparin-induced thrombocytopenia: effect of heparin platelet antibody on platelets. Br J Haematol 49:531–540, 1981.

Chong BH, Fawaz I, Chesterman CN, Berndt MC. Heparin-induced thrombocytopenia: mechanism of interaction of the heparin-dependent antibody with platelets. Br J Haematol 73:235–240, 1989a.

Chong BH, Castaldi PA, Berndt MC. Heparin-induced thrombocytopenia: effect of rabbit IgG, and its Fab and Fc fragments on antibody–heparin–platelet interaction. Thromb Res 55:291–295, 1989b.

Chong BH, Burgess J, Ismail F. The clinical usefulness of the platelet aggregation test for the diagnosis of heparin-induced thrombocytopenia. Thromb Haemost 69:344–350, 1993a.

Chong BH, Pilgrim RL, Cooley MA, Chesterman CN. Increased expression of platelet IgG Fc receptors in immune heparin-induced thrombocytopenia. Blood 81:988–993, 1993b.

Clark MR, Clarkson SB, Ory PA, Stollman N, Goldstein IM. Molecular basis for a polymorphism involving Fc receptor II on human monocytes. J Immunol 143:1731–1734, 1989.

Clark MR, Stuart SG, Kimberly RP, Ory PA, Goldstein IM. A single amino acid distinguishes the high-responder from the low-responder form of Fc receptor II on human monocytes. Eur J Immunol 21:1911–1916, 1991.

Cines DB, Tomaski A, Tannenbaum S. Immune endothelial-cell injury in heparin-associated thrombocytopenia. N Engl J Med 316:581–589, 1987.

Denomme GA, Warkentin TE, Horsewood P, Sheppard J-A I, Warner MN, Kelton JG. Activation of platelets by sera containing IgG1 heparin-dependent antibodies: an explanation for the predominance of the FcγRIIa "low responder" (his_{131}) gene in patients with heparin-induced thrombocytopenia. J Lab Clin Med 130:278–284, 1997.

Duits AJ, Bootsma H, Derksen RHWM, Spronk PE, Kater L, Kallenberg CGM, Capel PJA, Westerdaal NAC, Spierenburg GT, Gmelig-Meyling FHJ, van de Winkel JGJ. Skewed distribution of IgG Fc receptor IIa (CD32) polymorphism is associated with renal disease in systemic lupus erythematosus patients. Arthritis Rheum 39: 1832–1836, 1995.

Flesch BK, Bauer F, Neppert J. Rapid typing of the human Fcγ receptor IIA polymorphism by polymerase chain reaction amplification with allele-specific primers. Transfusion 38:174–176, 1998.

Fratantoni JC, Pollet R, Gralnick HR. Heparin-induced thrombocytopenia: confirmation of diagnosis with in vitro methods. Blood 45:395–401, 1975.

Gachet C, Astier A, de la Salle H, de la Salle C, Fridman WH, Cazenave J-P, Hanau D, Teillaud J-L. Release of FcγRIIa2 by activated platelets and inhibition of anti-CD9–mediated platelet aggregation by recombinant FcγRIIa2. Blood 85:698–704, 1995.

Gessner JE, Heiken H, Tamm A, Schmidt RE. The IgG Fc receptor family. Ann Hematol 76:231–248, 1998.

Green D, Harris K, Reynolds N, Roberts M, Patterson R. Heparin immune thrombocytopenia: evidence for a heparin–platelet complex as the antigenic determinant. J Lab Clin Med 91:167–175, 1978.

Greinacher A, Michels I, Kiefel V, Mueller-Eckhardt C. A rapid and sensitive test for diagnosing heparin-associated thrombocytopenia. Thromb Haemost 66:734–736, 1991.

Greinacher A, Pötzsch B, Amiral J, Dummel V, Eichner A, Mueller-Eckhardt C. Heparin-associated thrombocytopenia: isolation of the antibody and characterization of a multimolecular PF4–heparin complex as the major antigen. Thromb Haemost 71: 247–251, 1994a.

Greinacher A, Liebenhoff U, Kiefel V, Presek P, Mueller-Eckhardt C. Heparin-associated thrombocytopenia: the effects of various intravenous IgG preparations on antibody mediated platelet activation—a possible new indication of high dose i.v. IgG. Thromb Haemost 71:641–645, 1994b.

Herrmann DJ, Hamilton RG, Barington T, Frasch CE, Arakere G, Mäkelä O, Mitchell LA, Nagel J, Rijkers GT, Zegers B, Danve B, Ward JI, Brown CS. Quantitation of human IgG subclass antibodies to *Haemophilus influenzae* type b capsular polysaccharide. J Immunol Methods 148:101–114, 1992.

Horsewood P, Hayward CPM, Warkentin TE, Kelton JG. Investigation of the mechanisms of monoclonal antibody-induced platelet activation. Blood 78:1019–1026, 1991.

Hulett MD, Witort E, Brinkworth RI, McKenzie IFC, Hogarth PM. Multiple regions of human FcγRII (CD32) contribute to the binding of IgG. J Biol Chem 270:21188–21194, 1995.

Jiang X-M, Arepally G, Poncz M, McKenzie SE. Rapid detection of the FcγRIIA–H/R131 ligand-binding polymorphism using an allele-specific restriction enzyme digestion (ASRED). J Immunol Methods 199:55–59, 1996.

Karas SP, Rosse WF, Kurlander RJ. Characterization of the IgG–Fc receptor on human platelets. Blood 60:1277–1282, 1982.

Keller MA, Cassel DL, Rappaport EF, McKenzie SE, Schwartz E, Surrey S. fluorescence-based RT PCR analysis: determination of the ratio of soluble to membrane-bound forms of FcγRIIA transcripts in hematopoietic cell lines. PCR Methods Appl 3: 32–38, 1993.

Kelton JG, Smith JW, Santos AV, Murphy WG, Horsewood P. Platelet IgG Fc receptor. Am J Hematol 25:299–310, 1987.

Kelton JG, Sheridan D, Santos A, Smith J, Steeves K, Smith C, Brown C, Murphy WG. Heparin-induced thrombocytopenia: laboratory studies. Blood 72:925–930, 1988.

Kelton JG, Smith JW, Warkentin TE, Hayward CPM, Denomme GA, Horsewood P. Immunoglobulin G from patients with heparin-induced thrombocytopenia binds to a complex of heparin and platelet factor 4. Blood 83:3232–3239, 1994.

King M, McDermott P, Schreiber AD. Characterization of the Fc-gamma receptor on human platelets. Cell Immunol 128:462–479, 1990.

Koene HR, Kleijer M, Algra J, Roos D, von dem Borne AEGK, de Haas M. FcγRIIIa–158V/F polymorphism influences the binding of IgG by natural killer cell FcγRIIIa, independently of the FcγRIIIa–48L/R/H phenotype. Blood 90:1109–1114, 1997.

Koene HR, Kleijer M, Roos D, de Haas M, von dem Borne AEGK. FcγRIIIB gene duplication: evidence for presence and expression of three distinct FcγRIIIB genes in NA(1+,2+)SH(+) individuals. Blood 91:673–679, 1998.

Lebrazi J, Helft G, Abdelouahed M, Elalamy I, Mirshahi M, Samama MM, Lecompte T. Human anti-streptokinase antibodies induce platelet aggregation in an Fc receptor (CD32) dependent manner. Thromb Haemost 74:938–942, 1995.

Lehrnbecher T, Foster CH, Zhu S, Leitman S, Huppi K, Chanock S. Analysis of biologically significant variant alleles of the low affinity Fc gamma receptor cluster in healthy population: a foundation for genetic annotation studies that further defines the recently identified SH-FcgR3b as an independent locus. Blood 92(suppl 1):162a, 1998.

McCrae KR, Shattil SJ, Cines DB. Platelet activation induces increased Fcγ receptor expression. J Immunol 144:3920–3927, 1990.

Norris CF, Pricop L, Millard SS, Taylor SM, Surrey S, Schwartz E, Salmon JE, McKenzie SE. A naturally occurring mutation in FcγRIIA: a Q to K127 change confers unique IgG binding properties to the R131 allelic form of the receptor. Blood 91:656–662, 1998.

Ory PA, Clark MA, Kwoh EE, Clarkson SB, Goldstein IM. Sequences of complementary DNAs that encode the NA1 and NA2 forms of Fc receptor III on human neutrophils. J Clin Invest 84:1688–1691, 1989.

Osborne JM, Chacko GW, Brandt JT, Anderson CL. Ethnic variation in frequency of an allelic polymorphism of human FcγRIIa determined with allele specific oligonucleotide probes. J Immunol Methods 173:207–217, 1994.

Parren PWHI, Warmerdam PAM, Boeije LCM, Arts J, Westerdaal NAC, Vlug A, Capel PJA, Aarden LA, van de Winkel JGJ. On the interaction of IgG subclasses with the low affinity Fc gamma RIIa (CD32) on human monocytes, neutrophils, and platelets. Analysis of a functional polymorphism to human IgG2. J Clin Invest 90: 1537–1546, 1992.

Pfueller SL, David R. Different platelet specificities of heparin-dependent platelet aggregating factors in heparin-associated immune thrombocytopenia. Br J Haematol 64: 149–159, 1986.

Polgàr J, Eichler P, Greinacher A, Clemetson KJ. Adenosine diphosphate (ADP) and ADP receptor play a major role in platelet activation/aggregation induced by sera from heparin-induced thrombocytopenia patients. Blood 91:549–554, 1998.

Qiu WQ, de Bruin D, Brownstein BH, Pearse R, Ravetch JV. Organization of the human and mouse low-affinity FcγR genes: duplication and recombination. Science 248: 732–735, 1990.

Rappaport EF, Cassel DL, Walterhouse DO, McKenzie SE, Surrey S, Keller MA, Schreiber AD, Schwartz E. A soluble form of the human Fc receptor FcγRIIa: cloning, transcript analysis and detection. Exp Hematol 21:689–696, 1993.

Rascu A, Repp R, Westerdaal NAC, Kalden JR, van de Winkel JGJ. Clinical relevance of Fcγ receptor polymorphisms. Ann NY Acad Sci 815:282–295, 1997.

Rhodes GR, Dixon RH, Silver D. Heparin induced thrombocytopenia with thrombotic and hemorrhagic manifestations. Surg Gynecol Obstet 136:409–416, 1973.

Roberts B, Rosato FE, Rosato EF. Heparin: a cause of arterial emboli? Surgery 55:803–808, 1964.

Roitt I, Brostoff J, Male D, eds. Immunology. London: Gower Medical Publishing, 1985.
Rosenfeld SI, Looney RJ, Leddy JP, Phipps DC, Abraham GN, Anderson CL. Human platelet Fc receptor for immunoglobulin G. Identification as a 40,000-molecular-weight membrane protein shared by monocytes. J Clin Invest 76:2317–2322, 1985.
Rosenfeld SI, Ryan DH, Looney RJ, Anderson CL, Abraham GN, Leddy JP. Human Fcγ receptors: stable inter-donor variation in quantitative expression on platelets correlates with functional responses. J Immunol 144:3920–3927, 1987.
Rubinstein E, Boucheix C, Worthington RE, Carroll RC. Anti-platelet antibody interactions with Fcγ receptor. Semin Thromb Hemost 21:10–22, 1995.
Saffroy R, Bachelot-Loza C, Fridman WH, Aiach M, Teullaud J-L, Rendu F. Plasma levels of soluble Fcγ receptors II (sCD32) and III (sCD16) in patients with heparin-induced thrombocytopenia. Thromb Haemost 78:970–971, 1997.
Salem HH, Van der Weyden MB. Heparin-induced thrombocytopenia. Variable platelet-rich plasma reactivity to heparin-dependent aggregating factor. Pathology 15:297–299, 1983.
Salmon JE, Edberg JC, Kimberly RP. Fcγ receptor III on human neutrophils. J Clin Invest 85:1287–1295, 1990.
Salmon JE, Edberg JC, Brogle NL, Kimberly RP. Allelic polymorphism of human Fcγ receptor IIA and Fcγ receptor IIIB. Independent mechanisms for differences in human phagocyte function. J Clin Invest 89:1274–1281, 1992.
Sanders LAM, van de Winkel JGJ, Rijkers GT, Voorhorst-Ogink MM, de Haas M, Capel PJA, Zegers BJM. Fc gamma receptor IIa (CD32) heterogeneity in patients with recurrent bacterial respiratory tract infections. J Infect Dis 170:854–861, 1994.
Sedmak DD, Davis DH, Singh U, van de Winkel JG, Anderson CL. Expression of IgG Fc receptor antigens in placenta and on endothelial cells in humans. An immunohistochemical study. Am J Pathol 138:175–181, 1991.
Sheridan D, Carter C, Kelton JG. A diagnostic test for heparin-induced thrombocytopenia. Blood 67:27–30, 1986.
Suh J-S, Malik MI, Aster RH, Visentin GP. Characterization of the humoral response in heparin-induced thrombocytopenia. Am J Hematol 54:196–201, 1997.
Tax WJM, Williams HW, Reckers PPM, Capel PJA, Keone RAP. Polymorphism in mitogenic effect of IgG1 monoclonal antibodies against T3 antigen on human T cells. Nature 304:445, 1983.
Tax WJM, Hermes FFM, Willems RW, Capel JA, Koene RAP. Fc receptors for mouse IgG 1 on human monocytes: polymorphism and role in antibody-induced T cell proliferation. J Immunol 133:1185–1189, 1984.
Tomiyama Y, Kunicki TJ, Zipf TF, Ford SB, Aster RH. Response of human platelets to activating monoclonal antibodies: importance of FcγRII (CD32) phenotype and level of expression. Blood 80:2261–2268, 1992.
van de Winkel JGJ, Capel PJA. Human IgG Fc receptor heterogeneity: molecular aspects and clinical implications. Immunol Today 14:215–221, 1993.
Visentin GP, Ford SE, Scott JP, Aster RH. Antibodies from patients with heparin-induced thrombocytopenia/thrombosis are specific for platelet factor 4 complexed with heparin or bound to endothelial cells. J Clin Invest 93:81–88, 1994.
Warkentin TE, Hayward CPM, Smith CA, Kelly PM, Kelton JG. Determinants of donor

platelet variability when testing for heparin-induced thrombocytopenia. J Lab Clin Med 120:371–379, 1992.

Warkentin TE, Hayward CPM, Boshkov LK, Santos AV, Sheppard JI, Bode AP, Kelton JG. Sera from patients with heparin-induced thrombocytopenia generate platelet-derived microparticles with procoagulant activity: an explanation for the thrombotic complications of heparin-induced thrombocytopenia. Blood 84:3691–3699, 1994a.

Warkentin TE, Sheppard JI. Generation of platelet-derived microparticles and procoagulant activity by heparin-induced thrombocytopenia IgG/serum and other IgG platelet agonists: a comparison with standard platelet agonists. Platelets 10:319–326, 1999.

Warkentin TE, Levine MN, Hirsh J, Horsewood P, Roberts RS, Tech M, Gent M, Kelton JG. Heparin-induced thrombocytopenia in patients treated with low-molecular-weight heparin or unfractionated heparin. N Engl J Med 332:1330–1335, 1995.

Warmerdam PAM, van de Winkel JGJ, Gosselin EJ, Capel PJA. Molecular basis for a polymorphism of human Fcγ receptor II (CD32w). J Exp Med 172:19–25, 1990.

Warmerdam PAM, van de Winkel JGJ, Vlug A, Westerdaal NAC, Capel PJA. A single amino acid in the second domain of the human Fcγ receptor II is critical for human IgG2 binding. J Immunol 147:1338–1343, 1991.

Weismann RE, Tobin RW. Arterial embolism occurring during systemic heparin therapy. Arch Surg 76:219–227, 1958.

Wu J, Edberg JC, Redecha PB, Bansal V, Guyre PM, Coleman K, Salmon JE, Kimberly RP. A novel polymorphism of FcγRIIIa (CD16) alters receptor function and predisposes to autoimmune disease. J Clin Invest 100:1059–1070, 1997.

10
Immune Vascular Injury in Heparin-Induced Thrombocytopenia

Gowthami M. Arepally
University of New Mexico Health Sciences Center, Albuquerque, New Mexico

Mortimer Poncz
University of Pennsylvania School of Medicine and Children's Hospital of Philadelphia, Philadelphia, Pennsylvania

Douglas B. Cines
University of Pennsylvania School of Medicine, Philadelphia, Pennsylvania

I. INTRODUCTION

The most important complication of HIT is thrombosis. Clinically overt arterial or venous thrombi have been observed in 50% or more of thrombocytopenic patients with HIT in some series (see Chaps. 3 and 4), a frequency that far exceeds any other drug-induced immune platelet disorder. The propensity for thrombosis has been attributed to platelet activation through FcγIIA receptors by IgG-containing complexes that comprise heparin and platelet factor 4 (PF4) (see Chap. 9). However, studies indicate that the ''nonpermissive'' FcγIIA phenotype affords limited protection against thrombosis (Arepally et al., 1997; Bachelot-Loza et al., 1998; Denomme et al., 1997; Carlsson et al., 1998). Furthermore, the occasional patient in whom only IgM or IgA HIT antibodies are detected (Amiral et al., 1996) suggests that additional factors, acting at the level of the platelet or elsewhere, must contribute to the thrombotic diathesis. In addition, thrombi usually occur at a limited number of vessel sites, typically large arteries and veins (Boshkov et al., 1993) (see Chap. 3), even though circulating HIT antibodies and activated platelets can be readily detected in asymptomatic patients. These considerations point to injury to the local vascular milieu in influencing the clinical expression of disease.

There are several other reasons to suspect that immune complex-mediated injury of the vasculature may contribute to the thrombotic complications of HIT. First, the endothelium helps maintain the balance between blood fluidity and clotting. Second, the endothelium expresses heparan sulfate-containing proteoglycans that help regulate coagulation and contribute to the metabolism of PF4. Third, antiendothelial cell antibodies have been identified in patients with other disorders characterized by thrombosis and thrombocytopenia. And fourth, there is some direct evidence that patients with HIT form antibodies that recognize heparin–PF4 complexes on the endothelium, and thereby promote prothrombotic reactions.

II. THE ENDOTHELIUM IN HEMOSTASIS

The role of the endothelium in regulating blood fluidity and trafficking of circulating hematopoietic cells has been the subject of recent reviews (Bassenge, 1996; Bombeli et al., 1997; Cadroy et al., 1997; Lüscher and Barton, 1997; Cines et al., 1998). Endothelial cells (ECs) express a variety of factors that inhibit coagulation. These include soluble substances, such as nitric oxide and prostacyclin (acting to inhibit platelet activation), and tissue-type plasminogen activator (t-PA, acting to promote fibrinolysis), among many others. Endothelial cell surface-bound molecules with anticoagulant activity include heparan sulfate-containing proteoglycans (see later discussion), thrombomodulin, complement regulatory proteins, as well as receptors for activated protein C, urokinase, and plasminogen.

Unperturbed ECs also do not express several moieties that promote platelet and leukocyte adhesion, such as endothelial leukocyte adhesion molecule (ELAM), P-selectin, and platelet-activating factor (PAF). These can be induced, however, when the cells are stimulated by agonists, such as cytokines or endotoxin (Drake et al., 1993), or when the cells are injured by immune factors, atherosclerosis, or shear stress. Additionally, ECs exposed to such factors express a reduced content of heparan sulfate, internalize and degrade activated protein C, elaborate tissue factor, and secrete abundant plasminogen activator inhibitor, each of which may promote thrombus formation (Cines et al., 1998). Histochemical studies of the endothelium in murine models of inflammation have confirmed many of these observations, which have been predicated on cell culture data (Fries et al., 1993), affirming the notion that the endothelium undergoes a multifaceted change from an antithrombotic to a procoagulant phenotype in response to injury.

Also relevant to the pathogenesis of HIT is the remarkable heterogeneity of ECs, within and among different vascular beds, owing to genetic differences and acquired changes in phenotype (for review see Cines, 1998). For example, only a small fraction of ECs constitutively express t-PA or urokinase-type plasminogen activator in vivo (Levin et al., 1994), whereas a different subset express tissue factor when exposed to endotoxin (Drake et al., 1993). ECs from different organs express tissue-specific promoters that regulate the expression of von Willebrand factor (vWF) in vivo (Aird et al., 1997). ECs also show regional variation in the synthesis of prostacyclin, expression of leukocyte adhesion molecules and Fcγ receptors, among many other phenotypic differences.

There is also recent evidence to indicate that protein C activation on macrovascular ECs is mediated predominantly through the protein C receptor, whereas thrombomodulin (TM) may be the dominant system in the microvasculature (Laszik et al., 1997; Fukudome et al., 1998). TM changes thrombin from a procoagulant to an anticoagulant enzyme (i.e., TM-bound thrombin activates the natural anticoagulant zymogen, protein C) (Esmon, 1989). The anticoagulant function of TM in the microvasculature may contribute to the pathogenesis of warfarin-associated venous limb gangrene that can complicate HIT. This syndrome has been attributed to the coincidence of persistent thrombin generation and acquired protein C deficiency that may occur during the first few days of anticoagulation with warfarin (Warkentin et al., 1997; see Chaps. 3 and 12).

The behavior of ECs can also be modified during the evolution of vascular disease. For example, atherosclerotic vessels produce less nitric oxide in response to a variety of stimuli than do healthy vessels (Gryglewski, 1995). Atherosclerotic vessels may also undergo alterations in their expression of glycosaminoglycans (GAGs) (Williams and Tabas, 1995) and an increase in expression of various cell adhesion molecules (for review see Fuster et al., 1998). The binding of advanced glycation end products to specific EC receptors during normal aging and diabetes mellitus, increases vascular permeability, exposing the subendothelial matrix to lipoproteins and other injurious substances (Schmidt et al., 1994). It is also likely that genetic variation in EC behavior contributes to the host response to antibody- or platelet-mediated EC injury, although the methods to identify or monitor such risk factors remain to be developed. Thus, any inquiry into the reason why only a subset of patients who develop antiheparin–PF4 antibodies develop thrombosis, or why thrombi occur at restricted vascular sites, must take into consideration the specific attributes of a particular endothelial vascular bed.

III. IMMUNE ENDOTHELIAL CELL INJURY

Endothelial cell-reactive antibodies have been found in patients suffering from disorders characterized by vasculitis or thrombosis (for review see Meroni et al., 1996). The best-studied example is allograft rejection, a setting in which there is extensive evidence for antiendothelial cell antibodies (AECA), in part directed at carbohydrate antigens that regulate procoagulant activity in vitro (Saadi and Platt, 1995; Siegel et al., 1997). AECA have also been identified in patients with hyperacute and acute graft rejection, systemic lupus erythematosus (Cines et al., 1984), antiphospholipid antibody syndrome (McCrae et al., 1991), and hemolytic–uremic syndrome (Leung et al., 1988). What is curious is the extraordinary diversity of the clinical syndromes associated with AECA. Also of interest, the target cells used in most assays (i.e., endothelial cells derived from human umbilical vein [HUVEC]), are not known to be affected by immune vascular injury in the clinical setting. This suggests that the expression of the target antigen(s) is highly restricted in vivo, perhaps being expressed only at sites of injury or inflammation. Alternatively, these AECA could represent a surrogate marker for other pathogenic antibodies, or the capacity of the affected vasculature is a critical determinant of whether thrombosis develops.

Several effects of AECA that could contribute to thrombosis include cell lysis or apoptosis (Bordron et al., 1998; Nakamura et al., 1998), induction of cytokine secretion and promotion of leukocyte adhesion (Del Papa et al., 1997), enhancement of vascular permeability (Saadi and Platt, 1995), acceleration of procoagulant reactions (Saadi et al., 1995; Tannenbaum et al., 1986), and reduction in the expression of heparan sulfate (Platt et al., 1991). The reason why some antibodies promote thrombosis (e.g., HIT antibodies), whereas others induce primarily a necrotizing vasculitis, remains unresolved, but may relate directly to the biological functions of heparin and PF4 (Fig. 1).

IV. HEPARAN SULFATE–CONTAINING PROTEOGLYCANS, HEPARIN, AND THE ENDOTHELIUM

The expression and anticoagulant function of heparan sulfate-type proteoglycans (HSPGs) by ECs may be central to the pathogenesis of vascular thrombosis in patients with HIT. The biochemistry and function of these GAGs and proteoglycans to which they bind has been the subject of extensive study (for review see Ruoslahti, 1988; Rosenberg et al., 1997); the involvement of heparan sulfate in the development of HIT is considered elsewhere (see Chap. 8). HSPGs expressed by ECs bind antithrombin in vitro and in vivo, and accelerate the inactivation of thrombin and factor Xa approximately 20-fold (Marcum et al., 1984), an effect that is biologically equivalent to 0.1–0.5 U/mL of heparin (Marcum and Rosenberg, 1987). Yet less than 1% of the HSPGs isolated from cultured ECs express anticoagulant activity (Marcum and Rosenberg, 1984). Active species are characterized by an approximately twofold enrichment in glucuronyl 3-*O*-sulfated glucosamine residues, compared with inactive species (Marcum and Rosenberg, 1987), but the mechanisms that control the synthesis and postsynthetic modifications of HSPG remain poorly characterized.

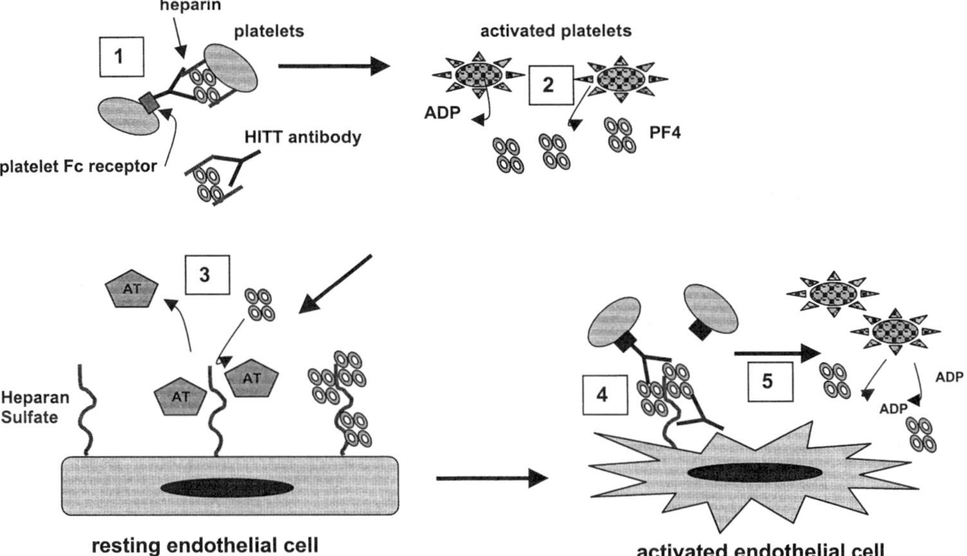

Figure 1 Model of HIT antibody interactions with endothelial cells: (1) HIT antibodies bind to circulating antigen that becomes localized to platelets. (2) Platelet activation occurs after Fc receptor binding, leading to platelet granule release. ADP is released from platelet dense granules and PF4 is released from platelet α-granules. (3) Released PF4 binds to platelets and endothelial cell heparan sulfate (HS), displacing antithrombin (AT) from endothelial cells. (4) Antigen complexes on endothelial cells bind HIT antibodies. (5) HIT antibody binding to endothelial cells leads to endothelial cell activation, resulting in further platelet activation.

Microheterogeneity in the composition of HSPG in arteries, veins, and capillaries has been noted (Lowe-Krentz and Joyce, 1991), but the significance of these differences is unknown. Expression of HSPG by ECs undergoes developmental changes (David et al., 1992), and its composition varies after the cells are exposed to thrombin (Benezra et al., 1993), homocysteine (Nishinage et al., 1993), heparin (Nader et al., 1989), wounding and migration (Kinesella and Wight, 1986), and after induction by activated platelets (Yahalom et al., 1984), among other stimuli. ECs also bind heparin (for review see Patton et al., 1995), which alters EC proliferation, matrix composition and many other vascular functions. It has also been reported that antithrombin is displaced from ECs by heparin, and its binding is inhibited by PF4 (Stern et al., 1985). Whether HIT antibodies promote the capacity of PF4 to neutralize antithrombin activity has not been reported.

V. PLATELET FACTOR 4 AND THE ENDOTHELIUM

The biochemistry of PF4 and its involvement in HIT is reviewed elsewhere (see Chap. 7). The metabolism of the protein is regulated by its interactions with the endothelium. PF4 is stored in the α-granules of platelets as a tetramer bound to chondroitin sulfate (Barber et al., 1972). The tetramer may dissociate from the glycosaminoglycan as the platelets are activated, but more likely, dissociation occurs subsequent to binding to EC HSPG, which contains a higher charge density. [^{125}I]PF4 is cleared from the circulation with an α-elimination phase approximating 2 min, which primarily represents binding to the endothelium, and a β-elimination phase approximating 40 min, corresponding to uptake and degradation, predominantly by hepatocytes (Rucinski et al., 1986, 1990).

The ECs bind about 50 pmol PF4/10^5 cells (Rybak et al., 1989). Several classes of binding sites have been identified, including a high-capacity, low-affinity site on HSPG, as well as higher-affinity–binding sites involving specific chemokine receptors and certain coagulant proteins (see later discussion). Binding of PF4 to the endothelium is attenuated by pretreatment with heparinase (Marcum et al., 1984), and plasma concentrations are increased 10- to 20-fold after heparin is infused intravenously (Dawes et al., 1982). Binding of PF4 to EC GAGs is electrostatic (Wu and Cohen, 1984), and is independent of the pentasaccharide involved in the binding of antithrombin (Loscalzo et al., 1985). The affinity of PF4 binding to ECs is lower than to purified heparin (K_d = 2 nM vs. 2–3 μM, respectively) (Rybak et al., 1989), consistent with the biochemical heterogeneity of vascular matrix. PF4 has a 10- to 100-fold greater affinity for EC HSPG than does antithrombin (Jordan et al., 1982) and markedly attenuates its antiprotease cofactor activity on intact vessels (Busch et al., 1980; Stern et al., 1985).

PF4 also binds to the chemokine receptor, Duffy (Hadley et al., 1994), which has been identified on ECs in postcapillary venules and in the splanchnic bed, even in individuals who do not express the antigen on their erythrocytes (Peiper et al., 1995). The distribution of Duffy on ECs in other vascular beds is less well studied. The binding site on PF4 for Duffy has not been deduced, and the capacity of Duffy-bound PF4 to bind heparin or HIT antibodies has not been reported. PF4 does not appear to bind to any of the other members of the chemokine receptor family (for review see Baggiolini et al., 1997), including CXCR4, the only other related receptor yet identified on ECs (Volin et al., 1998). However, PF4 exposed to leukocyte lysates is cleaved between Thr-16 and Ser-17 to yield a peptide with 30-fold greater biological activity than its parent molecule (Gupta et al., 1995). Such proteolysis may enable modified PF4 to bind to CXCR1 or R2 (formerly called IL-8R-α and -β, respectively) (for review see Baggiolini et al., 1997), but no evidence has been presented that ECs express either receptor, nor has binding of modified PF4 to CXCR4 been shown.

The CXC chemokines that contain a Glu-Leu-Arg (ELR) NH_2-terminal sequence induce angiogenesis, whereas those that do not, such as PF4 and γIP-10, inhibit angiogenesis (Baggiolini and Moser, 1997). The molecular basis by which PF4 inhibits angiogenesis is unclear. Considering that ECs lack CXCR1 and CXCR2, the effect of PF4 may be indirect. PF4 interrupts the binding of heparin-binding proteins, such as vascular endothelial cell growth factor (VEGF) and basic fibroblast growth factor (βFGF) to their receptors (Gengrinovitch et al., 1995; Peng et al., 1997). However, PF4 also inhibits angiogenesis stimulated by a truncated version of VEGF that lacks the heparin-binding domain (Gengrinovitch et al., 1995). Whether PF4 influences the behavior of ECs from disordered vessels in other ways, or whether the PF4-mediated signal transduction through chemokine receptors is modulated by HIT antibodies, deserves additional study.

PF4 binds preferentially to ECs at sites of angiogenesis (Hansell et al., 1995). For example, in a hamster cheek pouch model, [^{125}I]PF4 is taken up preferentially by ECs within the neovasculature where its binding is inhibited by the related CXC chemokine, γIP-10 (Luster et al., 1995). PF4 inhibits cell proliferation in vitro (Gupta and Singh, 1994; Maione et al., 1991; Sharpe et al., 1990) and tumor-induced neovascularization (Maione et al., 1991; Sharpe et al., 1990) in vivo. Both the heparin-binding domain (Gupta and Singh, 1994; Maione et al., 1990) and other portions of the molecule (Gupta et al., 1995; Gupta and Singh, 1994; Lecomte-Raclet et al., 1998; Maione et al., 1991) have been implicated. These concepts have yet to be tested in vivo. Furthermore, little else is known about the regional distribution and regulation of CXC receptors in normal or abnormal vessels. PF4 is endocytosed and is degraded in lysosomes (Rybak et al., 1989), but can permeate the subendothelium of damaged vessels, where it may retain its capacity to regulate chemotaxis and angiogenesis (Goldberg et al., 1980).

PF4 also binds to thrombomodulin (TM), a 60.3-kDa protein constitutively expressed on the surface of ECs. Binding of thrombin to TM alters its substrate specificity, such that proteolytic cleavage of protein C is accelerated 20,000-fold (Esmon, 1989). TM is posttranslationally modified by association with a chondroitin sulfate A-like GAG, which invests it with the capacity to bind cationic peptides at physiological pH. The binding of eosinophilic cationic protein, major basic protein, and histidine-rich glycoprotein to these GAG residues inhibits the function of TM (Slungaard and Key, 1994), whereas the binding of PF4 (but not β-thromboglobulin or thrombospondin) increases protein C cofactor activity 25-fold (Dudek et al., 1997). However, the physiological significance of this effect has not been established, although HIT antibodies have been implicated in the pathogenesis of warfarin-associated venous limb gangrene (see foregoing). With additional study, it is likely that other binding sites for this cationic peptide will be uncovered.

VI. EVIDENCE FOR ENDOTHELIAL CELL ANTIBODIES IN HIT

There are limited experimental data to indicate that EC-reactive antibodies or immune complexes contribute to the development of thrombosis in patients with HIT. Over 10 years ago, one group reported that sera from essentially all patients with HIT deposit increased amounts of IgG, IgM, or IgA on HUVEC (Cines et al., 1987). Binding was reduced when the cells were pretreated with enzymes that degrade heparin or heparan sulfate, whereas addition of chondroitinase was without effect. HIT sera induced ECs to express the procoagulant tissue factor, and the expression of procoagulant activity was enhanced further in the presence of platelets. These observations were confirmed and extended by Visentin and colleagues (1994), who demonstrated that the binding of HIT antibodies of HUVEC was dependent on PF4, but not on exogenous heparin, in contrast to the requirement for both to be added for antibody binding to platelets (Fig. 2). This is consistent with the concept that PF4, released from activated platelets, can form a competent antigenic complex on the pericellular matrix of the endothelium.

The role of EC-reactive antibodies was also explored in an animal model that simulates certain aspects of HIT (Blank et al., 1997). Mice injected with IgG fractions obtained from HIT patients developed anti-idiotypic antibodies that recognized complexes between human PF4 and heparin. Furthermore, the anti-idiotypic antibodies competed with the immunizing antibodies for binding to the antigenic complex. These effects were noted when antibodies obtained from mice immunized with control IgG were studied (Fig. 3a). Additionally, mice immunized with HIT–IgG developed thrombocytopenia when exposed to heparin. Affinity-purified antiheparin–PF4 antibodies bound to murine endothelioma cells in the presence of PF4, but not β_2GP I (Fig. 3b). Of interest, immunized mice did not develop overt thrombi on exposure to heparin, possibly because of insufficient circulating PF4, intrinsic differences in the balance between the procoagulant and fibrinolytic systems compared with humans, or differences in signal transduction through murine and human platelet Fcγ receptors. However, it is also possible that the difference lies in a reduced capacity of otherwise healthy mouse ECs to respond to the procoagulant stimulus induced by these antibodies, compared with the responsiveness of patients with HIT who, in the main, comprise a more elderly population with underlying vascular disorders.

More recently, antibody-mediated platelet activation has been implicated in the activation of ECs (Hebert et al., 1998). Sera from patients with HIT induced various changes in the behavior of HUVEC in the presence of platelets, including increased expression of E-selectin, VCAM, ICAM-1, and tissue factor, release of IL-1β, IL-6, TNF-α, and PAI-1, and adhesion of platelets to the activated ECs. EC activation was inhibited by SR121566A, a platelet glycoprotein IIb/IIIa antagonist, and, to some extent, by apyrase and ATPγS, implicating expression

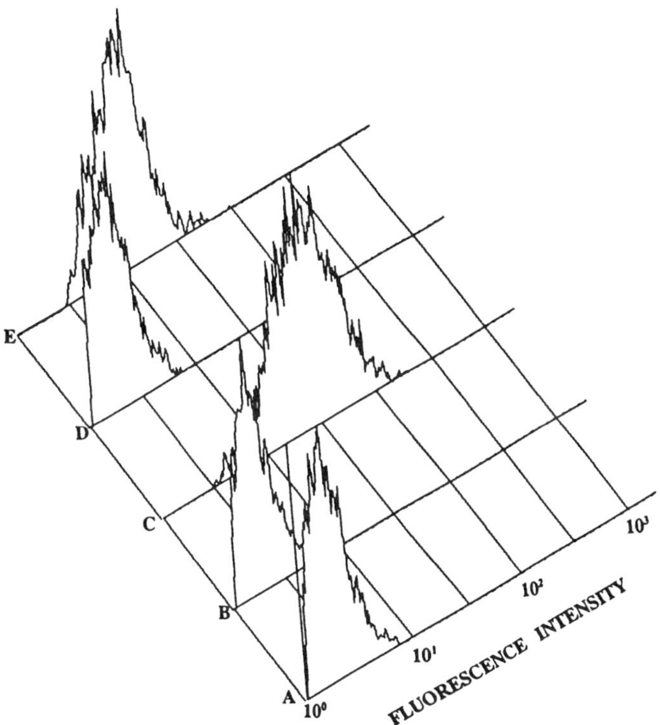

Figure 2 Binding of IgG (A–D) and IgM (E) from the plasma of a patient with HIT to cultured human umbilical vein endothelial cells (HUVEC): (A) Plasma alone; (B) plasma plus 0.05 U/mL heparin; (C) plasma plus 10 μg/mL PF4; (D) plasma plus 0.05 U/mL heparin plus 10 μg/mL PF4; (E) binding of IgM from plasma containing 10 μg/mL PF4. Both IgG (C) and IgM (E) bound to HUVEC in the presence of PF4 alone. The binding of each was completely inhibited by heparin. (From Visentin et al., 1994.)

of endogenous platelet fibrin(ogen) and release of ADP in the process. HIT sera exerted little effect on the behavior of HUVEC in the absence of platelets, even in the presence of exogenous PF4. These studies support the notion that platelet activation promotes their adhesion to the endothelium and the induction of procoagulant activity. Furthermore, these studies point toward a potentially important locus of control amenable to pharmacological intervention. However, the data do not explain why platelet activation caused by HIT antibodies predisposes to thrombosis, whereas stimulation by other potent antiplatelet antibodies does not. It is also unclear whether the intensity of platelet activation can distinguish HIT patients who develop thrombosis from those who do not.

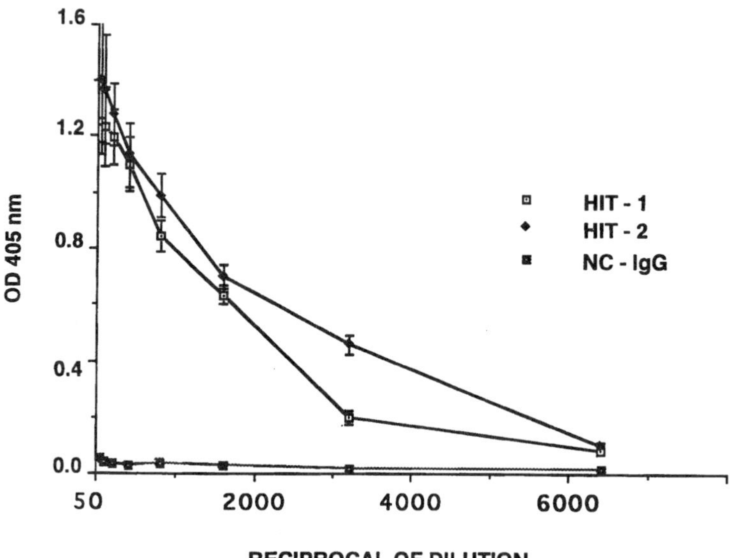

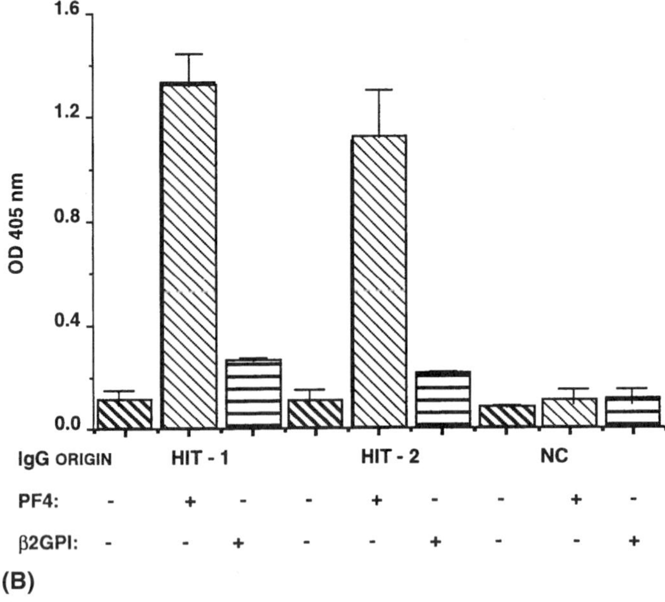

Figure 3 Antiendothelial antibodies in sera of mice immunized with HIT-IgG: (A) Sera from mice immunized with IgG fractions of two patients with heparin-induced thrombocytopenia, HIT-1 (□) and HIT-2 (○) or IgG from an individual not exposed to heparin, NC (■), were tested for binding to murine endothelial cells by ELISA. (B). Antiendothelial cell binding of affinity-purified anti-PF4/heparin IgG from sera of immunized mice. Affinity purified IgG (10 μg/mL) was tested for endothelial cell binding in the absence or presence of 10 μg PF4 or β_2-glycoprotein-1 (β_2-GP I). (From Blank et al., 1997.)

VII. PERSPECTIVE AND FUTURE DIRECTIONS

Heparin-induced thrombocytopenia continues to pose several enigmas including the fundamental issue of how heparin induces the formation of self-reactive antibodies to a native protein in such a high proportion of immunologically competent individuals (Visentin et al., 1996; Bauer et al., 1997). It also remains unclear why only a subset of patients with antiheparin–PF4 antibodies develop thrombocytopenia, and fewer still develop thrombosis. It is possible that characteristics of HIT antibodies, such as their subtype, specificity, and affinity for portions of the PF4 molecule, may provide some of the answers. However, it is also likely that part of the propensity for thrombosis, and the localization of clotting observed in HIT, relate to antigen expression and response to injury at the level of the vessel wall itself.

REFERENCES

Aird WC, Edelberg JM, Weiler-Guettler H, Simmons WW, Smith TW, Rosenberg RD. Vascular bed-specific expression of an endothelial cell gene is programmed by the tissue microenvironment. J Cell Biol 138:1117–1124, 1997.

Amiral J, Wolf M, Fischer A-M, Boyer-Neumann C, Vissac A-M, Meyer D. Pathogenicity of IgA and/or IgM antibodies to heparin–PF4 complexes in patients with heparin-induced thrombocytopenia. Br J Haematol 92:954–959, 1996.

Arepally G, McKenzie SE, Jiang X-M, Poncz M, Cines DB. FcγRIIA H/R[131] polymorphism, subclass-specific IgG anti-heparin/platelet factor 4 antibodies and clinical course in patients with heparin-induced thrombocytopenia and thrombosis. Blood 89:370–375, 1997.

Bachelot-Loza C, Saffroy R, Lasne D, Chatellier G, Aiach M, Rendu F. Importance of the FcγRIIa–Arg/His-131 polymorphism in heparin-induced thrombocytopenia diagnosis. Thromb Haemost 79:523–528, 1998.

Baggiolini M, Moser B. Blocking chemokine receptors. J Exp Med 186:1189–1191, 1997.

Baggiolini M, Dewald B, Moser B. Human chemokines: an update. Annu Rev Immunol 15:675–705, 1997.

Barber AJ, Käser-Glanzmann R, Jakábová M, Lüscher EF. Characterization of a chondroitin 4-sulfate proteoglycan carrier for heparin neutralizing activity (platelet factor 4) released from human blood platelets. Biochim Biophys Acta 286:312–329, 1972.

Bassenge E. Endothelial function in different organs. Prog Cardiovasc Dis 39:209–228, 1996.

Bauer TL, Arepally G, Konkle BA, Mestichelli B, Shapiro SS, Cines DB, Poncz M, McNulty S, Amiral J, Hauck WW, Edie RN, Mannion JD. Prevalence of heparin-associated antibodies without thrombosis in patients undergoing cardiopulmonary bypass. Circulation 95:1242–1246, 1997.

Benezra M, Vlodavsky I, Ishai-Michaeli R, Neufeld G, Bar-Shavit R. Thrombin-induced release of active basic fibroblast growth factor–heparan sulfate complexes from subendothelial extracellular matrix. Blood 81:3324–3331, 1993.

Blank M, Cines DB, Arepally G, Eldor A, Afek A, Shoenfeld Y. Pathogenicity of human anti-platelet factor 4 (PF4)/heparin in vivo: generation of mouse anti-PF4/heparin and induction of thrombocytopenia by heparin. Clin Exp Immunol 108:333–339, 1997.

Bombeli T, Mueller M, Haeberli A. Anticoagulant properties of the vascular endothelium. Thromb Haemost 77:408–423, 1997.

Bordron A, Dueymes M, Levy Y, Jamin C, Leroy J-P, Piette J-C, Shoenfeld Y, Youinou PY. The binding of some human antiendothelial cell antibodies induces endothelial cell apoptosis. J Clin Invest 101:2029–2035, 1998.

Boshkov LK, Warkentin TE, Hayward CP, Andrew M, Kelton JG. Heparin-induced thrombocytopenia and thrombosis: clinical and laboratory studies. Br J Haematol 84:322–328, 1993.

Busch C, Dawes J, Pepper DS, Wasteson A. Binding of platelet factor 4 to cultured human umbilical vein endothelial cells. Thromb Res 19:129–137, 1980.

Cadroy Y, Diquélou A, Dupouy D, Bossavy JP, Sakariassen KS, Sié P, Boneu B. The thrombomodulin/protein C/protein S anticoagulant pathway modulates the thrombogenic properties of the normal resting and stimulated endothelium. Arterioscler Thromb Vasc Biol 17:520–527, 1997.

Carlsson LE, Santoso S, Baurichter G, Kroll H, Papenberg S, Eichler P, Westerdaal NAC, Kiefel V, van der Winkel JGL, Graincher A. Heparin-induced thrombocytopenia: new insights into the impact of the FcγRIIa–R-H131 polymorphism. Blood 92: 1526–1531, 1998.

Cines DB, Lyss AP, Reeber M, Bina M, DeHoratius RJ. Presence of complement-fixing anti-endothelial cell antibodies in systemic lupus erythematosus. J Clin Invest 73: 611–625, 1984.

Cines DB, Tomaski A, Tannenbaum S. Immune endothelial-cell injury in heparin-associated thrombocytopenia. N Engl J Med 316:581–589, 1987.

Cines DB, Pollak ES, Buck CA, Loscalzo J, Zimmerman GA, McEver RP, Pober JS, Wick TM, Konkle BA, Schwartz BS, Barnathan ES, McCrae KR, Hug BA, Schmidt A-M, Stern DM. Endothelial cells in physiology and in the pathophysiology of vascular disorders. Blood 91:3527–3561, 1998.

David G, Bai XM, van der Schueren B, Cassiman JJ, van den Berghe H. Developmental changes in heparan sulfate expression: in situ detection with MAbs. J Cell Biol 119:961–975, 1992.

Dawes J, Pumphrey CW, McLaren KM, Prowse CV, Pepper DS. The in vivo release of human platelet factor 4 by heparin. Thromb Res 27:65–76, 1982.

Del Papa N, Guidali L, Sala A, Buccellati C, Khamashta MA, Ichikawa K, Koike T, Balestrieri G, Tincani A, Hughes GRV, Meroni PL. Endothelial cells as target for antiphospholipid antibodies. Human polyclonal and monoclonal anti-β_2-glycoprotein I antibodies react in vitro with endothelial cells through adherent β_2-glycoprotein I and induce endothelial activation. Arthritis Rheum 40:551–561, 1997.

Denomme GA, Warkentin TE, Horsewood P, Sheppard J-AI, Warner MN, Kelton JG. Activation of platelets by sera containing IgG1 heparin-dependent antibodies: an explanation for the predominance of the FCγRIIa ''low responder'' (his_{131}) gene in patients with heparin-induced thrombocytopenia. J Lab Clin Med 130:278–284, 1997.

Drake TA, Cheng J, Chang A, Taylor FB Jr. Expression of tissue factor, thrombomodulin, and E-selectin in baboons with lethal *Escherichia coli* sepsis. Am J Pathol 142: 1458–1470, 1993.

Dudek AZ, Pennell CA, Decker TD, Young TA, Key NS, Slungaard A. Platelet factor 4 binds to glycanated forms of thrombomodulin and to protein C. A potential mechanism for enhancing generation of activated protein C. J Biol Chem 272:31785–31792, 1997.

Esmon CT. The roles of protein C and thrombomodulin in the regulation of blood coagulation. J Biol Chem 264:4743–4746, 1989.

Fries JWU, Williams AJ, Atkins RC, Newman W, Lipscomb MF, Collins T. Expression of VCAM-1 and E-selectin in an in vivo model of endothelial activation. Am J Pathol 143:725–37, 1993.

Fukudome K, Ye X, Tsuneyoshi N, Tokunaga O, Sugawara K, Mizokami H, Kimoto M. Activation mechanism of anticoagulant protein C in large blood vessels involving the endothelial cell protein C receptor. J Exp Med 187:1029–1035, 1998.

Fuster V, Poon M, Willerson JT. Learning from the transgenic mouse. Endothelium, adhesive molecules, and neointimal formation. Circulation 97:16–18, 1998.

Gengrinovitch S, Greenberg SM, Cohen T, Gitay-Goren H, Rockwell P, Maione TE, Levi B-Z, Neufeld G. Platelet factor-4 inhibits the mitogenic activity of $VEGF_{121}$ and $VEGF_{165}$ using several concurrent mechanisms. J Biol Chem 270:15059–15065, 1995.

Goldberg ID, Stemerman MB, Handin RI. Vascular permeation of platelet factor 4 after endothelial injury. Science 209:611–612, 1980.

Gryglewski RJ. Endothelial nitric oxide, prostacyclin (PGI_2) and tissue plasminogen activator (t-PA): alliance or neutrality? Pol J Pharmacol 47:467–472, 1995.

Gupta SK, Singh JP. Inhibition of endothelial cell proliferation by platelet factor-4 involves a unique action on S phase progression. J Cell Biol 127:1121–1127, 1994.

Gupta SK, Hassel T, Singh JP. A potent inhibitor of endothelial cell proliferation is generated by proteolytic cleavage of the chemokine platelet factor 4. Proc Natl Acad Sci USA 92:7799–7803, 1995.

Hadley TJ, Lu Z-H, Wasniowska K, Martin AW, Peiper SC, Hesselgesser J, Horuk R. Postcapillary venule endothelial cells in kidney express a multispecific chemokine receptor that is structurally and functionally identical to the erythroid isoform, which is the Duffy blood group antigen. J Clin Invest 94:985–991, 1994.

Hansell P, Maione TE, Borgström P. Selective binding of platelet factor 4 to regions of active angiogenesis in vivo. Am J Physiol 269:H829–H836, 1995.

Hebert JM, Savi P, Jeske WP, Walenga JM. Effect of SR121566A, a potent GP IIb–IIIa antagonist, on the HIT serum/heparin-induced platelet-mediated activation of human endothelial cells. Thromb Haemost 80:326–331, 1998.

Jordan RE, Favreau LV, Braswell EH, Rosenberg RD. Heparin with two binding sites for antithrombin or platelet factor 4: J Biol Chem 257:400–406, 1982.

Kinsella MG, Wight TN. Modulation of sulfated proteoglycan synthesis by bovine aortic endothelial cells during migration. J Cell Biol 102:679–687, 1986.

Laszik Z, Mitro A, Taylor FB Jr, Ferrell G, Esmon CT. Human protein C receptor is present primarily on endothelium of large blood vessels: implications for the control of the protein C pathway. Circulation 96:3633–3640, 1997.

Lecomte-Raclet L, Alemany M, Sequeira-Le Grand A, Amiral J, Quentin G, Vissac AM, Caen JP, Han ZC. New insights into the negative regulation of hematopoiesis by chemokine platelet factor 4 and related peptides. Blood 91:2772–2780, 1998.

Leung DYM, Moake JL, Havens PL, Kim M, Pober JS. Lytic anti-endothelial cell antibodies in haemolytic-uraemic syndrome. Lancet 2:183–186, 1988.

Levin EG, Del Zoppo GJ. Localization of tissue plasminogen activator in endothelium of a limited number of vessels. Am J Pathol 144:855–861, 1994.

Loscalzo J, Melnick B, Handin RI. The interaction of platelet factor four and glycosaminoglycans. Arch Biochem Biophys 240:446–455, 1985.

Lowe-Krentz LJ, Joyce JG. Venous and aortic porcine endothelial cells cultured under standard conditions synthesize heparan sulfate chains which differ in charge. Anal Biochem 193:155–163, 1991.

Lüscher TF, Barton M. Biology of the endothelium. Clin Cardiol 20(suppl 2):II-3–II-10, 1997.

Luster AD, Greenberg SM, Leder P. The IP-10 chemokine binds to a specific cell surface heparan sulfate site shared with platelet factor 4 and inhibits endothelial cell proliferation. J Exp Med 182:219–231, 1995.

Maione TE, Gray GS, Petro J, Hunt AJ, Donner AL, Bauer SI, Carson HF, Sharpe RJ. Inhibition of angiogenesis by recombinant human platelet factor-4 and related peptides. Science 247:77–79, 1990.

Maione TE, Gray GS, Hunt AJ, Sharpe RJ. Inhibition of tumor growth in mice by an analogue of platelet factor 4 that lacks affinity for heparin and retains potent angiostatic activity. Cancer Res 51:2077–2083, 1991.

Marcum JA, Rosenberg RD. Anticoagulantly active heparin-like molecules from vascular tissue Biochemistry 23:1730–1737, 1984.

Marcum JA, Rosenberg RD. Anticoagulantly active heparan sulfate proteoglycan and the vascular endothelium. Semin Thromb Hemost 13:464–474, 1987.

Marcum JA, McKenney JB, Rosenberg RD. The acceleration of thrombin–antithrombin complex formation in rat hindquarters via heparinlike molecules bound to the endothelium. J Clin Invest 74:341–350, 1984.

McCrae KR, DeMichele A, Samuels P, Roth D, Kuo A, Meng Q-H, Rauch J, Cines DB. Detection of endothelial cell-reactive immunoglobulin in patients with antiphospholipid antibodies. Br J Haematol 79:595–605, 1991.

Meroni PL, Del Papa N, Borghi MO. Antiphospholipid and antiendothelial antibodies. Int Arch Allergy Immunol 111:320–325, 1996.

Nader HB, Buonassisi V, Colburn P, Dietrich CP. Heparin stimulates the synthesis and modifies the sulfation pattern of heparan sulfate proteoglycan from endothelial cells. J Cell Physiol 140:305–310, 1989.

Nakamura N, Ban T, Yamaji K, Yoneda Y, Wada Y. Localization of the apoptosis-inducing activity of lupus anticoagulant in an annexin V-binding subset. J Clin Invest 101:1951–1959, 1998.

Nishinaga M, Ozawa T, Shimada K. Homocysteine, a thrombogenic agent, suppresses anticoagulant heparan sulfate expression in cultured porcine aortic endothelial cells. J Clin Invest 92:1381–1386, 1993.

Patton WA II, Granzow CA, Getts LA, Thomas SC, Zotter LM, Gunzel KA, Lowe-Krentz LJ. Identification of a heparin-binding protein using monoclonal antibodies that block heparin binding to porcine aortic endothelial cells. Biochem J 311:461–469, 1995.

Peiper SC, Wang Z-X, Neote K, Martin AW, Showell HJ, Conklyn MJ, Ogborne K, Hadley TJ, Lu Z-H, Hesselgesser J, Horuk R. The Duffy antigen/receptor for chemokines (DARC) is expressed in endothelial cells of Duffy negative individuals who lack the erythrocyte receptor. J Exp Med 181:1311–1317, 1995.

Peng H, Wen TC, Igase K, Tanaka J, Matsuda S, Aburaya J, Sakanaka M. Suppression by platelet factor 4 of the myogenic activity of basic fibroblast growth factor. Arch Histol Cytol 60:163–174, 1997.

Platt JL, Lindman BJ, Geller RL, Noreen HJ, Swanson JL, Dalmasso AP, Bach FH. The role of natural antibodies in the activation of xenogenic endothelial cells. Transplantation 52:1037–1043, 1991.

Rosenberg RD, Shworak NW, Liu J, Schwartz JJ, Zhang L. Heparan sulfate proteoglycans of the cardiovascular system. Specific structures emerge but how is synthesis regulated? J Clin Invest 100(suppl):S67–S75, 1997.

Rucinski B, Knight LC, Niewiarowski S. Clearance of human platelet factor 4 by liver and kidney: its alteration by heparin. Am J Physiol 251:H800–H807, 1986.

Rucinski B, Niewiarowski S, Strzyzewski M, Holt JC, Mayo KH. Human platelet factor 4 and its C-terminal peptides: heparin binding and clearance from the circulation. Thromb Haemost 63:493–498, 1990.

Ruoslahti E. Structure and biology of proteoglycans. Annu Rev Cell Biol 4:229–255, 1988.

Rybak ME, Gimbrone MA Jr, Davies PF, Handin RI. Interaction of platelet factor four with cultured vascular endothelial cells. Blood 73:1534–1539, 1989.

Saadi S, Platt JL. Transient perturbation of endothelial integrity induced by natural antibodies and complement. J Exp Med 181:21–31, 1995.

Saadi S, Holzknecht RA, Patte CP, Stern DM, Platt JL. Complement-mediated regulation of tissue factor activity in endothelium. J Exp Med 182:1807–1814, 1995.

Schmidt AM, Mora R, Cao R, Yan SD, Brett J, Ramakrishnan R, Tsang TC, Simionescu M, Stern D. The endothelial cell binding site for advanced glycation end products consists of a complex: an integral membrane protein and a lactoferrin-like polypeptide. J Biol Chem 269:9882–9888, 1994.

Sharpe RJ, Byers HR, Scott CF, Bauer SI, Maione TE. Growth inhibition of murine melanoma and human colon carcinoma by recombinant human platelet factor 4. J Natl Cancer Inst 82:848–853, 1990.

Siegel JB, Grey ST, Lesnikoski B-A, Kopp CW, Soares M, am Esch JS II, Bach FH, Robson SC. Xenogeneic endothelial cells activate human prothrombin. Transplant 64:888–896, 1997.

Slungaard A, Key NS. Platelet factor 4 stimulates thrombomodulin protein C-activating cofactor activity. A structure-function analysis. J Biol Chem 269:25549–25556, 1994.

Stern D, Nawroth P, Marcum J, Handley D, Kisiel W, Rosenberg R, Stern K. Interaction of antithrombin III with bovine aortic segments. Role of heparin in binding and enhanced anticoagulant activity. J Clin Invest 75:272–279, 1985.

Tannenbaum SH, Finko R, Cines DB. Antibody and immune complexes induce tissue factor production by human endothelial cells. J Immunol 137:1532–1537, 1986.

Visentin GP, Ford SE, Scott JP, Aster RH. Antibodies from patients with heparin-induced thrombocytopenia/thrombosis are specific for platelet factor 4 complexed with heparin or bound to endothelial cells. J Clin Invest 93:81–88, 1994.

Visentin GP, Malik M, Cyganiak KA, Aster RH. Patients treated with unfractionated heparin during open heart surgery are at high risk to form antibodies reactive with heparin:platelet factor 4 complexes. J Lab Clin Med 128:376–383, 1996.

Volin MV, Joseph L, Shockley MS, Davies PF. Chemokine receptor CXCR4 expression in endothelium. Biochem Biophys Res Commun 242:46–53, 1998.

Warkentin TE, Elavathil LJ, Hayward CPM, Johnston MA, Russett JI, Kelton JG. The pathogenesis of venous limb gangrene associated with heparin-induced thrombocytopenia. Ann Intern Med 127:804–812, 1997.

Williams KJ, Tabas I. The response-to-retention hypothesis of early atherogenesis. Arterioscler Thromb Vasc Biol 15:551–558, 1995.

Wu V-Y, Cohen MP. Platelet factor 4 binding to glomerular microvascular matrix. Biochim Biophys Acta 797:76–82, 1984.

Yahalom J, Eldor A, Fuks Z, Vlodavsky I. Degradation of sulfated proteoglycans in the subendothelial extracellular matrix by human platelet heparitinase. J Clin Invest 74:1842–1849, 1984.

11

Laboratory Testing for Heparin-Induced Thrombocytopenia

Theodore E. Warkentin
McMaster University and Hamilton Health Sciences Corporation, Hamilton, Ontario, Canada

Andreas Greinacher
Ernst-Moritz-Arndt University, Greifswald, Germany

I. INTRODUCTION

Heparin-induced thrombocytopenia (HIT) is caused by heparin-dependent antibodies that usually recognize multimolecular complexes of platelet factor 4–heparin (PF4–H). HIT can be viewed as a *clinicopathologic syndrome* (Warkentin et al., 1998). This implies that a diagnosis of HIT should be based on two criteria: (1) clinically evident abnormalities, most commonly, thrombocytopenia with or without thrombosis (see Chap. 3), and (2) detection of HIT antibodies. In some ways, HIT resembles another clinicopathologic disorder, the antiphospholipid antibody (lupus anticoagulant) syndrome (Table 1).

Two major classes of assays—activation (functional) and antigen—have been developed to detect HIT antibodies (Table 2). A third (miscellaneous) group of assays will be discussed briefly at the end of this chapter.

II. ACTIVATION ASSAYS FOR HIT ANTIBODIES

A. Washed Platelet Assays

The classic washed platelet assay for HIT is the serotonin-release assay, or SRA (Sheridan et al., 1986; Warkentin et al., 1992). This assay was a modification of

Table 1 Two Clinicopathologic Syndromes: HIT and Antiphospholipid Antibody Syndrome

Laboratory features	Heparin-induced thrombocytopenia	Antiphospholipid antibody syndrome
Structure of the major antigen	'Cryptic' autoepitope on PF4 expressed when complexed with heparin (see Chaps. 6–8)	'Cryptic' autoepitope on β_2-GPI expressed when bound to anionic phospholipid (Pengo et al., 1995)
Nonspecific nature of anionic component of antigen (cross-reactivity)	Variable reactivity when heparin substituted by LMWH, danaparoid, pentosan polysulfate, and others	Variable reactivity when cardiolipin[a] substituted by phosphatidylserine[b] or other molecules (e.g., irradiated plastic)
Sequestered location of antigen	PF4 within platelet α-granules	Anionic phospholipids of inner leaflet of bilipid membranes
Functional assay	Heparin-dependent activation of platelets by patient serum or plasma	Prolongation of phospholipid-dependent coagulation assay by patient's plasma
Inhibition of functional assay	Inhibition by high-dose heparin	Inhibition of lupus anticoagulant assays by excess phospholipid
Antigen assay	PF4–H–EIA	Anticardiolipin EIA
Relative sensitivity of assays for antibodies	Antigen > functional	Antigen > functional
Relative specificity of assays for disease state	Functional > antigen	Functional > antigen

Information on relative sensitivity and specificity of functional and antigens assays for HIT and antiphospholipid antibody syndrome are provided elsewhere (Visentin et al., 1994; Ginsberg et al., 1995; Berube et al., 1998; Warkentin et al., 1999).

Abbreviations: EIA, enzyme immunoassay; β_2-GP I, beta$_2$-glycoprotein I; LMWH, low molecular weight heparin; PF4–H, platelet factor 4–heparin.

[a] Cardiolipin is found primarily in the inner leaflet of the mitochondrial membrane.

[b] Phosphatidylserine is located in the inner leaflet of platelet membranes, thus, antiphospholipid antibodies with antiphosphatidylserine activity could be relatively more important in the pathogenesis of thrombocytopenia.

Table 2 Classification of Laboratory Tests for HIT

Activation (functional) assays
- Washed platelet assays
  - Heparin-induced platelet activation (HIPA) test: visual assessment of platelet aggregation (Greinacher et al., 1991)
  - Serotonin-release assay (SRA): quantitation of ^{14}C-radiolabeled serotonin released from dense granules of activated platelets (Sheridan et al., 1986); chemical detection of serotonin also described (Schnell et al., 1998)
  - ATP release detected by luminography (Stewart et al., 1995)
  - Platelet microparticle assay: quantitation of platelet-derived microparticles by flow cytometry (Lee et al., 1996)
- Platelets in citrated platelet-rich plasma (c-PRP)
  - Platelet aggregation test (PAT): assessment of platelet aggregation using conventional aggregometry (Fratantoni et al., 1975; Chong et al., 1993a)
  - Annexin V-binding assay: quantitation by flow cytometry of annexin V binding to anionic phospholipids expressed by activated platelets (Tomer, 1997; Tomer et al., 1999)

Antigen assays
- Target antigen: platelet factor 4–heparin complexes
  - PF4–heparin enzyme immunoassay (PF4–H–EIA)
  - Surface-bound antigen (Amiral et al., 1992)
  - Fluid-phase antigen (Newman et al., 1998)
- Target antigen: platelet factor 4–polyvinylsulfonate complexes
  - PF4–polyvinylsulfonate-EIA (Collins et al., 1997; Visentin et al., 1997)

platelet-washing techniques in use at McMaster University that resuspended washed platelets in buffer containing physiological concentrations of calcium. The purpose was to avoid platelet activation artifacts associated with low calcium concentrations (Mustard et al., 1972; Kinlough-Rathbone et al., 1983; see Chap. 1). The use of washed platelets is also central to certain other functional assays, such as the heparin-induced platelet activation (HIPA) assay (Greinacher et al., 1991). Figure 1 summarizes washed platelet assays for HIT.

Preparation of Platelets for Washed Platelet Assays

1. Collect 8.4 volumes of blood from a normal donor into 1.6 volumes of acid–citrate–dextrose (ACD).

Comment. Aspirin-free normal blood donors whose platelets are known to respond well to HIT sera should be selected, as there is considerable heterogeneity to platelet activation by HIT sera among platelets obtained from different normal individuals (Warkentin et al., 1994). In Hamilton, platelets from two donors are combined. In Greifswald, platelets from four different donors selected randomly

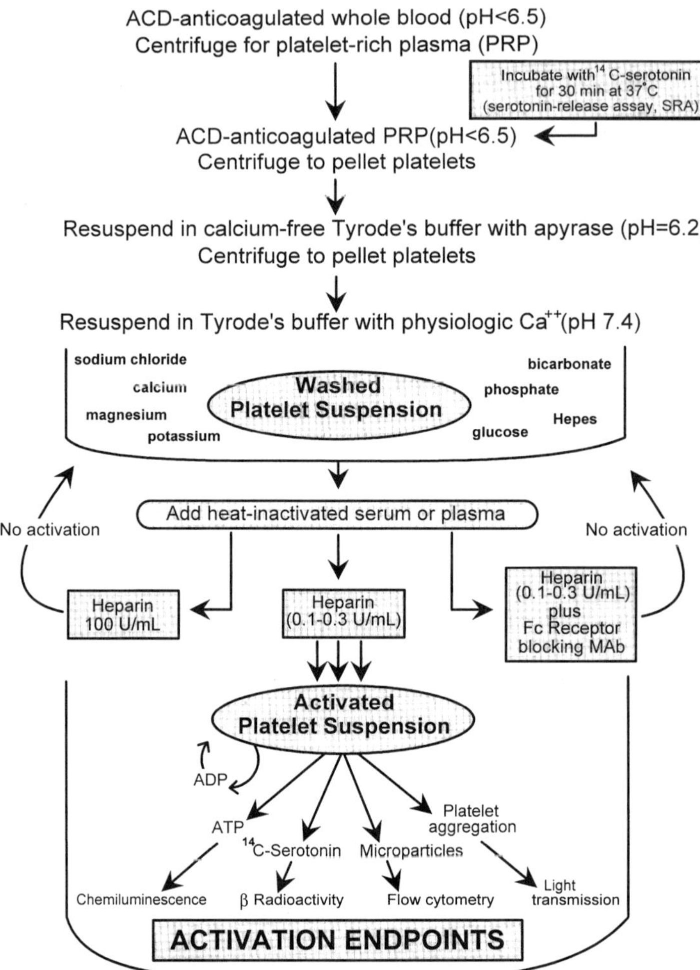

Figure 1 Schematic overview of washed platelet assays: HIT serum causes platelet activation at therapeutic (0.1- to 0.3-U/mL) heparin concentrations, but not in the presence of Fc receptor-blocking monoclonal antibody or high (100-U/mL) heparin concentrations. Platelet activation by HIT serum is potentiated by ADP release from platelet dense granules. Various platelet activation endpoints can be used. False-positive results can be avoided if typical reaction profiles of non-HIT platelet activation triggers are recognized [e.g., (1) residual thrombin (activation at low- but not high-heparin concentrations, including activation in the presence of Fc receptor-blocking monoclonal antibody; (2) immune complexes (activation at low- and high-heparin concentrations, both of which are inhibited by Fc receptor-blocking monoclonal antibody; and (3) thrombotic thrombocytopenic purpura (TTP) serum (variable activation in the presence of heparin that is not inhibited by Fc receptor-blocking monoclonal antibody)]. Abbreviations: ACD, acid–citrate–dextrose; ATP, adenosine triphosphate; PRP, platelet-rich plasma.

are prepared and tested individually. ABO blood group discrepancies do not affect the results of these assays (Greinacher et al., 1991).

2. Perform differential centrifugation to obtain ACD-anticoagulated platelet-rich plasma.

Comment. Low-speed centrifugation prepares ACD-anticoagulated platelet-rich plasma (PRP). Additional ACD (111 μL/mL PRP) is added (Greifswald) to ensure that the pH of the PRP is sufficiently low ($\leq$ 6.5) to prevent platelet aggregation that otherwise would occur during platelet pelleting: the platelet release reaction is triggered by close platelet contact in low-calcium concentrations at physiological pH (Kinlough-Rathbone et al., 1983). If the serotonin-release method is used, the PRP is incubated at 37°C for 30 min. with [^{14}C]serotonin (0.1 μCi/mL of PRP added from a stock solution of 50 μCi/mL of [^{14}C]serotonin) (Lee et al., 1996).

3. Wash the platelets by pelleting them from PRP, then gently resuspend the platelets in calcium- and magnesium-free Tyrode's buffer, pH 6.3, containing glucose (5.6 mmol/L) and apyrase (2.5 U/mL).

Comment. Tyrode's buffer consists of physiological concentrations of sodium chloride (NaCl, 137 mmol/L), potassium chloride (2.7 mmol/L), calcium chloride ($CaCl_2$, 2 mmol/L), magnesium chloride ($MgCl_2$, 1.0 mmol/L), and sodium dihydrogen phosphate (NaH_2PO_4, 3.3 mmol/L); however, calcium-free and magnesium-free Tyrode's is used in this wash step to avoid activating the coagulation factors and platelets. The low pH prevents platelets from aggregating during pelleting. Apyrase is an enzyme that degrades adenine nucleotides (i.e., accumulation of the ADP from the platelets is prevented). Azide-free bovine serum albumin (3.5 mg/mL) and hirudin (1 U/mL) are included in the wash buffer in Greifswald, but not Hamilton, although HEPES (5 mmol/L) is added to this buffer in Hamilton. Following resuspension, the platelets are incubated for 15 min. at 37°C (Greifswald).

4. Pellet the washed platelets as before, and then gently resuspend the platelets into calcium- and magnesium-containing Tyrode's buffer, pH 7.4, without apyrase or hirudin.

Comment. Following resuspension, the platelets should ''rest'' for 45 min. at 37°C (Greifswald). The final resuspension buffer (Tyrode's buffer at physiological pH) contains calcium (2 mmol/L) and magnesium (1 mmol/L Hamilton; 2 mmol/L Greifswald). The platelet count is adjusted to a minimum of 300×10^9/L; thus, after addition of washed platelets (75 μL) to the microtiter wells containing test serum (20 μL) and heparin–buffer (5 μL in Hamilton, 10 μL in Greifswald), the final platelet concentration will be at least 215×10^9/L. Apyrase must not be included in this buffer, as the ADP released during assessment of

HIT-induced platelet activation is an important potentiator of the platelet Fc receptor-mediated platelet activation (Polgár et al., 1998).

Test Conditions of Heparin-Dependent Platelet Activation: Perform Platelet Activation Studies Under Various Test Conditions

Comment. In Hamilton, sera are studied using six different reaction conditions: (1) buffer; (2) unfractionated heparin (UFH), 0.1 U/mL; (3) UFH, 0.3 U/mL; (4) UFH, 100 U/mL; (5) low molecular weight heparin (LMWH), enoxaparin, 0.1 U/mL; and (6) UFH, 0.3 U/mL plus a monoclonal antibody (IV.3) that inhibits platelet Fc receptor-mediated platelet activation. In Greifswald, routine testing is performed using (1) buffer; (2) LMWH (reviparin), 0.2 U/mL; (3) UFH, 100 U/mL; and (4) danaparoid, 0.2 U/mL (to assess cross-reactivity); (5) sometimes LMWH 0.2 U/mL plus IV.3 is performed to resolve unclear results. In Greifswald, the LMWH preparation, reviparin (Clivarine) is used because of its narrow molecular weight (MW) range (80% of its chains have molecular mass between 2.4–7.2 kDa; i.e., 4–12 disaccharide units) (Jeske et al., 1997); this results in more consistent formation of PF4–heparin complexes. Platelets are incubated with various test and positive and negative control sera under these various reaction conditions for up to 45 min (Greifswald) or 60 min (Hamilton). The order of pipetting is important in optimizing assay results (Eichler et al., 1999; see Table 3).

Interpretation of the Obtained Test and Control Data

Comment. Several techniques can be used to assess activation of washed platelets (see Fig. 1). The actual method of detection of platelet activation is probably less important than the technique of platelet preparation itself, including the selection of suitable platelet donors.

A positive test result is one in which heparin-dependent platelet activation occurs at therapeutic concentrations of heparin (0.1–0.3 U/mL), but is inhibited at very high (100 U/mL) heparin concentrations and in the presence of platelet Fc receptor-blocking monoclonal antibody. By assessing activation in the presence of different LMWH compounds or danaparoid, studies of in vitro cross-reactivity can be performed (discussed subsequently). It is important to ensure that control HIT sera, including one or more weak positive controls, react as expected. Given the experience from a workshop on testing for HIT antibodies (Eichler et al., 1999), we recommend exchange of weak positive control sera among laboratories for quality control.

Platelet Activation Endpoints

Carbon 14-serotonin release was the first activation endpoint described using washed platelets (Sheridan et al., 1986). In this method, the washed platelets are

Table 3 Pipette Scheme for the HIPA Test

	Add first	Add second	Add third	Add last		
	Heat-inactivated patient or control serum	UFH 1050 U/mL = 100 U/mL (final)	Washed platelet suspension (300,000 platelets/μL)	Suspension buffer	LMWH (2.1 anti-Xa U/mL) = 0.2 U/mL (final)	Danaparoid (2.1 anti-Xa U/mL) = 0.2 U/mL (final)
Control with buffer	20 μL		75 μL	10 μL		
Low heparin concentration	20 μL		75 μL		10 μL	
High heparin concentration	20 μL	10 μL	75 μL			
Cross-reactivity with danaparoid	20 μL		75 μL			10μL

The order of pipetting is important. After adding serum to the microtiter plate wells, high LMWH concentrations are added to the appropriate wells: this will disrupt PF4–heparin complexes that may be present in the serum. After adding washed platelets, buffer, LMWH (low concentrations), and danaparoid (for cross-reactivity testing) are added. If inhibition by monoclonal antibody IV.3 is tested, this reagent is added before addition of the washed platelet suspension. In Hamilton, the pipetting order for the SRA is (1) addition of buffer–heparin, (2) serum, and (3) platelets.

incubated with test and control serum or plasma and heparin–buffer in flat-bottomed polystyrene microtiter wells (in duplicate or triplicate), performed on a platelet shaker (shaken, not stirred). After 1 h, the reaction is halted with 100 μL of 0.5% EDTA in phosphated-buffered saline (PBS). The microtiter plates are centrifuged at 1000 *g* for 5 min, and 50 μL of supernatant fluid is transferred to tubes containing scintillation fluid for detection of [^{14}C]serotonin released during platelet activation.

Carbon-14 is a radioisotope with a long half-life (5730 years) that emits β-particles (electrons). Laboratories require special licenses to handle radioisotopes, thus limiting widespread use of this platelet-activation marker. However, it is also possible to quantitate serotonin by nonradioactive analysis (Schnell et al., 1998). Results are expressed as percentage of serotonin released. This is calculated based on comparison with maximal possible release (determined following detergent-induced platelet lysis), adjusted for background release (determined by quantitating serotonin release from a sample incubated with buffer alone). Acceptable experiments should have less than 5% background release, with both buffer and negative control serum testing negative for HIT antibodies.

Aggregation of Washed Platelets A convenient and useful activation endpoint—platelet aggregation—was reported in the heparin-induced platelet activation (HIPA) assay (Greinacher et al., 1991; Eichler et al., 1999). Test serum and heparin–buffer are placed in U-bottomed polystyrene microtiter wells containing two stainless steel spheres, and the platelets are stirred at approximately 500 rpm, using a magnetic stirrer. At 5-min. intervals, the wells are examined against an indirect light source: a change in appearance of the reaction mixture from turbidity (nonaggregated platelets) to transparency (aggregated platelets) is a positive result. Although the activation endpoint is evaluated subjectively, interobserver agreement is good. A further advantage of this technique is its repeated evaluation of platelet activation over time. Thus, strong HIT sera that cause the typical activation profile of HIT (i.e., activation at low, but not high, heparin concentrations) within 15–30 min are readily identified. In contrast, such a strong HIT serum might eventually cause platelet activation even at the high heparin concentration, and thus cause an ‘‘indeterminate’’ reaction pattern (activation at both low and high heparin concentrations) if activation is assessed at a later time point only. Occasionally, there is interference with visual interpretation (e.g., a lipemic serum).

Luminography Stewart et al. (1995) reported luminography to detect platelet activation, using a commercially available lumiaggregometer. Adenosine triphosphate (ATP) is released from platelet dense granules during platelet activation. In the presence of luciferin–luciferase reagent, a light flash is generated in the presence of ATP, which is detected and quantitated. Another group reported similar results using a standard scintillation counter (Teitel et al., 1996). It is uncertain how the sensitivity and specificity of these assays compare with other markers of platelet activation.

Platelet-Derived Microparticle Generation Generation of platelet-derived microparticles occurs when washed platelets are activated by HIT sera (Warkentin et al., 1994). With use of a fluorescein-labeled anti-GPIbα murine monoclonal antibody, a method for quantitating microparticles using flow cytometry was reported by Lee and co-workers (1996). Although both platelets and microparticles bind fluorescein-labeled anti-GPIbα monoclonal antibody, they can be distinguished by their size and scatter parameters using flow cytometry, with microparticles quantitated in relation to platelet numbers (Lee et al., 1996).

Heat-Inactivation of Patient Serum or Plasma

To avoid thrombin-induced platelet activation in buffer containing physiological calcium, steps are taken to inactivate residual thrombin. Thus, plasma and serum must first be heat-inactivated before use in these assays. Heating at 56°C for 30–45 min inactivates thrombin and complement. Fibrin and other precipitates are removed by high-speed centrifugation (8000 *g* for 5 min). More intense heating of serum (63°C for 20 min) forms platelet-activating immune complexes (Warkentin et al., 1994); thus, if a patient sample shows heparin-independent platelet activation (indeterminate result), another sample aliquot should be heat-inactivated, and the HIT assay repeated. Often, this will result in disappearance of the initial artifact that presumably was caused by too intense heat inactivation. Serum is preferred for use in functional HIT assays by the laboratories in Greifswald and Hamilton.

Biological Basis for High Sensitivity of Washed Platelets to Activation by HIT Antibodies

Table 4 lists differences between using washed platelets and platelets suspended in citrate-anticoagulated plasma to study HIT antibody-mediated platelet activation. Some of these differences may be important in explaining the greater sensitivity and specificity of washed platelets to detect HIT antibodies.

1. Baseline platelet activation, including platelet granule release, occurs during preparation of washed platelets. This enhances the platelet-binding capacity for heparin (Horne and Chao, 1989) and may also increase the availability of PF4 to form the target antigen.
2. Apyrase is used to prevent accumulation of ADP during platelet washing. This prevents platelets from becoming refractory to subsequent

Table 4 Comparison Between Citrated Platelet-Rich Plasma and Washed Platelet Assays

Technical aspects	Washed platelet assay	Platelet-rich plasma assay	Comments
Platelet preparation	High *g* centrifugation during washing: increased baseline platelet activation	Low *g* centrifugation: less baseline platelet activation	Availability of PF4 may be higher using washed platelets (greater formation of PF4–heparin antigen complexes)
Apyrase	Apyrase added to wash solution, but not to the final resuspension (reaction) buffer	No apyrase used (no wash steps)	Apyrase degrades ADP, and prevents its accumulation; thus, platelet refractoriness to ADP-mediated potentiation of HIT serum-induced platelet activation is avoided by apyrase
Reaction milieu	Physiological calcium concentration (2 mmol/L)	Low (micromolar) calcium owing to citrate	IgG-mediated platelet activation optimal with physiological calcium concentrations
IgG levels	Reduced IgG levels during final reaction	Normal plasma IgG levels	Reduced inhibition of Fc receptor-mediated platelet activation by IgG in washed platelet assays
Plasma protein levels	Reduced plasma protein levels	Normal plasma protein levels	Reduced nonidiosyncratic platelet activation by heparin using washed platelets (?)
Temperature	Room temperature	37°C	Unknown significance
Reaction assessment	Microtiter plates	Conventional aggregometer	Many assays performed simultaneously using microtiter plates

See text for further details on differences between washed platelet and citrated platelet-rich plasma assays (pp. 219–222).

ADP-mediated platelet activation (Ardlie et al., 1990). Empirically, apyrase grade III (Sigma) is acceptable for use: grades I and II are too impure, and grades IV and higher are expensive.

3. Physiological calcium concentrations are present when washed platelets are used. Under these conditions, ADP produces only primary platelet aggregation. However, as observed by Packham et al. (1971), traces of immunoglobulin complexes in amounts too low to cause aggregation themselves will cause secondary aggregation to occur following the addition of ADP. Recently, the importance of ADP in mediating HIT antibody-induced platelet activation has been reported by Polgár and colleagues (1998). Thus, the reaction conditions that exist when washed platelets are used appear to maximize HIT antibody-induced platelet activation because the platelets retain sensitivity to ADP-mediated platelet activation.
4. Low concentrations of IgG are present in the final washed platelet reaction mixture: There is a fivefold reduction in IgG compared with citrated platelet-rich plasma (c-PRP) assays, because only IgG from the test serum is present in the final reaction mixture. Chong and colleagues (1993a) showed that high plasma IgG levels in one platelet donor's blood seemed to explain the discrepancy between studies using donor c-PRP (poor reactivity) and donor washed platelets (good reactivity). These and other investigators (Greinacher et al., 1994b) also observed that addition of IgG inhibits HIT serum-induced activation of washed platelets in a dose-dependent fashion.
5. Low concentrations of fibrinogen and other plasma proteins could reduce the potential for nonidiosyncratic heparin-induced platelet activation (Salzman et al., 1980; Chong et al., 1993a). In contrast, low concentrations of heparin rarely cause significant activation of washed platelets. It is possible that acute-phase reactant proteins such as fibrinogen could lead to false-positive activation assays for HIT using c-PRP.
6. Room temperature conditions are used for washed platelet assays; in contrast, c-PRP studies are performed at 37°C. Although this is a major difference between the assays, it is unknown whether there are advantages or disadvantages of performing washed platelet assays at room temperature. In Greifswald, all buffers are warmed to 37°C, and all incubation steps are performed at this temperature; only the final incubation on the microtiter plates is performed at room temperature.
7. Multiple serum–platelet reactions in microtiter plates can be performed, and even several hundred reactions studied in parallel. Quality control is thereby enhanced by the large number of control and test reaction conditions that can be analyzed, and the long incubation period

employed (up to 60 min). The incubation period in HIT assays should be at least 20–30 min (Stewart et al., 1995).

Quality Control in Washed Platelet Assays for HIT

The variable reactivity of donor platelets to HIT sera is an important issue in activation assays for HIT. It has long been recognized that inconsistent results can be obtained using these assays (Salem and van der Weyden, 1983; Pfueller and David, 1986; Warkentin et al., 1992).

Hierarchical Versus Idiosyncratic Platelet Activation by HIT Sera The results of a systematic investigation, summarized in Table 5, showed that both HIT sera and platelet donors exhibit variable reactivity in a hierarchical, rather than an idiosyncratic, manner. The strongest reactions were produced by strong HIT sera against strongly reactive platelet donors. All of the negative reactions occurred when the weakest sera were mixed with the weakest platelets. Importantly, no unexpected negative reactions occurred elsewhere in the 10 × 10 serum–platelet grid (see Table 5). Furthermore, the relative ranking of platelet donors appeared to be stable over time, an observation also reported by Chong and colleagues (1993a) in their study of platelet donor variability using c-PRP.

The finding of a hierarchical pattern of reactivity has important implications for quality control in diagnostic testing for HIT using activation assays. First, it indicates that platelets from certain donors who tend to respond well to HIT sera should be chosen. Second, relatively weak HIT sera should be included as positive controls (~20–50% serotonin release, or 25-min–lag time in the HIPA).

Heparin-Independent Platelet Activation: Indeterminate Results About 5% of test sera or plasma give an *indeterminate result* in an activation assay. This is defined as platelet activation that occurs at both therapeutic (0.1–0.3 U/mL) and supratherapeutic (10–100 U/mL) heparin concentrations. Often, an interpretable result is obtained when the assay is repeated using another heat-inactivated aliquot. This suggests that the first result may have been an artifact caused by heat-aggregated IgG generated ex vivo. However, some serum and plasma samples repeatedly demonstrate heparin-independent platelet activation. Biological explanations include circulating immune complexes (e.g., systemic lupus erythematosus), high-titer HLA class I alloantibodies and, possibly, other platelet-activating factors (e.g., thrombotic thrombocytopenic purpura). An antigen assay is required for further investigation when an indeterminate result is consistently obtained.

Inhibition by High Heparin Concentrations Sheridan and colleagues (1986) first emphasized that there was a relatively specific activation profile triggered by HIT sera and plasmas: activation at therapeutic heparin concentrations (maximal at 0.1–0.3 U/mL) that progressively diminished with increasing hepa-

Table 5 Reactivities of Ten HIT Sera with Platelets from Ten Normal Donors

HIT sera	Normal platelet donors: strongest (P1) to weakest (P10)									
(S1–S10)	P_1 84.3	P_2 71.2	P_3 68.4	P_4 53.6	P_5 52.5	P_6 41.3	P_7 39.7	P_8 38.9	P_9 36.9	P_{10} 29.9
S_1 85.4	++++	++++	++++	++++	++++	++++	+++	++++	++	+++
S_2 84.4	++++	++++	++++	++++	++++	+++	+++	++++	+++	+++
S_3 69.1	++++	++++	++++	+++	+++	++	+++	++	++	++
S_4 61.0	++++	++++	+++	+++	+++	++	++	++	++	+
S_5 56.4	++++	+++	+++	++	+++	++	++	+	+	+
S_6 50.7	+++	+++	+++	+++	++	++	++	++	+	+
S_7 44.1	++++	+++	+++	+	++	+	+	+	++	−
S_8 30.1	++++	++	+++	+	+	+	−	−	−	−
S_9 24.2	+++	++	+	++	+	−	−	−	−	−
S_{10} 11.3	++	+	+	−	−	−	−	−	−	−

Serum samples and platelet donors are ranked from strongest to weakest (S_1–S_{10} and P_1–P_{10}, respectively), according to the mean percentage of [^{14}C]serotonin release when considering all 100 serum–platelet donor pairs (ten pairs corresponding to each HIT serum and each normal platelet donor). For each serum–platelet donor pair, the individual amount of serotonin release is summarized as follows: 80–100%, ++++; 60–79% release, +++; 40–59% release, ++; 20–39% release, +; < 20% release, −.

Overall, there is a graded pattern of reactivity among the individual reaction pairs that is *hierarchical* (i.e., there are no unexpected weak or strong reactions among the pairs). All negative reactions (< 20% release) were found in the lower right portion of the table. Conversely, the strongest reactions (≥ 80% release) were found in the upper left portion of the table.

Source: Warkentin et al., 1992.

rin concentrations, typically falling to background activation at very high (100 U/mL) heparin concentrations. Classically, a *positive test* was defined as greater than 20% serotonin release at 0.1 U/mL heparin, and less than 20% serotonin release at 100 U/mL heparin. These criteria should not be applied indiscriminately, however. For example, a very strong HIT serum could produce more than a 90% release at 0.1 U/mL heparin, and 25% release at 100 U/mL heparin. Alternatively, a serum or plasma sample that was not adequately heat-inactivated could produce a similar reaction profile (i.e., residual thrombin is inhibited by the high, but not low, heparin concentration). The strength of reactivity caused by patient serum can be helpful: clinically significant HIT antibodies almost always cause more than 50% serotonin release using optimally reactive platelets. In the HIPA test, differences in the lag time to platelet aggregation provide useful information.

Inhibition by Fc Receptor Blockade Platelet activation by HIT antibodies is inhibited in the presence of a murine IgG2b monoclonal antibody (IV.3) that recognizes the platelet FcγIIa receptor (Kelton et al., 1988; Chong et al., 1989) and can be used to enhance test specificity.

Interpretation of Platelet Activation by HIT Serum in the Absence of Added Heparin

With activation assays, it is not uncommon for HIT serum or plasma to cause platelet activation, even in the absence of added heparin. Usually, even greater platelet activation occurs in the presence of added heparin. When strong serum-dependent platelet activation occurs with buffer and at a 0.1- to 0.3-U/mL–heparin, concentration, it is important to ensure that the other reactions (at 100 U/mL heparin, and 0.1–0.3 U/mL heparin together with Fc receptor blockade) are as expected. This is because residual thrombin could produce strong platelet activation in both the absence and presence of low heparin concentration, thereby causing the potential for a false-positive result.

There are at least two potential explanations for strong platelet activation in the absence of added heparin. First, there may be residual heparin in the sample (White et al., 1992; Pötzsch et al., 1996). However, this phenomenon can persist despite attempts to remove heparin using binding resins. A second explanation is that some HIT antibodies recognize platelet-bound PF4 in the absence of an exogenous source of heparin, perhaps by PF4 bound to platelet glycosaminoglycans. This phenomenon has implications for the interpretation of tests of cross-reactivity of LMWH and danaparoid (Pötzsch et al., 1996), as discussed later.

Disadvantages of Washed Platelet Assays

The major disadvantage of washed platelet assays to detect HIT antibodies is that they are technically demanding and labor-intensive. A workshop that compared a washed platelet assay (the HIPA test) and an antigen assay showed greater variability in activation assay results among the participating laboratories (Eichler et al., 1999). Washed platelet activation assays are best suited for reference laboratories assessing many HIT sera, as this facilitates acquisition of sufficient technical experience to perform the assay successfully on a consistent basis. Assay-specific disadvantages include the requirement for radioactivity (SRA), the use of a subjective, visual endpoint (HIPA), and expensive equipment (flow cytometry-based assays).

B. Activation Assays Using Citrate-Anticoagulated Blood

The first reports describing the use of normal donor c-PRP to detect platelet activation caused by HIT serum or plasma appeared in the 1970s (Rhodes et al., 1973; Fratantoni et al., 1975; Babcock et al., 1976). A ratio of serum (or plasma) to c-PRP between 0.66 and 1.0 was used (e.g., 200 μL serum added to 200–300 μL c-PRP). No standardized method has evolved, however, although a survey of 54 laboratories in France (Nguyên et al., 1994) found some practices to be more common. For example, most laboratories test patient citrated platelet-poor plasma (c-PPP) rather than heat-inactivated serum. Variable heparin concentrations are used, most commonly between 0.5 and 1.0 U/mL. The ratio of patient c-PPP to donor c-PRP is usually 1 : 1, and ABO discrepancies are usually ignored. About 75% of the laboratories use at least two platelet donors for diagnostic testing.

Testing for HIT Antibodies Using c-PRP

The following description of the assay taken from Chong and colleagues (1989, 1993a) has the highest reported sensitivity and specificity among c-PRP methods. Blood is obtained from normal blood donors whose platelets respond well to serum or plasma from HIT patients, and c-PRP is prepared. Testing involves addition of 150 μL of patient heat-inactivated c-PPP or serum to 340 μL of c-PRP (final platelet concentration, 250–350 × 10^9/L) at 37°C. The platelets are monitored for a few minutes to exclude nonspecific platelet aggregation. After addition of 10 μL heparin–saline, aggregation is monitored over the next 15 min or until aggregation has occurred. A positive result is an increase in light transmission of more than 25% above baseline in the presence of therapeutic-dose heparin (0.5 U/mL) and patient serum or c-PPP, and inhibition of aggregation in the presence of patient serum or plasma and supratherapeutic-dose heparin (100 U/mL). Use of such a two-point assay reduced the false-positive rate, as serum or plasma from some patients without HIT caused platelet aggregation at all heparin concentrations tested. To ensure that the platelets are functional, platelets are also tested with collagen (2 μg/mL). Details on methodology of c-PRP assays are also given elsewhere (Kapsch and Silver, 1981; Almeida et al., 1998).

Some workers report that platelets from a patient with HIT are very reactive to heparin-dependent activation by their own serum or plasma (Kappa et al., 1987; Chong et al., 1993b). Use of autologous c-PRP can sometimes be limited by the patient's thrombocytopenia, however. Potential explanations for the high sensitivity of autologous platelets include persisting high Fc receptor expression on platelets of patients with acute HIT (Chong et al., 1993b) and baseline platelet activation (Chong et al., 1994), with the potential for higher PF4 availability.

Disadvantages of c-PRP Aggregation Assays

Problems with these assays include (1) potential for false-positive interpretation if heparin produces nonspecific aggregation of donor platelets, an effect that could be enhanced nonspecifically by proaggregatory factors in the patient serum or plasma; and (2) risk for false-negative interpretation if HIT serum-induced platelet aggregation begins even before addition of heparin.

Nonspecific activation of platelets by heparin occurs with some normal donor c-PRP (Chong et al., 1993a), rendering these donors unsuitable for diagnostic testing. It is also possible that plasma from very sick patients may be more likely to cause nonspecific aggregation of platelets in c-PRP in the presence of heparin (Goodfellow et al., 1998).

An important practical disadvantage is that only a limited number of platelet aggregation tracings can be performed using conventional aggregometers. Thus, relatively few reactions with a limited number of patient and control samples can be evaluated.

Other Assays Using Citrated-Anticoagulated Whole Blood or Platelet-Rich Plasma

Tomer (1997) reported a c-PRP activation assay for HIT antibodies in which the activation endpoint is quantitation of binding of fluorescein-labeled recombinant annexin V to platelets, as detected using flow cytometry. Annexin V, a placental protein, interacts with the prothrombinase-binding anionic phospholipids expressed on the surface of activated platelets, and correlates with platelet procoagulant activity. It is uncertain whether the reaction conditions employed (e.g., 30-min incubation at 26°C) or the high sensitivity of annexin V binding (300-fold increase over baseline) overcomes the inherent limitations of sensitivity observed with other assays using c-PRP.

C. Comparison of Washed Platelet and c-PRP Activation Assays

It became evident during the mid-1980s that the sensitivity of c-PRP aggregation assays for HIT was relatively poor (Kelton et al., 1984; Pfueller et al., 1986). Favaloro and colleagues (1992) first compared the c-PRP aggregation assay with the washed platelet SRA. They observed that only 6 of 13 HIT sera or plasmas that tested positive in the SRA also tested positive in the c-PRP aggregation assay. In contrast, no sample was identified that tested positive only in the aggregation assay. Chong and colleagues (1993a) also found a higher sensitivity for the SRA method. However, considerable variability in sensitivity for HIT antibodies among the various platelet donors was seen, ranging from 39–81% (c-PRP assay) to 65–94% (washed platelet SRA).

Strong evidence in favor of a higher sensitivity for washed platelet assays was provided by direct comparison using platelets prepared and tested in parallel that were obtained simultaneously from the same platelet donors (Greinacher et al., 1994a). Only 23 of 70 HIT sera that tested positive by the HIPA assay also tested positive using c-PRP aggregation. In contrast, all but 1 of 24 sera testing positive in the c-PRP aggregation assay also tested positive in the HIPA test.

III. ANTIGEN ASSAYS FOR HIT ANTIBODIES

A. Solid-Phase Enzyme Immunoassay

The solid-phase, enzyme immunoassay (EIA) has been described in detail (Amiral et al., 1992; Visentin et al., 1994; Greinacher et al., 1994a; Amiral et al., 1995; Horsewood et al., 1996). Methods differ in the way that PF4–heparin complexes are coated to the microtiter wells. A general scheme is shown in Fig. 2. In this assay, stoichiometric concentrations of PF4 and heparin (e.g., 50 μL each of 20 μg/mL PF4 and 1 U/mL UFH) dissolved in phosphate buffer are added together to the wells of a microtiter plate, and incubated at 4°C overnight.

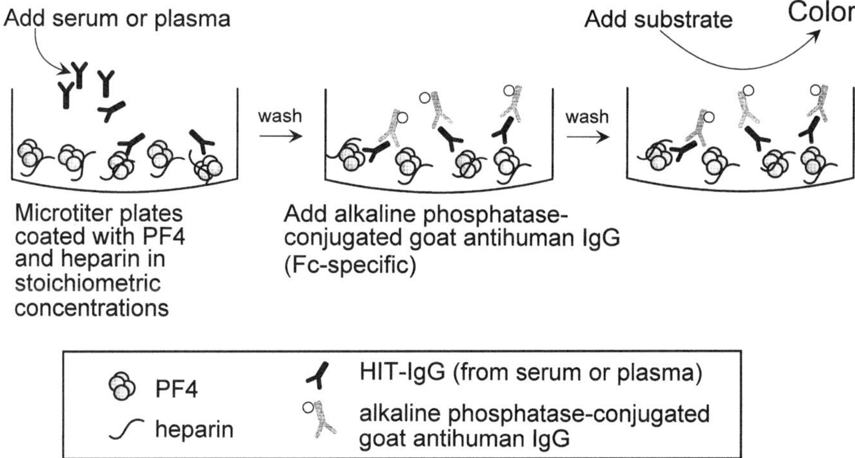

Figure 2 Schematic figure of solid-phase PF4–heparin–EIA.

After washing with phosphate buffer saline–Tween 20 (PBS–Tw), the wells are ''blocked'' with a protein-containing solution such as PBS–Tw containing either 10% normal goat serum (NGS) or 20% fetal calf serum, followed by washing with PBS–Tw. To perform the assay, 50–100 μL of test or control plasma or serum diluted 1:50 in PBS containing 2% normal goat serum is added to duplicate wells for 1 h at room temperature. After thorough washing with PBS–Tw, bound immunoglobulin is detected by adding alkaline phosphatase-conjugated goat antihuman immunoglobulin (e.g., affinity-purified goat antihuman IgG Fc diluted 1:1000 in PBS–Tw–(2% NGS), followed by incubation for 1 h at room temperature. After through washing, incubation with *p*-nitrophenyl phosphate in 1 M diethanolamine buffer is added. After incubation in the dark, the reaction is stopped with 1 N NaOH, and absorbance is read at 405 nm using an automated microplate reader. The upper limit of the normal range is usually set at the mean plus 3 SD obtained using normal sera. Some laboratories set an indeterminate range for samples that are only minimally above the upper normal range.

B. Fluid-Phase EIA

The fluid-phase EIA for HIT antibodies (Newman et al., 1998) is an adaption of a staphylococcal protein A antibody-capture EIA method (Nagi et al., 1993). By permitting antibody–antigen interactions to occur in a fluid phase, problems of protein (antigen) denaturation inherent in solid-phase assays are avoided.

Platelet factor 4 (5% biotinylated) is mixed with an optimal concentration of heparin, and this antigen mixture is incubated with diluted patient serum or plasma (Fig. 3). Subsequently, the antigen–antibody mixture is incubated with protein G–Sepharose in a microcentrifuge tube. Biotinylated antigen–antibody complexes become bound to the protein G–Sepharose by antibody Fc, and the complexes are separated from unbound antigen by centrifugation and washing. The amount of biotin–PF4–heparin–antibody complexes immobilized to the beads is measured using peroxidase substrate after initial incubation with streptavidin-conjugated peroxidase.

The fluid-phase EIA appears to have a lower rate of false-positive reactions. This may be because in the solid-phase EIA, nonspecific binding of IgG to the microtiter wells can occur. Furthermore, the cryptic antigen site of PF4 can be exposed when the molecule comes into close contact with the plastic surface, even in the absence of heparin. The fluid-phase assay avoids these problems by first precipitating all reactive IgG antibodies, then detecting the antigen specifically bound to the IgG. Thus, higher concentrations of patient serum or plasma can be tested without increasing nonspecific reactivity. The advantages of this assay in performing in vitro cross-reactivity are discussed later. Because antibody is bound using protein G–Sepharose, IgM and IgA anti-PF4–heparin antibodies are not detected in this assay.

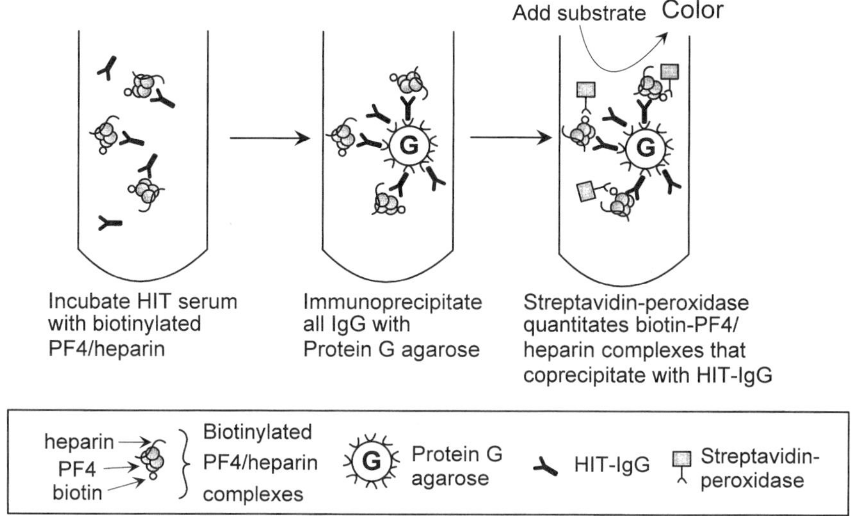

Figure 3 Schematic figure of fluid-phase PF4–heparin–EIA.

C. PF4–Polyvinylsulfonate Antigen Assay

Several negatively charged substances can cause the cryptic autoepitope within PF4 to become recognizable to HIT antibodies (see Chaps. 6–8). Indeed, a commercial assay for HIT using PF4 complexed with polyvinylsulfonate has been developed (Collins et al., 1997; Visentin et al., 1997). Sensitivity and reproducibility were high using polyvinylsulfonate that had been fractionated to a relatively uniform molecular weight (5000 ± 500 Da). Some technical advantages of this assay include the observation that the ratio of PF4/PVS is not critical (cf. PF4–heparin), with acceptable concentrations of PVS ranging from 0.1 to 100 μmol/L for a corresponding concentration of 10 μg/mL PF4. The antigen complex is also stable for long periods.

D. Comparison of Activation and Antigen Assays

Both PF4–heparin–EIA and washed platelet activation assays have approximately equal sensitivity for clinical HIT (Greinacher et al., 1994a; Warkentin et al., 1999). For serum or plasma samples that are known to be positive by one sensitive washed platelet activation assay (e.g., SRA or HIPA), the corresponding probability of the PF4–heparin–EIA for confirming the positive result is at least 75–90% (Greinacher et al., 1994a; Arepally et al., 1995). Conversely, a similar percentage of referred samples that test positive in the EIA will also test positive using a washed platelet activation assay (Greinacher et al., 1994a). The sensitivity

Table 6 Discrepancies in Results of HIT Antibody Testing: Possible Explanations and Implications

c-PRP aggregation assay	Washed platelet activation assay (SRA or HIPA)	PF4–H-EIA	Interpretation (assumes clinical picture compatible with HIT)	Possible explanations and implications
Neg	Neg	Neg	Not HIT	Continue or resume heparin
Pos	Pos	Pos	HIT	Stop heparin and give alternative anticoagulant
Pos	Neg	Neg	Not HIT	False-positive aggregation assay (see text); continue or resume heparin
Pos	Pos	Neg	HIT caused by antibodies against ''minor'' antigen	Stop heparin and give alternative anticoagulant
Neg	Pos	Pos	HIT (weak-moderate antibodies)	Stop heparin and give alternative anticoagulant
Neg	Neg	Pos	Weak HIT-IgG antibodies; IgM/IgA anti-PF4–H antibodies	Stop heparin and give alternative anticoagulant if clinical picture warrants; otherwise, maintain heparin
Neg	Pos	Neg	Possible thrombin artifact or HIT caused by antibodies against ''minor'' antigen	Repeat assay with a new heat-inactivated serum aliquot; stop heparin and give alternative anticoagulant if clinical picture warrants
Pos	Neg	Pos	HIT (false-negative washed platelet assay)	Stop heparin and give alternative anticoagulant; check washed platelet activation assay method

Pos, positive test result; Neg, negative test result.

of both EIA and SRA was even higher (> 90%) for detecting antibodies that caused HIT in prospectively studied postoperative patients (Warkentin et al., 1999).

Although both antigen and activation assays have similar high sensitivity for clinical HIT, there is evidence that antigen assays have greater sensitivity for detecting HIT antibodies not associated with thrombocytopenia or other clinical events (Amiral et al., 1995; Arepally et al., 1995; Bauer et al., 1997; Warkentin et al., 1999). Data reported by Visentin and colleagues (1994) also support this difference in sensitivity between the assays. These workers studied 12 HIT plasmas that tested positive in both SRA and PF4–heparin–EIA. However, at a 1:100 sample dilution, only 2 of the 12 samples still tested positive in the activation assay. In contrast, even at a 1:200 dilution, all 12 plasmas still tested positive in the EIA. Bachelot and colleagues (1998) observed that HIT plasmas that tested only weakly positive in the PF4–heparin–EIA tended to give negative washed platelet SRA results when using platelets with the least reactive FcγIIA receptor genotype, Arg^{131} (see Chap. 9).

The difference in sensitivity for HIT antibodies between the PF4–heparin–EIA and aggregation studies using c-PRP is considerable. Only about 33–40% of samples that test positive in the PF4–heparin–EIA also test positive using c-PRP aggregation (Greinacher et al., 1994a; Nguyên et al., 1995). Although one laboratory reported a greater sensitivity using c-PRP aggregation than the EIA (Look et al., 1997), these workers did not employ a two-point method, and so may have observed false-positive results using the aggregation assay.

Table 6 summarizes possible explanations for discrepancies in results of activation and antigen assays for HIT.

IV. INTERPRETATION OF HIT TEST RESULTS

It is important to incorporate clinical information into the interpretation of any laboratory result for HIT. This is because thrombocytopenia, whether or not caused by HIT, is common in hospitalized patients receiving heparin, and because nonpathogenic HIT antibodies are often detected by sensitive assays in patients who have received heparin for 5 or more days.

A. Rapid Versus Typical Onset of Thrombocytopenia

Diagnostic algorithms taking into account the pretest probability of HIT are shown in Fig. 4A (activation assay screen) and 4B (antigen assay screen). We have organized the diagnostic approach based on the timing of onset of thrombocytopenia, either rapid (< 5 days) or typical (≥ 5 days; see Chap. 3).

In general, there are two broad pretest probabilities for patients with rapid

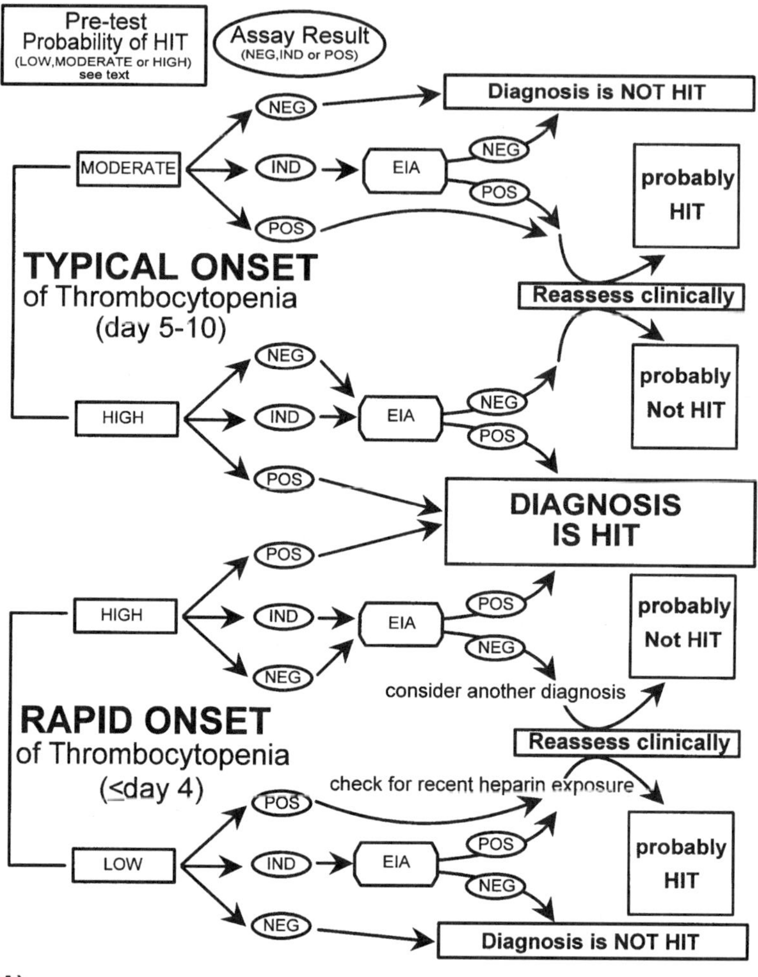

Figure 4 (A) Diagnostic algorithm using a washed platelet activation assay as a screening test for HIT, either the serotonin-release assay (SRA) or the heparin-induced platelet activation (HIPA) test. (B) Diagnostic algorithm using PF4/H-EIA as a screening test for HIT. Abbreviations: IND, indeterminate test result; NEG, negative test result; POS, positive test result. The asterisk (*) in B indicates that a washed platelet activation assay could be useful in a patient with moderate pretest probability for HIT and a positive PF4–heparin–EIA, as a positive activation assay has a higher specificity for clinical HIT (see Table 7).

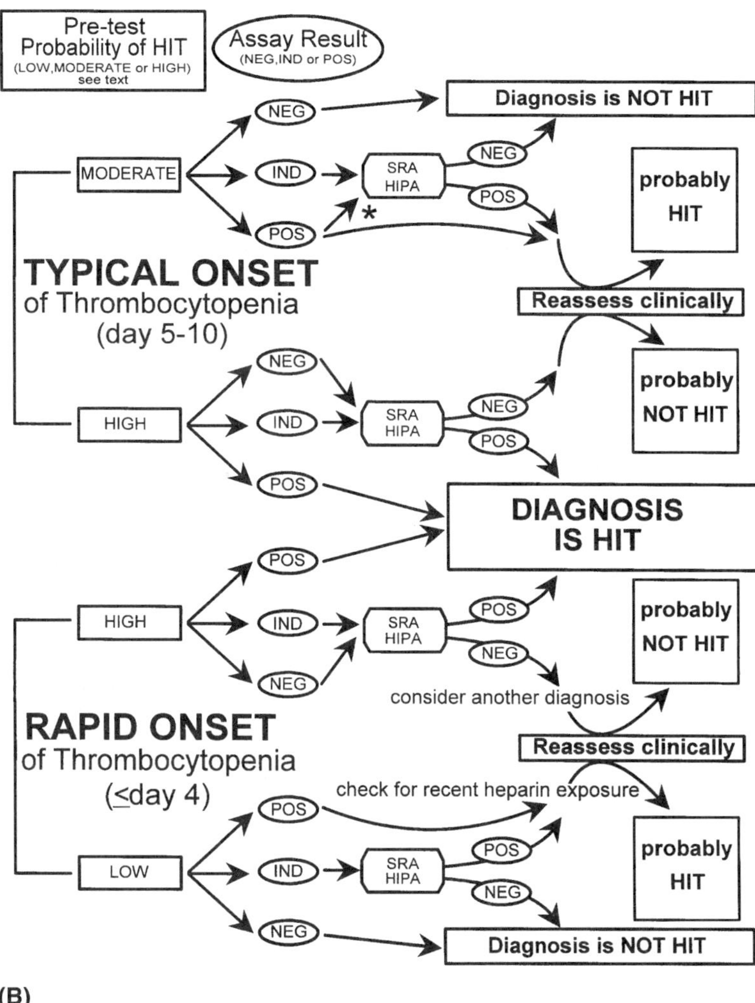

(B)

thrombocytopenia: low and high. Patients with low pretest probability for HIT are those who have not recently been exposed to heparin (thus, they would not be expected to have circulating HIT antibodies, or to have generated them so quickly), or who have another good explanation for thrombocytopenia. (An important caveat is that sometimes a recent heparin exposure is not known to the patient or has not been documented in the medical records.) With a low pretest

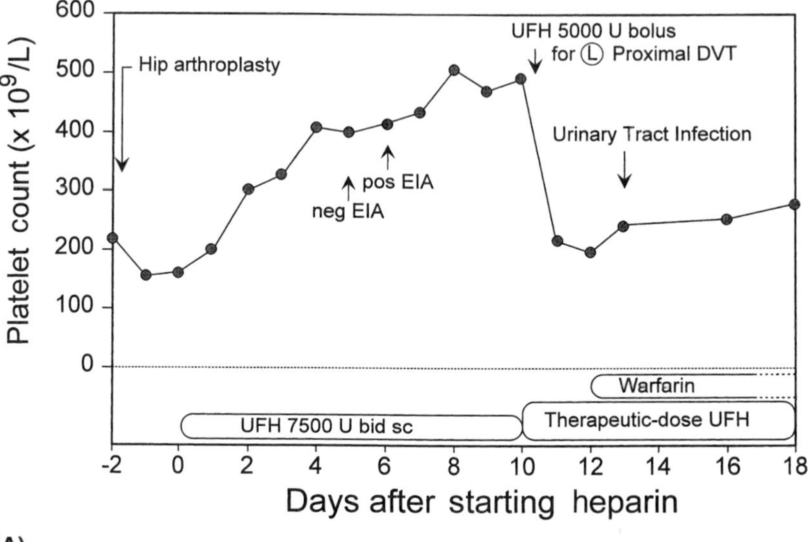

(A)

Figure 5 Two patients with moderate pretest probability of HIT: Although both patients had positive laboratory testing for HIT antibodies, the clinical courses indicate difficulty in ascertaining the actual role HIT played in the thrombocytopenia and thrombotic events. (A) This 74-year-old female patient, identified in a clinical trial (Warkentin et al., 1995a,b), developed HIT antibodies by PF4–heparin–EIA (baseline to day 5, < 0.450 O.D.; day 6, O.D. = 0.783; day 10, O.D. = 1.734), but borderline-positive testing by SRA (~20% serotonin release). Clinical events suggesting HIT include the abrupt platelet count fall from 491 to 197 × 10^9/L after receiving therapeutic-dose UFH and the proximal deep venous thrombosis (DVT). However, urinary tract infection could also have explained the thrombocytopenia. (B) This 71-year-old female patient developed thrombocytopenia, beginning on day 5 of heparin treatment (nadir, 31 × 10^9/L, day 8), together with clinical and laboratory evidence for septicemia. Laboratory testing for HIT antibodies was strongly positive by activation assay (SRA, 90% release at 0.1 U/mL heparin, < 5% release at 100 U/mL heparin) and weakly positive by PF4–heparin–EIA: O.D. = 0.709). Clinical evidence for HIT includes the symptomatic DVT and (possible) pulmonary embolism; however, the dramatic increase in platelet count during therapeutic-dose heparin treatment, and the bacteremia, are strong evidence for septicemia, rather than HIT, as an explanation for the thrombocytopenia.

probability for HIT, either of the sensitive assays for HIT (washed platelet activation assay or antigen assay) can reliably rule out HIT. However, an unexpected negative result in a patient with a high pretest probability, or an unexpected positive result in a patient with a low pretest probability, should lead to repeating the test or performance of the complementary activation or antigen assay. Additionally, further clinical information should be sought (e.g., has another explana-

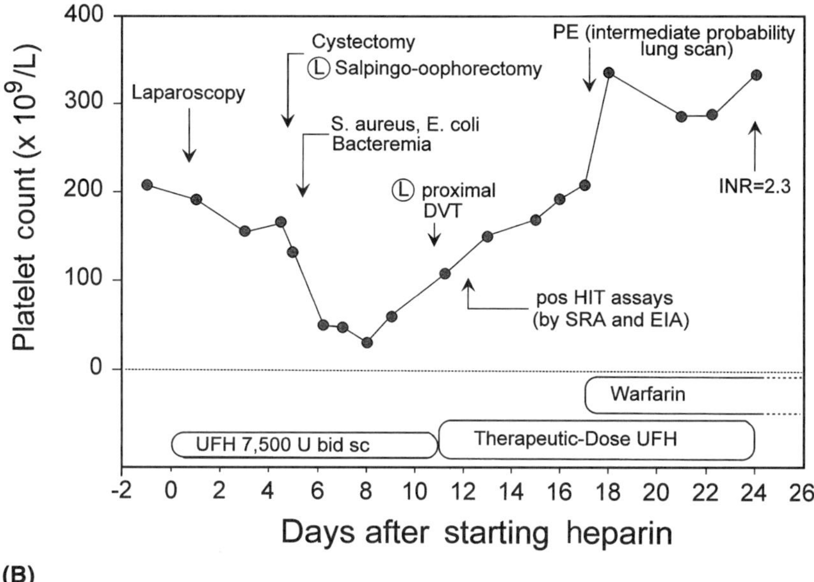

(B)

tion for the thrombocytopenia become apparent? could the patient have had an unrecognized recent heparin exposure?).

In contrast, for patients with the typical temporal onset of thrombocytopenia (i.e., a platelet count fall that begins 5–10 days after beginning heparin treatment), we believe that, in general, there are two different pretest probabilities for HIT: moderate and high. Because HIT is a relatively common explanation for thrombocytopenia that begins during this characteristic time period, it should be considered a plausible diagnosis even if another possible explanation for thrombocytopenia is identified (hence, a moderate pretest probability). In a patient without another apparent explanation for thrombocytopenia, or one in whom an unexplained new thrombotic event has occurred, the pretest probability for HIT would be considered to be high.

B. Diagnostic Interpretation of Laboratory Results

In patients with a high pretest probability of HIT who have a negative screening test, the test should be repeated and the complementary activation or antigen assay should be performed. The diagnosis of HIT is very unlikely if both activation and antigen assays are negative. In patients with a moderate pretest probability who have one or more positive tests for HIT, the final diagnosis may well rest on the overall clinical picture, rather than on the test result alone (Fig. 5A,B; see analysis in Table 7). This conclusion results from two clinical realities: (1)

Table 7 Interpretation of Laboratory Testing for HIT in Postoperative Cardiac and Orthopedic Surgical Patients with Late-Onset Thrombocytopenia

Postoperative patient population	Pretest probability for HIT[a]	Antigen assay (anti-PF4–H–EIA)				Activation assay (SRA or HIPA)			
		Sensitivity[b]	Specificity[b]	Posttest probability if result is: Pos	Neg	Sensitivity[b]	Specificity[b]	Posttest probability if result is: Pos	Neg
Cardiac	0.50 (moderate)	0.95	0.50	0.66	0.09	0.95	0.80	0.83	0.06
	0.90 (high)			0.94	0.47			0.98	0.36
Orthopedic	0.50 (moderate)	0.95	0.92	0.92	0.05	0.95	0.97	0.97	0.05
	0.90 (high)			0.99	0.33			0.997	0.32

[a] The pretest probability refers to the physician's estimate of the likelihood of HIT in a given clinical setting (e.g., a moderate probability (0.50) could be a patient whose timing of onset of thrombocytopenia suggests HIT, but in whom there is clinical evidence of septicemia (fever and chills, blood culture results pending). A high pretest probability could be a patient whose timing of onset of thrombocytopenia suggests HIT, and there is a thrombotic event.

[b] Assumptions for test sensitivity and specificity in the cardiac and orthopedic surgical populations are based on published data. The analysis shows that in a postoperative cardiac patient with moderate pretest probability for HIT, the posttest probability rises only to 0.66 if the EIA is positive, and to 0.83 if the SRA or HIPA are positive.

Sources: Greinacher et al., 1994a; Visentin et al., 1996; Bauer et al., 1997; Warkentin et al., 1999.

sensitive HIT assays frequently detect clinically insignificant HIT antibodies in patients who have received heparin for more than 5 days, and (2) thrombocytopenia—whether caused by HIT or not—is common in clinical practice (see Chap. 4). There is evidence that positive washed platelet activation assays for HIT have greater diagnostic specificity for clinical HIT (Warkentin et al., 1999), especially when strong, rapid platelet activation is produced by patient serum. Regardless, these considerations underscore the importance of conceptualizing HIT as a clinicopathologic syndrome, in which both clinical information and results of HIT antibody testing are used for diagnosis.

V. IN VITRO CROSS-REACTIVITY

A. Cross-Reactivity Using Activation Assays

Cross-reactivity studies have been performed most frequently using activation assays. However, there are no standard methods for, or even a standard definition of, in vitro cross-reactivity. In one study of LMWH and danaparoid cross-reactivity, an increase in platelet activation in the presence of the drug over baseline was used to determine cross-reactivity (Warkentin, 1996). This definition was used to avoid falsely attributing cross-reactivity to drug-independent platelet activation that is produced by some patients' sera. The reason for this definition was the common phenomenon that platelet activation can be caused by a patient's serum even in the absence of added heparin. In the HIPA test, comparison of the lag time to aggregation can be used to judge cross-reactivity: if a sample shows platelet aggregation with heparinoid or LMWH earlier than in the presence of buffer, then cross-reactivity is present. In general, in vitro cross-reactivity with danaparoid is usually clinically insignificant (Warkentin, 1996; Newman et al., 1998; see Chap. 14).

Comparison of c-PRP Versus Washed Platelet Assays

Sensitive washed platelet assays generally show almost 100% cross-reactivity of HIT antibodies for LMWH (Greinacher et al., 1992; Warkentin et al., 1995a). Indeed, UFH and LMWH are essentially indistinguishable in these assays. However, very different results have been reported by investigators using c-PRP assays (Chong et al., 1989; Makhoul et al., 1986; Kikta et al., 1993; Vun et al., 1996). Here, LMWH consistently shows less cross-reactivity compared with UFH. It is possible that differences in nonidiosyncratic heparin-induced platelet activation underlie these observations (see Chap. 5): UFH is more likely to result in weak platelet activation, including some PF4 release, that leads to amplification of the platelet activation response in the presence of PF4–heparin-reactive HIT antibodies. In contrast, in washed platelet assays, IgG-mediated platelet activation, but not nonidiosyncratic heparin-induced platelet activation, occurs.

B. Cross-Reactivity Using Antigen Assays

Although it is theoretically possible to perform a solid-phase EIA to assess cross-reactivity (Amiral et al., 1995), this is complicated because the antigen has to be coated as a complex to the solid phase. This problem has been overcome in a fluid-phase EIA described by Newman and colleagues (1998). Because this assay detects binding to a defined quantity of labeled PF4-containing antigen, the assay is able to determine in vitro cross-reactivity more accurately than the solid-phase EIA. These investigators observed an in vitro cross-reactivity rate of 88% for LMWH; about half the HIT samples reacted weakly against danaparoid in their study.

VI. MISCELLANEOUS ASSAYS FOR HIT ANTIBODIES

A third group of assays detect heparin-dependent immunoglobulin binding to platelet membranes (Griffiths and Dzik, 1997). None of these assays appear to be sufficiently reliable to have gained widespread acceptance for the diagnosis of HIT. This may be related to the fundamental pathogenesis of HIT: the pathogenic platelet-activating properties of HIT antibodies appear to be mediated by relatively few antibodies. Thus, despite producing strong platelet activation, concomitant evaluation of heparin-dependent IgG binding to platelets by flow cytometry, for instance, was either no greater than background (Warkentin et al., 1994) or, in the presence of PF4, only an average of 5.6 times background (Visentin et al., 1994). Furthermore, only 7 of 12 sera exhibited any detectable IgG binding by flow cytometry, even though all 12 were positive using conventional activation or antigen assays (Visentin et al., 1994).

Assays have been developed that attempt to measure an increase in heparin-dependent platelet-bindable immunoglobulin in the presence of HIT serum (Howe and Lynch, 1985; Lynch and Howe, 1985; Gruel et al., 1991), but these whole-platelet EIA methods have been superceded by the more specific PF4–heparin-EIA described earlier. Immunofluorescence assays have also been reported (Wolf et al., 1983; Silberman and Kovarik, 1987).

A commercially available platelet-bindable IgG assay that uses anti–IgG-coated indicator red cells, known as the solid-phase red cell adherence assay (SPRCA), has been developed (Sinor et al., 1990; Sinor and Stone, 1994; Leach et al., 1994, 1995, 1997). Platelets are coated onto U-shaped microtiter platelet wells, and either heparin–serum (*immune complex* method), or heparin–albumin with subsequent addition of serum after a wash step (*hapten* method), is added.

After washing, red cells coated with anti-IgG are added to the wells. Following centrifugation, the appearance of the indicator red cells on the well bottoms is scored on a 10-point scale, ranging from negative (tight red cell button) to strongly positive (diffuse red cell binding on the well bottom). According to Leach and colleagues (1997), both immune complex and hapten reaction profiles are commonly seen with putative HIT sera (immune complex > both > hapten). However, only limited comparisons with conventional HIT assays have been performed, and the diagnostic usefulness of these assays is unknown. Disadvantages include the subjective scoring system, as well as the need to ensure that HLA and platelet-specific alloantibodies do not interfere with testing.

There have been attempts to identify specific binding of heparin-dependent antibodies to platelet glycoproteins using immunoblotting and immunoprecipitation (Lynch and Howe, 1985; Howe and Lynch, 1985; Greinacher et al., 1994c). However, no study has identified a consistent reaction profile diagnostic of HIT. There is thus no experimental evidence implicating the involvement of platelet glycoproteins as an immune target in the pathogenesis of HIT.

ACKNOWLEDGMENTS

Studies described in this chapter were supported by the Heart and Stroke Foundation of Ontario (operating grants A2449 and T2967), and by the Deutsche Forschungsgemeinschaft Gir 1096/2-1 and Gir 1096/2-2. Dr. Warkentin was a Research Scholar of the Heart and Stroke Foundation of Canada.

REFERENCES

Almedia JI, Coats R, Liem TK, Silver D. Reduced morbidity and mortality rates of the heparin-induced thrombocytopenia syndrome. J Vasc Surg 27:309–316, 1998.

Ardlie NG, Packham MA, Mustard JF. Adenosine diphosphate-induced platelet aggregation in suspensions of washed rabbit platelets. Br J Haematol 19:7–17, 1970.

Amiral J, Bridey F, Dreyfus M, Vissac AM, Fressinaud E, Wolf M, Meyer D. Platelet factor 4 complexed to heparin is the target for antibodies generated in heparin-induced thrombocytopenia. Thromb Haemost 68:95–96, 1992.

Amiral J, Bridey F, Wolf M, Boyer-Neumann C, Fressinaud E, Vissac AM, Peynaud-Debayle E, Dreyfus M, Meyer D. Antibodies to macromolecular platelet factor 4–heparin complexes in heparin-induced thrombocytopenia: a study of 44 cases. Thromb Haemost 73:21–28, 1995.

Arepally G, Reynolds C, Tomaski A, Amiral J, Jawad A, Poncz M, Cines DB. Comparison of the PF4/heparin ELISA assay with the ^{14}C-serotonin assay in the diagnosis of heparin-induced thrombocytopenia. Am J Clin Pathol 104:648–654, 1995.

Babcock RB, Dumper CW, Scharfman WB. Heparin-induced immune thrombocytopenia. N Engl J Med 295:237–241, 1976.

Bachelot-Loza C, Saffroy R, Lasne D, Chatellier G, Aiach M, Rendu F. Importance of the FcγRIIa–Arg/His-131 polymorphism in heparin-induced thrombocytopenia diagnosis. Thromb Haemost 79:523–528, 1998.

Bauer TL, Arepally G, Konkle BA, Mestichelli B, Shapiro SS, Cines DB, Poncz M, McNulty S, Amiral J, Hauck WW, Edie RN, Mannion JD. Prevalence of heparin-associated antibodies without thrombosis in patients undergoing cardiopulmonary bypass surgery. Circulation 95:1242–1246, 1997.

Berube C, Mitchell L, Silverman E, David M, Saint Cyr C, Laxer R, Adams M, Vegh P, Andrew M. The relationship of antiphospholipid antibodies to thromboembolic events in pediatric patients with systemic lupus erythematosus: a cross-sectional study. Pediatr Res 44:351–366, 1998.

Chong BH, Ismail F, Cade J, Gallus AS, Gordon S, Chesterman CN. Heparin-induced thrombocytopenia: studies with a new molecular weight heparinoid, Org 10172. Blood 73:1592–1596, 1989.

Chong BH, Burgess J, Ismail F. The clinical usefulness of the platelet aggregation test for the diagnosis of heparin-induced thrombocytopenia. Thromb Haemost 69:344–350, 1993a.

Chong BH, Pilgrim RL, Cooley MA, Chesterman CN. Increased expression of platelet IgG Fc receptors in immune heparin-induced thrombocytopenia. Blood 81:988–993, 1993b.

Chong BH, Murray B, Berndt MC, Dunlop LC, Brighton T, Chesterman CN. Plasma P-selectin is increased in thrombotic consumptive platelet disorders. Blood 83:1535–1541, 1994.

Collins JL, Aster RH, Moghaddam M, Piotrowski MA, Strauss TR, McFarland JG. Diagnostic testing for heparin-induced thrombocytopenia (HIT): an enhanced platelet factor 4 complex enzyme linked immunosorbent assay (PF4 ELISA) [abstr]. Blood 90(suppl 1):461a, 1997.

Eichler P, Budde U, Haas S, Kroll H, Loreth RM, Meyer O, Pachmann U, Pötzsch B, Schabel A, Albrecht D, Greinacher A. First workshop for detection of heparin-induced antibodies: validation of the heparin-induced platelet activation test (HIPA) in comparison with a PF4/heparin ELISA. Thromb Haemost 81:625–629, 1999.

Favaloro EJ, Bernal-Hoyos E, Exner T, Koutts J. Heparin-induced thrombocytopenia: laboratory investigation and confirmation of diagnosis. Pathology 24:177–183, 1992.

Fratantoni JC, Pollet R, Gralnick HR. Heparin-induced thrombocytopenia: confirmation of diagnosis with in vitro methods. Blood 45:395–401, 1975.

Ginsberg JS, Wells PS, Brill-Edwards P, Donovan D, Moffatt K, Johnston M, Stevens P, Hirsh J. Antiphospholipid antibodies and venous thromboembolism. Blood 86: 3685–3691, 1995.

Goodfellow KJ, Brown P, Malia RG, Hampton KK. A comparison of laboratory tests for the diagnosis of heparin-induced thrombocytopenia [abstr]. Br J Haematol 101(suppl 1):89, 1998.

Greinacher A, Michels I, Kiefel V, Mueller-Eckhardt C. A rapid and sensitive test for diagnosing heparin-associated thrombocytopenia. Thromb Haemost 66:734–736, 1991.

Greinacher A, Michels I, Mueller-Eckhardt C. Heparin-associated thrombocytopenia: the antibody is not heparin specific. Thromb Haemost 67:545–549, 1992.

Greinacher A, Amiral J, Dummel V, Vissac A, Kiefel B, Mueller-Eckhardt C. Laboratory diagnosis of heparin-associated thrombocytopenia and comparison of platelet aggregation test, heparin-induced platelet activation test, and platelet factor 4/heparin enzyme-linked immunosorbent assay. Transfusion 34:381–385, 1994a.

Greinacher A, Liebenhoff U, Kiefel V, Presek P, Mueller-Eckhardt C. Heparin-associated thrombocytopenia: the effects of various intravenous IgG preparations on antibody mediated platelet activation—a possible new indication for high dose i.v. IgG. Thromb Haemost 71:641–645, 1994b.

Greinacher A, Pötzsch B, Amiral J, Dummel V, Eichner A, Mueller-Eckhardt C. Heparin-associated thrombocytopenia: isolation of the antibody and characterization of a multimolecular PF4–heparin complex as the major antigen. Thromb Haemost 71: 247–251, 1994c.

Griffiths E, Dzik WH. Assays for heparin-induced thrombocytopenia. Transf Med 7:1–11, 1997.

Gruel Y, Rupin A, Darnige L, Moalic-Reverdiau P, Poumier-Gaschard P, Binet C, Bardos P, Leroy J. Specific quantitation of heparin-dependent antibodies for the diagnosis of heparin-associated thrombocytopenia using an enzyme-linked immunosorbent assay. Thromb Res 62:377–387, 1991.

Horne MK III, Chao ES. Heparin binding to resting and activated platelets. Blood 74: 238–243, 1989.

Horsewood P, Warkentin TE, Hayward CPM, Kelton JG. The epitope specificity of heparin-induced thrombocytopenia. Br J Haematol 95:161–167, 1996.

Howe SE, Lynch DM. An enzyme-linked immunosorbent assay for the evaluation of thrombocytopenia induced by heparin. J Lab Clin Med 105:554–559, 1985.

Jeske W, Fareed J, Eschenfelder V, Iqbal O, Hoppensteadt D, Ahsan A. Biochemical and pharmacologic characteristics of reviparin, a low-molecular-mass heparin. Semin Thromb Hemost 23:119–128, 1997.

Kappa JR, Fisher CA, Berkowitz HD, Cottrell ED, Addonizio VP Jr. Heparin-induced platelet activation in sixteen surgical patients: diagnosis and management. J Vasc Surg 5:101–109, 1987.

Kapsch D, Silver D. Heparin-induced thrombocytopenia with thrombosis and hemorrhage. Arch Surg 116:1423–1427, 1981.

Kelton JG, Sheridan D, Brain H, Powers PJ, Turpie AG, Carter CJ. Clinical usefulness of testing for a heparin-dependent platelet-aggregating factor in patients with suspected heparin-associated thrombocytopenia. J Lab Clin Med 103:606–612, 1984.

Kelton JG, Sheridan D, Santos A, Smith J, Steeves K, Smith C, Brown C, Murphy WG. Heparin-induced thrombocytopenia: laboratory studies. Blood 72:925–930, 1988.

Kikta MJ, Keller MP, Humphrey PW, Silver D. Can low molecular weight heparins and heparinoids be safely given to patients with heparin-induced thrombocytopenia syndrome? Surgery 114:705–710, 1993.

Kinlough-Rathbone RL, Packham MA, Mustard JF. Platelet aggregation. In: Harker LA, Zimmerman TS, eds. Methods in Hematology: Measurements of Platelet Function. Edinburgh: Churchill Livingstone, 1983:64–91.

Lee DP, Warkentin TE, Denomme GA, Hayward CPM, Kelton JG. A diagnostic test for heparin-induced thrombocytopenia: detection of platelet microparticles using flow cytometry. Br J Haematol 95:724–731, 1996.

Leach MF, Ammann J, AuBuchon JP. Comparison of solid-phase and standard techniques for detection of drug-dependent platelet antibodies [abstr]. Transfusion 34(suppl): 17S, 1994.

Leach MF, Cooper LK, AuBuchon JP. Detection of drug-dependent platelet antibodies by use of solid-phase red cell adherence techniques. Immunohematology 11:143–149, 1995.

Leach MF, Cooper LK, AuBuchon JP. Detection of drug-dependent, platelet-reactive antibodies by solid-phase red cell adherence assays. Br J Haematol 97:755–761, 1997.

Look KA, Sahud M, Flaherty S, Zehnder JL. Heparin-induced platelet aggregation vs. platelet factor 4 enzyme-linked immunosorbent assay in the diagnosis of heparin-induced thrombocytopenia–thrombosis. Am J Clin Pathol 108:78–82, 1997.

Lynch DM, Howe SE. Heparin-associated thrombocytopenia: antibody binding specificity to platelet antigens. Blood 66:1176–1181, 1985.

Makhoul RG, Greenberg CS, McCann RL. Heparin-induced thrombocytopenia and thrombosis: a serious clinical problem and potential solution. J Vasc Surg 4:522–528, 1986.

Mustard JF, Perry DW, Ardlie NG, Packham MA. Preparation of suspensions of washed platelets from humans. Br J Haematol 22:193–204, 1972.

Nagi PK, Ackermann F, Wendt H, Savoca R, Bosshard HR. Protein A antibody-capture ELISA (PACE): an ELISA format to avoid denaturation of surface-adsorbed antigens. J Immunol Methods 158:267–276, 1993.

Newman PM, Swanson RL, Chong BH. Heparin-induced thrombocytopenia: IgG binding to PF4–heparin complexes in the fluid phase and cross-reactivity with low molecular weight heparin and heparinoid. Thromb Haemost 80:292–297, 1998.

Nguyên P, Lecompte T, and Groupe d'Etude sur l'Hémostase et la Thromboses (GEHT) de la Société Française d'Hématologie. Nouv Rev Fr Hematol 36:353–357, 1994.

Nguyên P, Droullé C, Potron G. Comparison between platelet factor 4/heparin complexes ELISA and platelet aggregation test in heparin-induced thrombocytopenia [letter]. Thromb Haemost 74:793–810, 1995.

Packham MA, Guccione MA, Perry DW. ADP does not release platelet granule contents in a plasma-free system [abstr]. Fed Proc 30:201, 1971.

Pengo V, Biasiolo A, Fior MG. Autoimmune antiphospholipid antibodies are directed against a cryptic epitope expressed when β_2-glycoprotein I is bound to a suitable surface. Thromb Haemost 73:29–34, 1995.

Pfueller SL, David R. Different platelet specificities of heparin-dependent platelet aggregating factors in heparin-induced thrombocytopenia. Br J Haematol 64:149–159, 1986.

Polgár J, Eichler P, Greinacher A, Clemetson KJ. Adenosine diphosphate (ADP) and ADP receptor play a major role in platelet activation/aggregation induced by sera from heparin-induced thrombocytopenia patients. Blood 91:549–554, 1998.

Pötzsch B, Keller M, Madlener K, Müller-Berghaus G. The use of heparinase improves the specificity of crossreactivity testing in heparin-induced thrombocytopenia [letter]. Thromb Haemost 76:1118–1122, 1996.

Rhodes GR, Dixon RH, Silver D. Heparin induced thrombocytopenia with thrombotic and hemorrhagic manifestations. Surg Gynecol Obstet 136:409–416, 1973.

Salem HH, van der Weyden MB. Heparin induced thrombocytopenia. Variable platelet-rich plasma reactivity to heparin dependent platelet aggregating factor. Pathology 15:297–299, 1983.

Salzman EW, Rosenberg RD, Smith MH, Lindon JN, Favreau L. Effect of heparin and heparin fractions on platelet aggregation. J Clin Invest 65:64–73, 1980.

Schnell MK, Giordano KJ, Henry M, Munizza M, Nance S, Murphy S, Warkentin TE. Diagnosis of heparin-induced thrombocytopenia (HIT): comparison of methods. Transfusion 38(suppl):98S, 1998.

Sheridan D, Carter C, Kelton JG. A diagnostic test for heparin-induced thrombocytopenia. Blood 67:27–30, 1986.

Silberman S, Kovarik P. Heparin-induced thrombocytopenia: use of indirect immunofluorescence. Ann Clin Lab Sci 17:106–110, 1987.

Sinor LT, Stone DL, Plapp FV, Rachel JM, Thompson KS. Detection of heparin-IgG immune complexes on platelets by solid phase red cell adherence assays. Immunocorrespondence 4:1–6, 1990.

Sinor LT, Stone DL. Serological confirmation of heparin-induced thrombocytopenia. Clin Hemost Rev 8:9–10, 1994.

Stewart MW, Etches WS, Boshkov LK, Gordon PA. Heparin-induced thrombocytopenia: an improved method of detection based on lumi-aggregometry. Br J Haematol 91: 173–177, 1995.

Teitel JM, Gross P, Blake P, Garvey MB. A bioluminescent adenosine nucleotide release assay for the diagnosis of heparin-induced thrombocytopenia [letter]. Thromb Haemost 76:479, 1996.

Tomer A. A sensitive and specific functional flow cytometric assay for the diagnosis of heparin-induced thrombocytopenia. Br J Haematol 98:648–656, 1997.

Tomer A, Masalunga C, Abshire TC. Determination of heparin-induced thrombocytopenia: a rapid flow cytometric assay for direct demonstration of antibody-mediated platelet activation. Am J Hematol 61:53–61, 1999.

Visentin GP, Ford SE, Scott JP, Aster RH. Antibodies from patients with heparin-induced thrombocytopenia/thrombosis are specific for platelet factor 4 complexed with heparin or bound to endothelial cells. J Clin Invest 93:81–88, 1994.

Visentin GP, Moghaddam M, Collins JL, McFarland JG, Aster RH. Antibodies associated with heparin-induced thrombocytopenia (HIT) report conformational changes in platelet factor 4 (PF4) induced by linear polyanionic compounds [abstr]. Blood 90(suppl 1):460a, 1997.

Vun CH, Evans S, Chong BH. Cross-reactivity study of low molecular weight heparin and heparinoid in heparin-induced thrombocytopenia. Thromb Res 81:525–532, 1996.

Warkentin TE. Danaparoid (Orgaran) for the treatment of heparin-induced thrombocytopenia (HIT) and thrombosis: effects on in vivo thrombin and cross-linked fibrin generation, and evaluation of the clinical significance of in vitro cross-reactivity (XR) of danaparoid for HIT-IgG [abstr]. Blood 88(suppl 1):626a, 1996.

Warkentin TE. Heparin-induced thrombocytopenia: pathogenesis, frequency, avoidance and management. Drug Safety 17:325–341, 1997.

Warkentin TE, Hayward CPM, Smith CA, Kelly PM, Kelton JG. Determinants of platelet variability when testing for heparin-induced thrombocytopenia. J Lab Clin Med 120:371–379, 1992.

Warkentin TE, Hayward CPM, Boshkov LK, Santos AV, Sheppard JI, Bode AP, Kelton JG. Sera from patients with heparin-induced thrombocytopenia generate platelet-derived microparticles with procoagulant activity: an explanation for the thrombotic complications of heparin-induced thrombocytopenia. Blood 84:3691–3699, 1994.

Warkentin TE, Levine MN, Hirsh J, Horsewood P, Roberts RS, Gent M, Kelton JG. Heparin-induced thrombocytopenia in patients treated with low-molecular-weight heparin or unfractionated heparin. N Engl J Med 332:1330–1335, 1995.

Warkentin TE, Simpson PJ, Sheppard JI, Moore JC, Horsewood P, Kelton JG. Importance of patient population in the frequency of HIT: a comparison of activation and antigen assays [abstr]. Thromb Haemost 82(suppl):363–364, 1999.

White MM, Siders L, Jennings LK, White FL. The effect of residual heparin on the interpretation of heparin-induced platelet aggregation in the diagnosis of heparin-associated thrombocytopenia [letter]. Thromb Haemost 68:88, 1992.

Wolf H, Nowack H, Wick G. Detection of antibodies interacting with glycosaminoglycan polysulfate in patients treated with heparin or other polysulfated glycosaminoglycans. Int Arch Allergy Appl Immunol 70:157–163, 1983.

12
Pseudo-Heparin-Induced Thrombocytopenia

Theodore E. Warkentin
McMaster University and Hamilton Health Sciences Corporation, Hamilton, Ontario, Canada

I. INTRODUCTION

A. The Concept of Pseudo-HIT

Heparin-induced thrombocytopenia (HIT) is strongly associated with life- and limb-threatening venous and arterial thrombosis, including pulmonary embolism, venous limb gangrene, and large vessel arterial occlusion. However, HIT is by no means a unique explanation for the combination of thrombocytopenia and thrombosis (Table 1).

In these pseudo-HIT disorders, thrombocytopenia usually occurs early during the course of heparin treatment. This could reflect the prothrombotic process associated with the patient's primary diagnosis. Alternatively, heparin could exacerbate the platelet count fall by nonimmune proaggregatory effects on platelets (see Chap. 5). If the patient previously received heparin, physicians might consider HIT in the differential diagnosis of the platelet count fall.

However, one pseudo-HIT syndrome in particular closely resembles even the typical day 5 to 10 timing of thrombocytopenia characteristic of HIT: adenocarcinoma-associated disseminated intravascular coagulation (DIC). In these patients, the fall in platelet count begins soon after stopping heparin treatment. Because the patients usually will have received heparin for 5–10 days to treat adenocarcinoma-associated thrombosis, the timing of the onset of thrombocytopenia closely resembles immune HIT. Furthermore, the frequent occurrence of new or progressive thrombosis in this setting also suggests HIT.

This chapter draws attention to those clinical disorders that can mimic and, thereby, be confused with, HIT. This is not a trivial distinction: whereas heparin

Table 1 Pseudo-HIT Disorders Characterized by Thrombocytopenia and Thrombosis

Pseudo-HIT disorder	Pathogenesis of thrombocytopenia and thrombosis	Timing
Adenocarcinoma	DIC secondary to procoagulant material(s) produced by neoplastic cells	Late[a]
Pulmonary embolism	Platelet activation by clot-bound thrombin	Early[b] or late[c]
Diabetic ketoacidosis	Hyperaggregable platelets in ketoacidosis (?)	Early[d]
Antiphospholipid antibody syndrome	Multiple mechanisms described, including platelet activation by antiphospholipid antibodies (?)	Early
Thrombolytic therapy	Platelet activation by thrombin bound to fibrin degradation products (?)	Early[e]
Infective endocarditis	Infection-associated thrombocytopenia; ischemic events secondary to septic emboli	Early
Paroxysmal nocturnal hemoglobinuria	Platelets susceptible to complement-mediated damage; platelet hypoproduction	Early
Posttransfusion purpura (PTP)	'Pseudospecific' alloantibody-mediated platelet destruction (exception: bleeding, not thrombosis)	Late[f]

These pseudo-HIT disorders can mimic HIT by causing thrombocytopenia and thrombosis in association with heparin treatment. An exception is PTP, which causes bleeding, but not thrombosis; however, PTP can resemble HIT because both disorders usually occur about a week after major surgery requiring blood and postoperative heparin. The pseudo-HIT disorders can be categorized based on whether the onset of thrombocytopenia is typically "early" (< 5 days) or "late" (≥ 5 days) in relation to the heparin.

[a] See Fig. 1 for an example of pseudo-HIT caused by adenocarcinoma-associated DIC.

[b] See Fig. 2 for early thrombocytopenia associated with pulmonary embolism.

[c] See Fig. 3 for late thrombocytopenia associated with pulmonary embolism.

[d] See Fig. 4 for early thrombocytopenia associated with diabetic ketoacidosis.

[e] See Fig. 1 in Warkentin and Kelton (1994) for an example of thrombocytopenia caused by thrombolytic therapy.

[f] See Fig. 5 in Chap. 3 for an illustrative case in which PTP vs. HIT was the major differential diagnosis.

is contraindicated in patients with HIT, it often is the optimal treatment of patients with pseudo-HIT. Second, the close clinical parallels between HIT and certain pseudo-HIT disorders can provide insights into the pathogenesis of thrombosis. For example, the recognition that venous limb gangrene can complicate metastatic adenocarcinoma, and the clinical parallels with a similar syndrome in HIT patients, suggests that a common factor (coumarin anticoagulation) may play a crucial pathogenic role in both disorders (Warkentin, 1999). Likewise, similarities between HIT and the lupus anticoagulant syndrome suggest that they could also share common pathogenic mechanisms (Arnout, 1996).

II. PSEUDO-HIT SYNDROMES

A. Adenocarcinoma

Mucin-producing adenocarcinoma is an important cause of venous and arterial thrombosis that occurs in association with thrombocytopenia. In these patients, DIC is often the explanation for the thrombocytopenia. The diagnosis is suggested by reduced fibrinogen levels (or prolonged thrombin time), elevated prothrombin time, and elevated cross-linked (D-dimer) fibrin degradation products (or a positive protamine sulfate paracoagulation test).

Adenocarcinoma-associated DIC can strongly resemble HIT (Fig. 1). Typically, a patient presents with idiopathic deep vein thrombosis (DVT), sometimes with mild to moderate thrombocytopenia. During treatment with therapeutic-dose

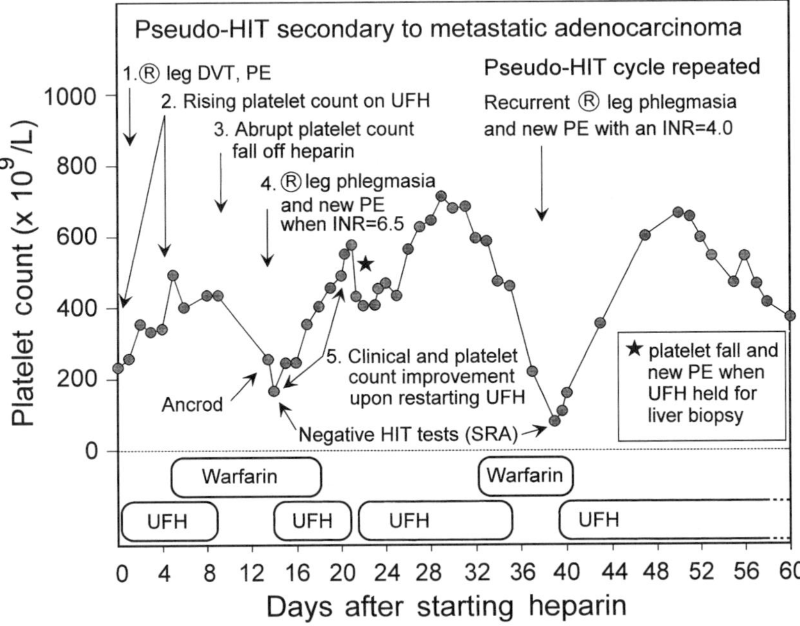

Figure 1 Pseudo-HIT: Adenocarcinoma with thrombocytopenia and phlegmasia cerulea dolens after stopping administration of unfractionated heparin (UFH). The late presentation of thrombocytopenia suggested HIT, prompting use of an alternative anticoagulant (ancrod). Heparin was restarted when HIT antibodies were not detected by serotonin-release assay (SRA). Subsequently, discontinuation of heparin led to recurrence of thrombocytopenia and warfarin-associated phlegmasia cerulea dolens (repeat of pseudo-HIT cycle). Abbreviations: DVT, deep venous thrombosis; INR, international normalized ratio; PE, pulmonary embolism.

heparin, the platelet count rises, likely because of improved control of DIC by the heparin. In my experience, this oftentimes dramatic rise in the platelet count during heparin treatment of ''idiopathic'' DVT is a clinically useful marker for adenocarcinoma-associated DIC. During the 5- to 10-day period of heparin treatment with overlapping warfarin anticoagulation, no problems are encountered. However, there is rapid recurrence of thrombocytopenia within hours or days of discontinuing the heparin, despite apparent therapeutic anticoagulation with warfarin, during which time the patient develops new or progressive venous, or even arterial, thrombosis. Thus, the onset of thrombocytopenia and thrombosis generally occurs within the 5- to 10-day ''window'' that suggests HIT.

Venous Limb Gangrene Complicating Adenocarcinoma

The venous thrombotic events complicating adenocarcinoma include DVT, phlegmasia cerulea dolens, and even venous limb gangrene (Everett and Jones, 1986; Adamson et al., 1993). Clinical and laboratory parallels between HIT and adenocarcinoma suggest that, paradoxically, coumarin treatment could contribute to the pathogenesis of venous gangrene in these patients through a disturbance in procoagulant–anticoagulant balance (Warkentin, 1996, 1999). Table 2 summarizes the proposed pathogenesis of this syndrome from the perspective of the characteristic clinical triad of venous limb gangrene: (1) thrombocytopenia

Table 2 Clinical Triad of Coumarin-Induced Venous Limb Gangrene

A: Underlying disorder associated with platelet and coagulation system activation	B: Active deep vein thrombosis (DVT)	C. Supratherapeutic International Normalized Ratio (INR)
Heparin-induced thrombocytopenia: HIT–IgG-induced platelet activation; activation of coagulation by procoagulant, platelet-derived microparticles	1. Direct propagation of thrombi from large to small vessels	1. High INR is a surrogate marker for severe reduction in protein C (activated protein C protects microvasculature from thrombin)
Adenocarcinoma: cancer-induced DIC resulting in thrombin-induced platelet activation	2. Stasis (predisposes to thrombosis distal to active DVT)	2. Persisting thrombin generation despite elevated INR

Features A, B, and C represent the clinical triad of coumarin-induced venous limb gangrene.
Source: Warkentin, 1996; 1999, Warkentin, et al., 1997.

caused by HIT or adenocarcinoma-associated DIC; (2) active DVT before the use of coumarin or the onset of venous limb gangrene; and (3) a supratherapeutic international normalized ratio (INR).

Venous limb gangrene appears to result from failure of the protein C anticoagulant pathway to regulate thrombin generation within the microvasculature (Warkentin 1996; Warkentin et al., 1997; see Chap. 3). Here, the elevated INR may represent a surrogate marker for marked reduction in functional protein C levels (by a parallel reduction in factor VII); the thrombocytopenia is a surrogate marker for uncontrolled thrombin generation associated either with HIT or adenocarcinoma (see Table 2). As venous limb gangrene occurs in a limb with preceding active DVT, this suggests that local factors, such as direct extension of thrombosis, as well as exacerbation of distal thrombosis by venous stasis, contribute to large- and small-vessel thrombosis characteristic of this syndrome.

Venous thrombosis complicating adènocarcinoma, especially when complicated by DIC or severe venous ischemia or necrosis, should be treated with heparin, rather than warfarin or other coumarin anticoagulants. Reversal of warfarin anticoagulation (with vitamin K and plasma infusion, but not with prothrombin complex concentrates, as these do not contain sufficient protein C) and prompt control of DIC with heparin, could salvage a limb with severe phlegmasia, or limit damage in a patient with venous gangrene. An effective agent often is low molecular weight heparin (Prandoni, 1997). I recommend intermittent monitoring using antifactor Xa levels, because some patients with heparin resistance require high doses of LMWH to achieve therapeutic anticoagulation.

Ironically, one of the problems of heparin in these patients is its efficacy: thus, if heparin is discontinued for any reason, rapid recurrence of thrombocytopenia and thrombosis can result. Figure 1 shows an example in which thrombocytopenia and pulmonary embolism occurred (day 21) when heparin was held for a few hours to permit a liver biopsy to diagnose metastatic carcinoma. I have also observed a patient with lung adenocarcinoma in whom heparin was held to permit limb amputation; postanesthesia, the patient was aphasic (intraoperative stroke). Often, recurrent thrombosis is as ''malignant'' as the cancer itself.

B. Pulmonary Embolism

Mild thrombocytopenia is common in patients with pulmonary embolism. Sometimes, the thrombocytopenia is severe, and associated with laboratory markers of DIC (Stahl et al., 1984; Mustafa et al., 1989; Fig. 2). The thrombocytopenia presumably results from thrombin-induced platelet activation. Large thromboemboli within the high-flow pulmonary vessels may act as a reservoir for clot-bound thrombin that is relatively protected from inhibition by antithrombin-dependent

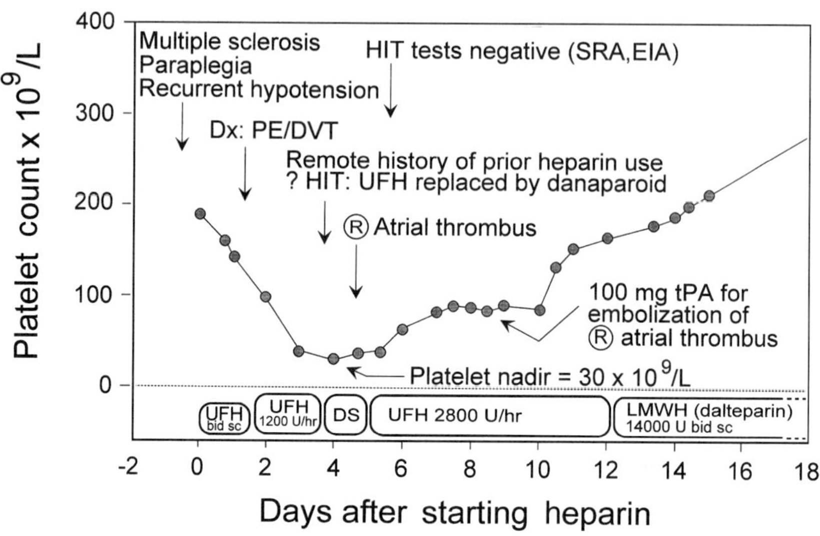

Figure 2 Pseudo-HIT secondary to pulmonary embolism and DIC: An obese, 50-year-old man with paraplegia was admitted for recurrent hypotension. He initially received twice-daily (b.i.d.) subcutaneous (sc), unfractionated heparin (UFH) for antithrombotic prophylaxis, as the initial diagnosis was septicemia. Deep vein thrombosis (DVT) and pulmonary embolism (PE) were then diagnosed (Dx), and therapy changed to intravenous UFH, 1200 U/h. The platelet count fell over 4 days to a nadir of 30×10^9/L; danaparoid sodium (DS) was given because of concern over possible HIT (there was a remote history of previous heparin use). An echocardiogram showed large right atrial thrombus (likely representing a leg vein embolus), and the patient was transferred to a cardiac surgical center. The platelet count fall was judged too rapid to be HIT (see Chap. 3), a viewpoint supported by negative testing for HIT antibodies by serotonin-release assay (SRA) and PF4–heparin enzyme-linked immunosorbent assay (EIA). UFH administration was restarted in higher doses with antifactor Xa monitoring to overcome heparin resistance. Recurrent hypotension occurred when the right atrial thrombus embolized; full hemodynamic and platelet count recovery occurred following tissue plasminogen activator (t-PA) administration, followed by UFH, then low molecular weight heparin (LMWH), and (later) warfarin treatment. The patient was well at 1-year follow-up, without evidence for carcinoma.

inhibitors (Weitz et al., 1990). This view is indirectly supported by the observation that thrombocytopenia commonly occurs in patients with pulmonary embolism, but not in patients with DVT alone (Monreal et al., 1991).

Because HIT also is strongly associated with pulmonary embolism (Warkentin et al., 1995), a diagnostic and therapeutic dilemma results when a patient presents with pulmonary embolism and thrombocytopenia 5 or more days after surgery managed with postoperative heparin prophylaxis (Fig. 3). Initiating therapeutic heparin could have catastrophic consequences for the patient who has circulating HIT antibodies, although in sufficient doses, it is effective for a patient with pulmonary embolism and DIC without HIT. Because these two possibilities cannot be readily distinguished on clinical grounds alone, one should manage such a patient with an alternative anticoagulant until the results of HIT antibody testing become available.

C. Diabetic Ketoacidosis

Diabetic ketoacidosis (DKA) can be associated with acute thromboembolic complications. Evidence for in vivo platelet activation was observed in one study of ten patients who had elevated plasma levels of platelet factor 4 and β-thromboglobulin during DKA that resolved following recovery (Campbell et al., 1985). Figure 4 illustrates a patient with ''white clots'' in the femoral artery, leading to amputation, who was initially thought to have HIT. However, HIT antibody testing and subsequent clinical events proved that the patient did not have HIT as the initial explanation for this dramatic clinical presentation of thrombocytopenia and thrombosis complicating DKA (although HIT occurred later in the clinical course). I am also aware of a patient with essential thrombocythemia who developed postoperative DKA, thrombocytopenia, and bilateral lower limb artery thrombosis that occurred too early during UFH prophylaxis (days 2–3) to have been caused by immune HIT.

D. Antiphospholipid Antibody Syndrome or Lupus Anticoagulant Syndrome

Clinical Features

Antiphospholipid antibodies can be detected either as ''lupus anticoagulants'' or as anticardiolipin antibodies (Ginsberg et al., 1995; Asherson et al., 1989; see Chap. 11). Antiphospholipid antibody syndrome (APLAS) is characterized by increased risk for thrombosis and recurrent fetal loss: limb or intra-abdominal vein thrombosis, dural sinus thrombosis, nonatheromatous arterial thrombosis, cardiac valvulitis, and microvascular thrombosis (e.g., acrocyanosis, digital ulceration or gangrene, livedo reticularis) are described (Hojnik et al., 1996; Gibson et al., 1997). Many patients have thrombocytopenia (Morgan et al., 1993; Galli et al., 1996), which is typically mild and intermittent. The explanation for thrombocytopenia is uncertain: some patients have platelet-reactive autoantibodies (Galli et al., 1994; Lipp et al., 1998), but platelet-activating effects of IgG are also suspected.

The explanation for the prothrombotic tendency of APLAS is also elusive.

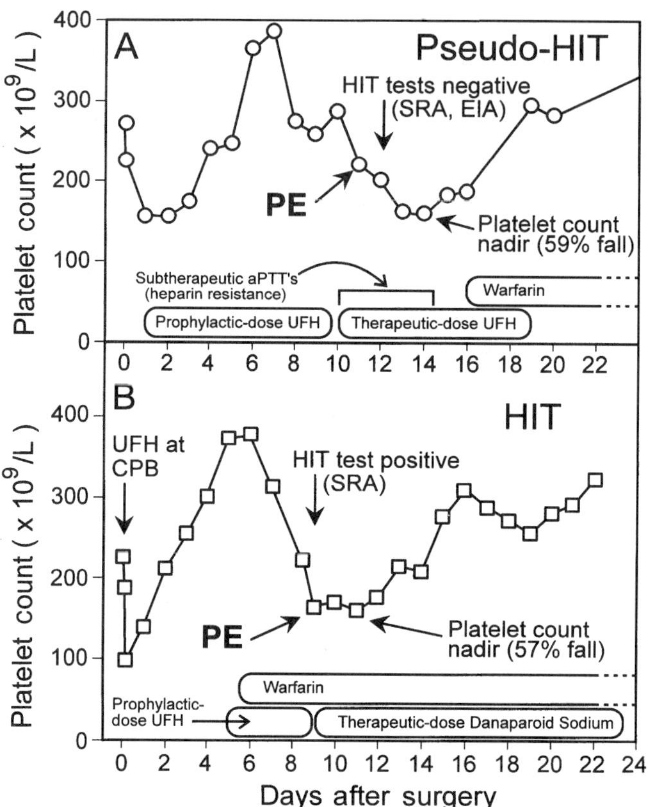

Figure 3 Pseudo-HIT associated with pulmonary embolism versus HIT: (A) A patient developed a platelet count fall from 387 to 159 × 10^9/L (59% fall) that began on day 7 of UFH prophylaxis following orthopedic surgery. Pulmonary embolism (PE) was diagnosed by pulmonary angiography on postoperative day 11. The platelet count fell during initial intravenous heparin therapy, rising only when sufficient UFH was given (2360 U/h) to overcome ''heparin resistance'' (as shown by subtherapeutic activated partial thromboplastin times, aPTTs). HIT antibodies were not detectable (day 12), either by serotonin-release assay (SRA, < 5% release) or PF4–heparin–EIA (optical density, 0.149; negative, < 0.450). (B) A platelet count profile similar to that seen in Fig. 3A also occurred in a patient who developed a platelet count fall from 378 to 161 × 10^9/L (57% fall) that began on day 7 after cardiac surgery in which unfractionated heparin (UFH) was given for cardiopulmonary bypass (CPB). The platelet count recovered on therapeutic-dose danaparoid. Only one clinical clue pointed to the diagnosis of HIT: erythematous skin lesions at the UFH injection sites were also observed on day 7 (not shown on figure). Testing for HIT antibodies was strongly positive in the SRA (98% release at 0.1 U/mL heparin; 0% release at 100 U/mL heparin and at 0.1 U/mL heparin in the presence of Fc receptor-blocking monoclonal antibody). The similar platelet count profiles between these patients illustrate the difficulty in determining on clinical grounds whether postoperative PE is caused by HIT or not.

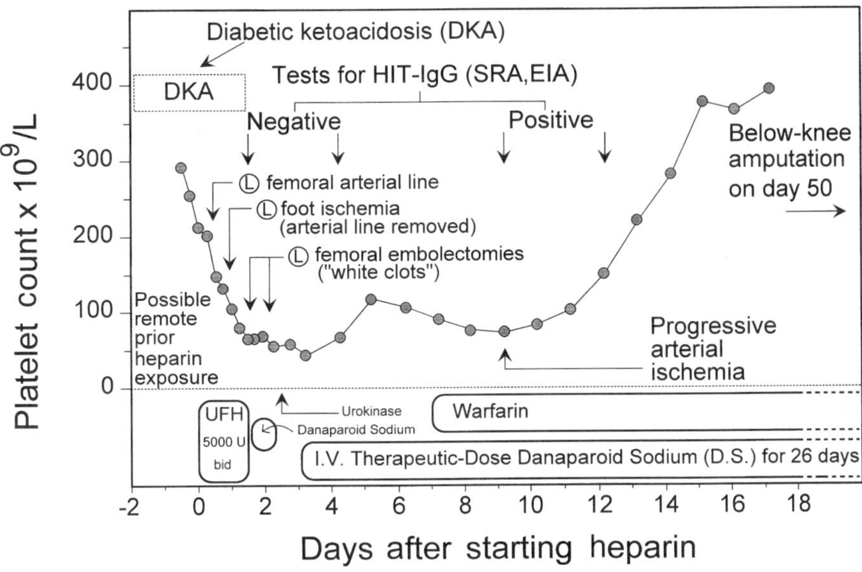

Figure 4 Pseudo-HIT during diabetic ketoacidosis (DKA), later complicated by HIT: A 27-year-old man developed rapid onset of thrombocytopenia and white clots in the left femoral artery (at a femoral artery catheter site) during management of DKA that included prophylactic-dose unfractionated heparin (UFH). HIT was suspected erroneously on the basis of a possible previous remote heparin exposure (gastric surgery 10 years earlier). The patient underwent two embolectomies as well as treatment with urokinase and intravenous (iv) danaparoid. The patient developed a second platelet count fall during danaparoid treatment that began on day 6 in relation to the initial course of UFH. Tests for HIT antibodies changed from negative (serotonin-release assay [SRA]: days 1 and 4, serotonin release $< 5\%$) to positive (days 9 and 12, serotonin release 92% and 80%, respectively). By PF4/heparin–EIA (set up to detect IgG antibodies), the day 1 sample also was negative (O.D., 0.262; negative, less than 0.450), the day 4 sample was weakly positive (0.804), and the day 9 and 12 samples were strongly positive (1.863 and 1.002, respectively). Although the possibility of in vivo cross-reactivity of danaparoid with the HIT antibodies is suggested by the thrombocytopenia and progression of limb ischemia, the platelet count subsequently rose during danaparoid treatment, and no additional thromboembolic events occurred. In vitro cross-reactivity was detected on the day 9, but not the day 12, blood sample.

A multifactorial pathogenesis is likely, because the antibodies recognize complexes of negatively charged phospholipid with many different protein cofactors, such as β_2-glycoprotein I (β_2GP I), prothrombin, protein C, protein S, and annexin V (Galli, 1996; Triplett, 1996; see Chap. 2). Indeed, interference with endothelial cell function, impaired fibrinolysis, disturbances in protein C anticoagulant pathway activities, and antibody-mediated platelet activation, all have been described (for review see Petri, 1997).

Parallels Between APLAS and HIT

Tablc 3 lists some common features of APLAS and HIT. Both clinicopathologic disorders are characterized by thrombocytopenia, a paradoxical risk for venous and arterial thrombosis, and associated antibodies that can be detected by either functional or antigen assays (see Chap. 11). The parallels between these disorders led Arnout (1996) to hypothesize that IgG-mediated platelet activation could explain thrombosis in APLAS. Supportive experimental data include the observations that antiphospholipid antibodies enhance platelet activation induced by other agonists (Martinuzzo et al., 1993). Furthermore, Arvieux et al. (1993) observed that murine monoclonal antibodies reactive against β_2GP I induced platelet activation in the presence of subthreshold concentrations of ADP and epineph-

Table 3 Clinical Parallels Between HIT and APLAS

	Heparin-induced thrombocytopenia (HIT)	Antiphospholipid antibody syndrome (APLAS)
Thrombotic paradox	Thrombosis despite thrombocytopenia	Thrombosis despite prolonged coagulation tests (± thrombocytopenia)
Spectrum of thrombotic events	Venous > arterial thrombosis; adrenal infarction, dural sinus thrombosis	Venous > arterial thrombosis; adrenal infarction, dural sinus thrombosis
Severity of thrombocytopenia	Mild to moderate thrombocytopenia	Mild to moderate thrombocytopenia
Laboratory diagnosis by (1) functional or (2) antigen assays	(1) Platelet activation assays (e.g., serotonin release assay, heparin-induced platelet activation test); (2) platelet factor 4–heparin–EIA	(1) Lupus anticoagulant (i.e., prolonged phospholipid-dependent coagulation assay in presence of patient plasma); (2) anticardiolipin–EIA
Pathogenesis	Platelet activation by platelet Fc receptors; endothelial activation by immune injury	Uncertain pathogenesis: immune platelet activation and endothelial injury are possible factors

Further laboratory parallels between HIT and APLAS are discussed in Chap. 11.
Abbreviations: EIA, enzyme-linked immunosorbent assay.

rine, an effect dependent on binding to platelet FcγIIa receptors. However, other workers were unable to demonstrate enhanced platelet activation in the presence of IgG antiphospholipid antibodies (Shi et al., 1993; Ford et al., 1998).

Thrombocytopenia in Patients with APLAS Receiving Heparin

In retrospective studies, Auger and colleagues (1995) reported that platelet counts typically fell by about 50% in patients with chronic thromboembolic disease and the lupus anticoagulant who were treated with heparin. Neither timing of the onset of thrombocytopenia, nor results of specific antigen or activation assays for HIT antibodies were reported, so it remains uncertain whether these patients had (immune) HIT. It is possible that nonidiosyncratic platelet activation caused by heparin could increase the thrombocytopenic potential of antiphospholipid antibodies in the absence of HIT antibodies. Alternatively, some patients with APLAS may have circulating HIT antibodies in the absence of recent heparin exposure (Lasne et al., 1997).

E. Thrombolytic Therapy

Acute thrombocytopenia is common in patients treated with streptokinase, especially when combined with heparin (Balduini et al., 1993). This could represent a direct, activating stimulus of heparin on platelets that perhaps is exacerbated by procoagulant effects of thrombolytic therapy. For example, fibrin degradation products generated by thrombolytic agents bind and protect thrombin from inhibition by heparin (Weitz et al., 1998). Such a mechanism could explain thrombocytopenia after use of any thrombolytic drug.

However, some investigators have reported that plasma containing antistreptokinase antibodies can activate platelets through their Fc receptors in the presence of streptokinase (Vaughan et al., 1988; Lebrazi et al., 1995). Thus, high-titer antistreptokinase antibodies found in some normal individuals could explain the occasional occurrence of thrombocytopenia and thrombosis following treatment with streptokinase.

F. Infective Endocarditis

Infective endocarditis is frequently complicated by thrombocytopenia. These patients are also at risk for septic emboli manifesting as stroke, myocardial infarction, renal infarction, or even acute limb ischemia (de Gennes et al., 1990). Thus, the profile of macrovascular thrombosis and thrombocytopenia characteristic of HIT can be mimicked, especially as heparin is often used to anticoagulate patients with septic endocarditis (Delahaye et al., 1990). Microembolization leading to multiple small infarcts or microabscesses, in such organs as muscles, adrenal glands, and spleen, is an additional feature of endocarditis (Ting et al., 1990) that is not seen in HIT.

G. Paroxysmal Nocturnal Hemoglobinuria

Paroxysmal nocturnal hemoglobinuria (PNH) is a clonal myeloid disorder characterized by an acquired defect in the X-linked phosphatidylinositol glycan class A (PIG-A) gene, leading to loss of cell surface glycosylphosphatidylinositol (GPI)-anchored proteins (for review see Rosse, 1997). Loss of the complement-regulating GP I-linked surface proteins, decay-accelerating factor, and membrane attack complex inhibitory factor), causes the red cells to be exquisitely sensitive to complement-mediated hemolysis. Some patients have thrombocytopenia, and an increased risk for unusual, life-threatening venous thrombotic events, such as hepatic vein thrombosis, occurs in some patients. Thus, the clinical profile of HIT potentially can be mimicked. The thrombocytopenia could be related either to decreased platelet production or to complement-mediated formation of procoagulant platelet microparticles (Wiedmer et al., 1993).

H. Posttransfusion Purpura

Posttransfusion purpura (PTP) is a rare syndrome characterized by severe thrombocytopenia and mucocutaneous bleeding that begins 5–10 days after blood transfusion, usually red cell concentrates. More than 95% of affected patients are older women, in keeping with its pathogenesis of an anamnestic recurrence of platelet-specific alloantibodies in women previously sensitized by pregnancy. Destruction of autologous platelets is believed to result from the pseudospecificity of the alloimmune response, e.g., the high-titer anti-HPA-1a alloantibodies (the most frequent cause of the syndrome) probably somewhat recognize the autologous HPA-1b alloantigen (see Chap. 2).

Because both PTP and HIT typically occur about a week after surgery managed with perioperative blood transfusions and postoperative heparin prophylaxis, a diagnostic dilemma can arise. A useful clinical clue is the presence or absence of petechiae: PTP almost invariably is characterized by this hallmark of severe thrombocytopenia, whereas patients with HIT generally do not develop petechiae, even if they have very severe thrombocytopenia (see Fig. 5, Chap. 3).

III. RECOGNITION AND TREATMENT OF PSEUDO-HIT

Many patients with pseudo-HIT can be distinguished from HIT because of the early onset of thrombocytopenia (see Table 1). Unless the patient received heparin within the past 100 days, the early platelet count fall is strong evidence against HIT (see Chap. 3). These patients with pseudo-HIT should be further anticoagulated with heparin.

However, for patients with adenocarcinoma-associated DIC, or postoperative pulmonary embolism, in whom the platelet count fall can occur after 5 days

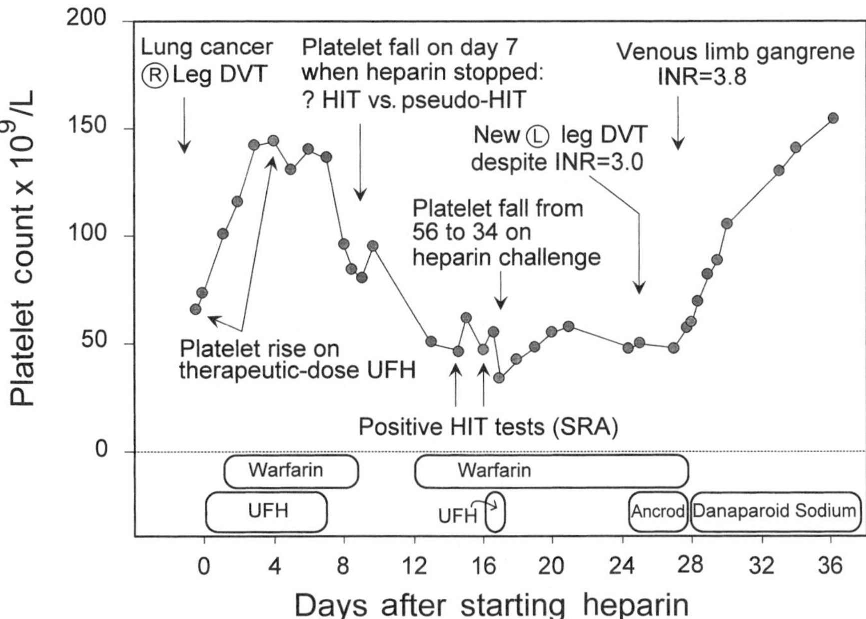

Figure 5 Pseudo-HIT complicated by HIT: A 78-year-old man, with right proximal lower limb deep venous thrombosis (DVT) and thrombocytopenia, developed progressive platelet count increase during therapeutic-dose UFH treatment. Recurrent thrombocytopenia developed after UFH was stopped, and when the patient was anticoagulated with warfarin. A liver biopsy on day 9 showed metastatic adenocarcinoma (primary lung neoplasm), and adenocarcinoma-associated disseminated intravascular coagulation (DIC) was diagnosed. However, a heparin challenge produced a further platelet count fall; HIT antibody testing was strongly positive (serotonin-release assay [SRA]: 88% serotonin release at 0.1 U/mL heparin; $<$ 15% release at 0 and 100 U/mL heparin). Subsequently, the patient developed new left-sided DVT, as well as venous gangrene of the left foot during treatment with warfarin and ancrod (peak INR = 3.8). Although the clinical course was initially identical with pseudo-HIT (rising platelet count on heparin therapy; abrupt platelet count fall after heparin administration was stopped), the subsequent heparin-induced fall in the platelet count, and strong positive HIT test results, indicate the patient also had HIT.

of heparin treatment, the diagnosis will be initially uncertain. As heparin can cause catastrophic complications if HIT is the underlying cause, and as two alternative anticoagulants (danaparoid and lepirudin) are available in most countries, treatment with one of these agents before obtaining results of HIT antibody testing should be considered. For patients with adenocarcinoma without HIT antibodies, longer-term management is often more successful with LMWH or UFH than with warfarin (Prandoni, 1997).

A. Pseudo-HIT Complicated by HIT

Heparin-induced thrombocytopenia is a relatively common complication of heparin therapy. It may be even more common in patients who have baseline platelet activation and PF4 release, as occurs in adenocarcinoma-associated DIC or diabetic ketoacidosis. Therefore, a patient with early thrombocytopenia attributable to a pseudo-HIT disorder may subsequently develop clinically significant HIT antibodies (see Fig. 4). Another example is that of a patient with lung cancer and DVT who developed a platelet count rise during intravenous heparin therapy, followed by recurrent thrombocytopenia and, ultimately, venous limb gangrene during anticoagulation with warfarin and ancrod (Fig. 5). In this situation, one might have expected platelet count recovery during a second course of heparin. However, an intravenous heparin challenge resulted in worsening of thrombocytopenia, and the patient had a strong positive assay for HIT antibodies. These patient cases emphasize the importance of a high clinical suspicion for HIT even in complex situations for which other explanations for thrombocytopenia are present. The wider availability of assays for HIT antibodies should help clinicians better diagnose and manage patients who develop thrombocytopenia and thrombosis during or shortly following heparin treatment.

REFERENCES

Adamson DJA, Currie JM. Occult malignancy is associated with venous thrombosis unresponsive to adequate anticoagulation. Br J Clin Pract 47:190–191, 1993.

Arnout J. The pathogenesis of the antiphospholipid antibody syndrome: a hypothesis based on parallelisms with heparin-induced thrombocytopenia. Thromb Haemost 75:536–541, 1996.

Arvieux J, Roussel B, Pouzol P, Colomb MG. Platelet activating properties of murine monoclonal antibodies to beta$_2$-glycoprotein I. Thromb Haemost 70:336–341, 1993.

Asherson RA, Khamashta MA, Ordi-Ros J, Derksen RH, Machin SJ, Barquinero J, Outt HH, Harris EN, Vilardell-Torres M, Hughes GR. The ''primary'' antiphospholipid syndrome: Major clinical and serological features. Medicine 68:366–374, 1989.

Auger WR, Permpikul P, Moser KM. Lupus anticoagulant, heparin use, and thrombocytopenia in patients with chronic thromboembolic pulmonary hypertension: a preliminary report. Am J Med 99:392–396, 1995.

Balduini CL, Noris P, Bertolino G, Previtali M. Heparin modifies platelet count and function in patients who have undergone thrombolytic therapy for acute myocardial infarction [letter]. Thromb Haemost 69:522–532, 1993.

Campbell RR, Foster KJ, Stirling C, Mundy D, Reckless JPD. Paradoxical platelet behaviour in diabetic ketoacidosis. Diabetic Med 3:161–164, 1985.

De Gennes C, Souilhem J, Du LTH, Chapelon C, Raguin G, Wechsler B, Blétry O, Godeau P. Embolie artérielle des membres au cours des endocardites infectieuses sur valves natives. Presse Méd 19:1177–1181, 1990.

Delahaye JP, Poncet P, Malquarti V, Beaune J, Garé JP, Mann JM. Cerebrovascular accidents in infective endocarditis: role of anticoagulation. Eur Heart J 11:1074–1078, 1990.

Everett RN, Jones FL Jr. Warfarin-induced skin necrosis. A cutaneous sign of malignancy? Postgrad Med 79:97–103, 1986.

Ford I, Urbaniak S, Greaves M. IgG from patients with antiphospholipid syndrome binds to platelets without induction of platelet activation. Br J Haematol 102:841–849, 1998.

Galli M. Non beta$_2$-glycoprotein I cofactors for antiphospholipid antibodies. Lupus 5:388–392, 1996.

Galli M, Daldossi M, Barbui T. Anti-glycoprotein Ib/IX and IIb/IIIa antibodies in patients with antiphospholipid antibodies. Thromb Haemost 71:571–575, 1994.

Galli M, Finazzi G, Barbui T. Thrombocytopenia in the antiphospholipid syndrome. Br J Haematol 93:1–5, 1996.

Gibson GE, Su WP, Pittelkow MR. Antiphospholipid syndrome and the skin. J Am Acad Dermatol 36(pt 1):970–82, 1997.

Ginsberg JS, Wells PS, Brill-Edwards P, Donovan D, Moffatt K, Johnston M, Stevens P, Hirsh J. Antiphospholipid antibodies and venous thromboembolism. Blood 86: 3685–3691, 1995.

Hojnik M, George J, Ziporen L, Shoenfeld Y. Heart valve involvement (Libman-Sacks endocarditis) in the antiphospholipid syndrome. Circulation 93:1579–1587, 1996.

Lasne D, Saffroy R, Bachelot C, Vincenot A, Rendu F, Papo T, Aiach M, Piette J-C. Tests for heparin-induced thrombocytopenia in primary antiphospholipid syndrome [letter]. Br J Haematol 97:939, 1997.

Lebrazi J, Helft G, Abdelouahed M, Elalamy I, Mirshahi M, Samama MM, Lecompte T. Human anti-streptokinase antibodies induce platelet aggregation in an Fc receptor (CD32) dependent manner. Thromb Haemost 74:938–942, 1995.

Lipp E, von Felten A, Sax H, Müller, D, Berchtold P. Antibodies against platelet glycoproteins and antiphospholipid antibodies in autoimmune thrombocytopenia. Eur J Haematol 60:283–288, 1998.

Martinuzzo ME, Maclouf J, Carreras LO, Lévy-Toledano S. Antiphospholipid antibodies enhance thrombin-induced platelet activation and thromboxane formation. Thromb Haemost 70:667–671, 1993.

Monreal M, Lafoz E, Casals A, Ruíz J, Arias A. Platelet count and venous thromboembolism. A useful test for suspected pulmonary embolism. Chest 100:1493–1496, 1991.

Morgan M, Downs K, Chesterman CN, Biggs JC. Clinical analysis of 125 patients with the lupus anticoagulant. Aust NZ J Med 23:151–156, 1993.

Mustafa MH, Mispireta LA, Pierce LE. Occult pulmonary embolism presenting with thrombocytopenia and elevated fibrin split products. Am J Med 86:490–491, 1989.

Petri M. Pathogenesis and treatment of the antiphospholipid antibody syndrome. Adv Rheumatol 81:151–77, 1997.

Prandoni P. Antithrombotic strategies in patients with cancer. Thromb Haemost 78:141–144, 1997.

Rosse WF. Paroxysmal nocturnal hemoglobinuria as a molecular disease. Medicine 76: 63–93, 1997.

Shi W, Chong BH, Chersterman CN. β_2-Glycoprotein I is a requirement for anticardiolipin antibodies binding to activated platelets: differences with lupus anticoagulants. Blood 81:1255–1262, 1993.

Stahl RL, Javid JP, Lackner H. Unrecognized pulmonary embolism presenting as disseminated intravascular coagulation. Am J Med 76:772–778, 1984.

Ting W, Silverman NA, Arzouman DA, Levitsky S. Splenic septic emboli in endocarditis. Circulation 82(5 suppl):IV105–109, 1990.

Triplett DA. Lupus anticoagulants/antiphospholipid-protein antibodies: the great imposters. Lupus 5:431–435, 1996.

Vaughan DE, Kirshenbaum JM, Loscalzo J. Streptokinase-induced, antibody-mediated platelet aggregation: a potential cause of clot propagation in vivo. J Am Coll Cardiol 11:1343–1348, 1988.

Warkentin TE. Heparin-induced thrombocytopenia: IgG-mediated platelet activation, platelet microparticle generation, and altered procoagulant/anticoagulant balance in the pathogenesis of thrombosis and venous limb gangrene complicating heparin-induced thrombocytopenia. Transfusion Med Rev 10:249–258, 1996.

Warkentin TE. Venous limb gangrene (VLG) complicating warfarin treatment of deep-vein thrombosis (DVT) in metastatic carcinoma (abstract). Blood 1999. In press.

Warkentin TE, Kelton JG. Interaction of heparin with platelets, including heparin-induced thrombocytopenia. In: Bounameaux H, ed. Low-Molecular-Weight Heparins in Prophylaxis and Therapy of Thromboembolic Diseases. New York: Marcel Dekker, 1994:75–127.

Warkentin TE, Elavathil LJ, Hayward CPM, Johnston MA, Russett JI, Kelton JG. The pathogenesis of venous limb gangrene associated with heparin-induced thrombocytopenia. Ann Intern Med 127:804–812, 1997.

Warkentin TE, Levine MN, Hirsh J, Horsewood P, Roberts RS, Gent M, Kelton JG. Heparin-induced thrombocytopenia in patients treated with low-molecular weight heparin or unfractionated heparin. N Engl J Med 332:1330–1335, 1995.

Weitz JI, Hudoba M, Massel D, Maraganore J, Hirsh J. Clot-bound thrombin is protected from inhibition by heparin-antithrombin III but is susceptible to inactivation by antithrombin III-independent inhibitors. J Clin Invest 86:385–391, 1990.

Weitz JI, Leslie B, Hudoba M. Thrombin binds to soluble fibrin degradation products where it is protected from inhibition by heparin-antithrombin but susceptible to inactivation by antithrombin-independent inhibitors. Circulation 97:544–552, 1998.

Wiedmer T, Hall SE, Ortel TL, Kane WH, Rosse WF, Sims PJ. Complement-induced vesiculation and exposure of membrane prothrombinase sites in platelets of paroxysmal nocturnal hemoglobinuria. Blood 82:1192–1196, 1993.

13
Treatment of Heparin-Induced Thrombocytopenia: An Overview

Andreas Greinacher
Ernst-Moritz-Arndt University, Greifswald, Germany

Theodore E. Warkentin
McMaster University and Hamilton Health Sciences Corporation, Hamilton, Ontario, Canada

I. INTRODUCTION

Heparin-induced thrombocytopenia (HIT) presents a unique situation: heparin causes the very problems its use was intended to prevent; namely, such complications as pulmonary embolism, stroke, and limb gangrene. Furthermore, there are several treatment paradoxes that pose serious management pitfalls (Table 1). This chapter summarizes our treatment approach, with emphasis on practical management issues. We view HIT as a syndrome of increased thrombin generation. Accordingly, we emphasize the use of rapidly acting anticoagulant drugs that control thrombin generation in HIT.

This chapter is not the outcome of a formal consensus conference, as defined elsewhere (McIntyre, 1998). Nevertheless, we have used an evidence-based approach to frame our recommendations. Because there are relatively few prospective comparative data available, almost all of our recommendations are "grade C" [i.e., predominantly based on observational, or "level III – V" evidence (Cook et al., 1995; Guyatt et al., 1998)]. We have graded our recommendations as C-1 if the treatment effect seems clear, and as C-2 if the treatment effect seems equivocal on current evidence (Guyatt et al., 1998).

Ranking of Evidence: Level I: one or more randomized controlled trials (RCTs) in which the lower limit of the confidence interval (CI) for the treatment

Table 1 Treatment Paradoxes of HIT Management

Treatment for HIT	Paradoxical effect of treatment	Comments
Discontinue heparin	High frequency of thrombosis despite stopping heparin	Consider use of alternative, rapidly-acting anticoagulant[a] when heparin is stopped because of suspected HIT
Coumarin (e.g., warfarin, phenprocoumon)	High frequency of thrombosis; potential for warfarin-induced venous limb gangrene syndrome	Control thrombin generation with alternative anticoagulant[a] and await partial or full resolution of HIT before starting coumarin for longer-term control of thrombosis
Low molecular weight heparin (LMWH)	High frequency of thrombocytopenia or thrombosis when given to patients with acute HIT	Although LMWH is less likely than unfractionated heparin (UFH) to cause HIT, LMWH is relatively likely to maintain or worsen acute HIT caused by UFH
Platelet transfusions	May increase risk for platelet-mediated thrombosis	Spontaneous bleeding is uncommon even in severe HIT; thus, prophylactic platelet transfusions are contraindicated
Vena cava filters	May increase risk for inferior vena cava thrombosis, DVT, or pulmonary embolism	Vena cava filters should be avoided in acute HIT; if used, concomitant anticoagulation should be given, if possible

[a] Rapidly acting alternative parenteral anticoagulants, such as danaparoid and lepirudin, are discussed in Table 2.

effect exceeds the minimal clinically important benefit; level II: one or more RCTs in which the CI for the treatment effect overlaps the minimal clinically important benefit; level III: nonrandomized concurrent cohort study; level IV: nonrandomized historic cohort study; level V: case-series. *Grades of recommendation*: grade A: based on level I evidence; grade B: based on level II evidence; grade C: based on level III–V evidence (Cook et al., 1995; Guyatt et al., 1998).

A. Disclaimer

There are several challenging aspects to treating patients with HIT. In particular, these patients are not clinically homogeneous: they represent a complex mix of varying initial indication for heparin, location and severity of HIT-associated thrombosis, and not infrequently, dysfunction of one or more vital organs. This presents difficulties both for performing clinical studies, as well as in the application of treatment recommendations for individual patients. Furthermore, there are important differences among countries in the approval or availability status of certain recommended treatment approaches. *The treatment recommendations we make cannot thus be indiscriminately applied to all patients with suspected HIT.*

A further practical problem is that the major treatment options for HIT include relatively new and, for many physicians, unfamiliar or even unapproved anticoagulant agents. (Indeed, the approval of lepirudin as a treatment for a thrombosis that complicates HIT, by the European Union in May 1997, represented the first time an anticoagulant drug obtained by recombinant technology became available for clinical use.) This presents extra challenges to physicians, and also to laboratories asked to monitor anticoagulant treatment effects, as the treatment ''learning curve'' may occur in emergency situations. Also, immediate results of reliable laboratory tests for HIT are usually unavailable. Difficult management decisions may be needed amid diagnostic uncertainty: a diagnosis of HIT that seems obvious in retrospect may not have been so clear during its early evolution.

As an iatrogenic illness that occurs unexpectedly, often in a setting of antithrombotic prophylaxis, medicolegal aspects must be considered (see Chap. 18). Thus, once HIT is entertained as part of a differential diagnosis, we suggest that physicians carefully document the various diagnostic and treatment considerations as events unfold.

As one of those *common, rare diseases* [We acknowledge Prof. R. Hull (Calgary, Canada) for his description of HIT as a ''common, rare disease.''] that physicians only occasionally manage, and only rarely enter into clinical studies, we need to acknowledge that no final answer for treatment is likely to emerge. Therefore, this chapter should be viewed as a starting point for further discussion and study of the treatment of HIT patients.

II. NONIMMUNE HEPARIN-ASSOCIATED THROMBOCYTOPENIA

In some patients, especially those with comorbid conditions associated with platelet activation (burns, anorexia nervosa), heparin treatment can result in a transient decrease in platelet count (Burgess and Chong., 1997; Reininger et al., 1996; see Chap. 5). Unfractionated heparin (UFH) activates platelets directly (Salzman et al., 1980), an effect observed less frequently with low-molecular weight heparin (LMWH) (Brace and Fareed, 1990). Known as nonimmune heparin-associated thrombocytopenia (nonimmune HAT), this direct proaggregatory effect of heparin occurs predominantly in patients receiving high-dose, intravenous UFH therapy. Typically, platelet counts decrease within the first 1–2 days of treatment, and then recover over the next 3–4 days. There are no data indicating that these patients are at increased risk for adverse outcomes, including thrombosis. Indeed, it is possible that inappropriate discontinuation of heparin for nonimmune HAT could increase the risk for thrombosis owing to the underlying clinical condition for which the heparin is being given.

> *Recommendation.* Heparin should not be discontinued in patients clinically suspected to have nonimmune heparin-associated thrombocytopenia (grade C-2).

III. THERAPY OF (IMMUNE) HIT

A. Pathogenesis of HIT: Treatment Implications

Heparin-induced thrombocytopenia is caused by antibodies that usually recognize multimolecular complexes of platelet factor 4 (PF4) and heparin. HIT can be viewed as a syndrome of in vivo thrombin generation that results from the activation of platelets, endothelium, and coagulation pathways (Fig. 1; see Chaps. 5–10; Warkentin and Kelton, 1994; Greinacher, 1995; Warkentin, 1997; Warkentin et al., 1998).

Given this model of pathogenesis, therapy for acute HIT should focus on the following issues: (1) interruption of the immune response (e.g., discontinuation of heparin); (2) rapid reduction of increased thrombin generation; and (3) treatment of HIT-associated thrombosis. In most patients with HIT, effective pharmacological therapy for thrombosis will involve an agent that rapidly controls thrombin generation, although, in some situations, additional adjunctive treatments may be necessary (e.g., surgical thromboembolectomy, medical thrombolysis).

A newly recognized treatment issue involves patients with detectable anti-PF4–heparin antibodies, but no platelet count reduction or other clinical evidence of HIT. With increased testing for HIT antibodies, it is now clear that many patients develop HIT antibodies without developing clinical HIT (see Chaps. 4 and 11). In these patients, it seems acceptable to continue heparin treatment, but to monitor the platelet counts carefully (''watch-and-wait'' strategy).

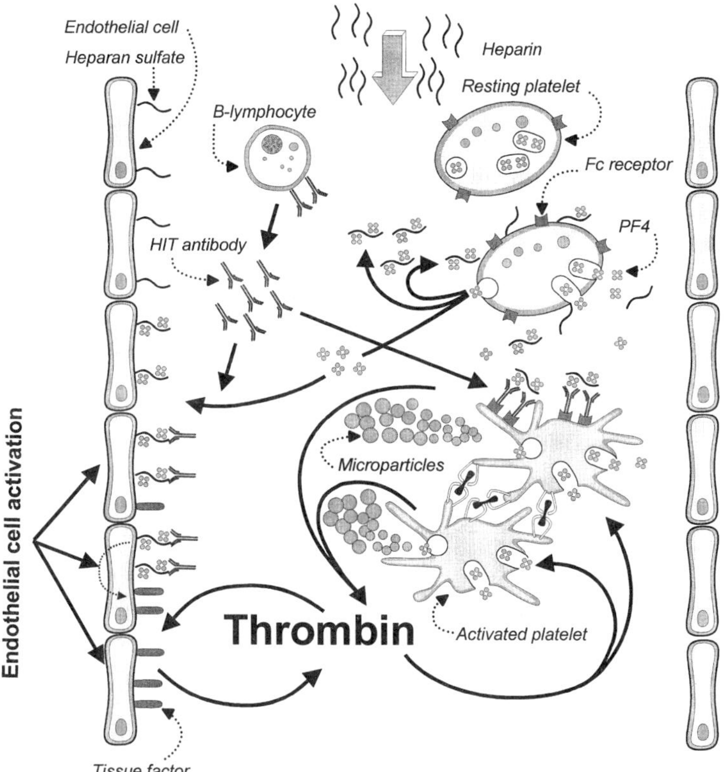

Figure 1 Pathogenesis of HIT; a central role for thrombin generation: HIT–IgG antibodies bind to several identical epitopes on the same antigen complex, thus forming immune complexes that become localized to the platelet surface. The IgG immune complexes can cross-link the platelet FcγRIIa receptors, resulting in FcγRIIa-dependent platelet activation (Kelton et al., 1988). The GP IIb/IIIa complex is not required for platelet activation (Greinacher et al., 1994a). The activated platelets trigger a cascade of events that ultimately lead to activation of the coagulation pathways, resulting in thrombin generation. Activated platelets release their α-granule proteins (Chong et al., 1994), including PF4, leading to formation of more multimolecular PF4–heparin complexes, setting up a vicious cycle of platelet activation, triggering even more platelet activation (Greinacher, 1995). The activated platelets bind fibrinogen, recruit other platelets, and begin to form a primary clot. During shape change, procoagulant, platelet-derived microparticles are released, providing a phospholipid surface for amplifying thrombin generation (Warkentin et al., 1994). The released PF4 also binds to endothelial cell heparan sulfate, forming local antigen complexes to which HIT antibodies bind (Cines et al., 1987; Visentin et al., 1994; Greinacher et al., 1994b). Tissue factor expression on activated endothelial cells further enhances thrombin generation.

B. Discontinuation of Heparin for Clinically Suspected HIT

Numerous case reports describe the occurrence of new, progressive, or recurrent thromboembolic events during continued or repeated use of heparin in patients with acute HIT. Moreover, the thrombocytopenia usually persists if the administration of heparin is not stopped. Thus, all heparin treatment should be discontinued in patients suspected of having HIT, with consideration for use of another anticoagulant (discussed subsequently), pending results of HIT antibody testing.

> *Recommendation.* All heparin administration should be discontinued in patients clinically suspected of having (immune) HIT (grade C-1).

The routine use of heparin (e.g., line flushing) is pervasive in hospitals. Thus, based on our experience it can be helpful to institute methods to reduce the risk for inadvertent heparin use in hospitalized patients with HIT.

> *Recommendation.* A clearly visible note should be placed above the patient's bed stating ''NO HEPARIN: HIT'' (grade C-2).

Not infrequently, patients in whom heparin administration has been stopped because of clinically suspected HIT subsequently are found to have negative laboratory tests for HIT antibodies. In our experience, it is reasonable and safe to restart heparin therapy in these patients, provided the intervening clinical events are consistent with an alternative explanation for thrombocytopenia (see Chaps. 2, 3, and 12), and provided the laboratory has adequately excluded the presence of HIT antibodies (see Chap. 11).

> *Recommendation.* Heparin can be safely restarted in patients proved not to have HIT antibodies by sensitive activation or antigen assay (grade C-1).

C. Anticoagulation of the HIT Patient with Thrombosis

The Need for Anticoagulation of HIT-Associated Thrombosis

Heparin-induced thrombocytopenia is a strong, independent risk factor for venous and arterial thrombosis (Warkentin et al., 1995). HIT can be complicated by thrombosis in several ways: (1) a preceding thrombosis, leading to the heparin treatment that caused HIT; (2) new, progressive, or recurrent thrombosis resulting from HIT itself; or (3) for both reasons.

For a HIT patient with thrombosis in whom heparin administration has been discontinued, there is, nevertheless, a very high risk for subsequent thrombosis. This was shown in two historically controlled prospective treatment cohort studies (Greinacher et al., 1999a,b), in which the incidence of thrombotic events ranged from 5–10% per patient day (see Chap. 15). This high event rate occurred after stopping heparin therapy, but before starting alternative anticoagulation, because the study protocol required that HIT be confirmed by laboratory assay before patient enrollment into the study (mean period of treatment delay, 1.7 days). This experience suggests that alternative anticoagulant therapy should not be delayed for results of HIT antibody testing in patients strongly suspected of having HIT.

Anticoagulants Evaluated for Treatment of HIT

Current treatment of HIT focuses on agents that rapidly control thrombin generation (Warkentin et al., 1998; Hirsh et al., 1998). Table 2 lists the available evidence on efficacy for three such agents: danaparoid, lepirudin, and argatroban. There is most experience with danaparoid and lepirudin, both of which are now widely available. Argatroban has also been evaluated for treating HIT, but published data are still limited, and the drug is not currently available.

Only one randomized controlled trial for the management of HIT has been performed: this study compared danaparoid with dextran for the treatment of HIT-associated thrombosis (Chong, 1996; Ortel and Chong, 1998; see Chap. 14). Only preliminary results of this level I evidence study have been published, as of December 1999. Therefore, we have listed the recommendation for use of danaparoid for treatment of HIT-associated thrombosis as grade C-1, although this recommendation has the potential to be upgraded to level B-1.

> *Recommendation.* Therapeutic-dose anticoagulation with a rapidly acting anticoagulant, e.g., danaparoid or lepirudin, should be given to a patient with thrombosis complicating acute HIT. Treatment should not be delayed for laboratory confirmation in a patient strongly suspected of having HIT (grade C-1).

Pharmacological and Pharmacokinetic Considerations: Danaparoid and Lepirudin

The lack of prospective comparative studies between danaparoid and lepirudin precludes definitive conclusions about relative efficacy and safety. However, there are several pharmacological and pharmacokinetic differences that physicians should consider when determining which drug may be preferred in an individual patient (Tables 3 and 4). For example, in a patient with vital organ or limb ischemia or infarction who might need urgent surgical intervention, an agent with a short half-life (e.g., lepirudin) may be preferred. On the other hand, in a patient with venous thromboembolism, in whom an uncomplicated overlap with (longer-term) warfarin anticoagulation is anticipated, or who requires outpatient treatment by subcutaneous injections, danaparoid may have certain advantages. Other factors to consider: drug availability to, and prior experience of, the physician; availability and turnaround time of laboratory monitoring; and so on.

Table 2 Rapidly Acting Anticoagulants for the Treatment of HIT: Summary of Main Evidence for Efficacy

Drug	Mechanism of action	Evidence of efficacy in HIT, ranked by level of evidence (I–V)[a]
Danaparoid sodium (Orgaran, formerly known as Org 10172 and Lomoparan	Mixture of glycosaminoglycans with anti-Xa activity ≫ anti-IIa (thrombin) activity	I: Randomized controlled trial (Chong, 1996) showed higher thrombosis resolution rate in patients receiving danaparoid plus warfarin, compared with dextran plus warfarin (mild thrombosis: 92 vs. 71%; $p = 0.04$; serious thrombosis: 92 vs. 33%; $p < 0.001$). III: No difference in time to platelet count recovery, or in thrombotic outcomes, in patients with or without in vitro cross-reactivity (Warkentin, 1996). IV: Lower frequency of thrombosis with danaparoid compared with ancrod treatment (6 vs 25%; $p = 0.04$) (Warkentin, 1996). V: A 91% success rate (defined as platelet count recovery without new or progressive thrombosis, and without complications that required discontinuation of danaparoid therapy) in 338 patients with acute HIT, in an uncontrolled, compassionate-release study (Magnani, 1993, 1997).
Recombinant hirudin (lepirudin, Refludan)	Recombinant protein derived from leeches that directly inactivates thrombin	IV: Lepirudin was associated with a lower composite event rate (new thrombosis, limb amputation, death) in patients with serologically confirmed HIT compared with historic control subjects: 25 vs. 52% at day 35 follow-up in the first study ($p = 0.014$), and a trend toward a lower composite endpoint in the second study (31 vs. 52%; $p = 0.12$) (Greinacher et al., 1999a,b).
Argatroban (Novastan)	Small molecule, direct thrombin inhibitor	IV: Argatroban was associated with a lower composite event rate (new thrombosis, limb amputation, death) in patients with clinically diagnosed HIT, compared with historic control subjects, for patients with isolated HIT (27 vs. 33%; $p = 0.08$; $p = 0.038$ for covariate-adjusted, time-to-event comparison) and for patients with HIT associated with thrombosis (43% vs. 54%; $p < 0.01$) (Lewis et al., 1997).

[a] See pp. 261–262 for description of ranking of level of evidence (grades I–V).

Table 3 Main Characteristics of Danaparoid Sodium

Mechanism of action, pharmacokinetics	Monitoring	Undesirable effects	Comments
Catalyzes the inactivation of factor Xa by AT, and of thrombin (IIa) by AT and HCII	AT levels at start of treatment	Cross-reactivity (XR) with HIT antibodies: in vitro XR usually not associated with adverse effects; patients should be monitored for in vivo XR (unexplained platelet count fall, progressive new TECs); in vivo XR is estimated to occur in ~3% of patients (Magnani, 1993)	Anticoagulant effect depends on adequate AT levels
Bioavailability after sc injection ~100%; peak anti-Xa levels, 4–5 h after injection (Danhof et al., 1992)	Anti-Xa levels during treatment by an amidolytic assay using danaparoid reference curve	Bleeding complications in compassionate-release study (Ortel and Chong, 1998): fatal (0.9%), major nonfatal bleeding (6.5%); no major bleeds in RCT (Chong, 1996)	Does not significantly prolong the aPTT, ACT, PT/INR (no interference with monitoring of overlapping oral anticoagulants)
Mean plasma distribution time following iv bolus, ~2.3 h	Monitoring recommended in patients with: (1) significant renal impairment; (2) body weight < 45 kg or > 110 kg; (3) life- or limb-threatening thrombosis; (4) unexpected bleeding; (5) critically ill or unstable patient	Skin hypersensitivity: very rare	Reduce dosage if serum creatinine > 265 µmol/L
Plasma $t_{1/2}$ of anti-Xa activity, 17–28 h (mean, 25 h); $t_{1/2}$ of anti-IIa activity, 2–4 h (Danhof et al., 1992)			*No antidote*: In case of overdosage, stop the drug and treat bleeding with blood products as indicated

Abbreviations: ACT, activated clotting time; aPTT, activated partial thromboplastin time; AT, antithrombin; HCII, heparin cofactor II; iv, intravenous; PT/INR, prothrombin time/international normalized ratio; RCT, randomized controlled trial; sc, subcutaneous; $t_{1/2}$, drug half-life.

Table 4 Main Characteristics of the r-Hirudin, Lepirudin

Mechanism of action, pharmacokinetics	Monitoring	Undesirable effects	Comments
Direct, noncovalent, irreversible inhibitor of free and clot-bound thrombin Bioavailability after sc injection, ~100%; peak effect, 2–3 h Mean plasma distribution time after iv bolus, ~2 h Mean plasma $t_{1/2}$, 1.3 h; $t_{1/2}$ greatly prolonged in renal failure (~200 h in nephrectomized patients)	aPTT during treatment; a more precise monitoring is possible by the ECT (see Chaps. 15, 17) Daily aPTT monitoring is recommended in all patients (see Comments re: antihirudin antibodies) Monitoring by ECT recommended: 1. During cardiopulmonary bypass surgery; 2. Unexpected bleeding	Development of antihirudin antibodies in ~40% of patients. In about 3% of patients, these antibodies enhance the anticoagulant effect of hirudin, and require a substantial dose reduction. Allergic reactions: very rare Skin hypersensitivity: very rare Bleeding complications in HIT patients in prospective studies: major bleeding in two prospective studies, 13.4, 17% (see Chap. 15)	~40% of patients develop antihirudin antibodies on day 5 or later of treatment; in only ~5% of these patients is a dose reduction needed for prolonged $t_{1/2}$ Variable effect on PT/INR (potential for interference with monitoring of overlapping oral anticoagulants) Reduce dosage if serum creatinine >120 μmol/L *No antidote:* In case of overdosage, stop the drug and treat bleeding with blood products as indicated (hemofiltration with a high-flux membrane is a possible treatment for life-threatening bleeding) Combination with antiplatelet drugs may enhance bleeding risk

Abbreviations: aPTT, activated partial thromboplastin time; ECT, ecarin-clotting time; sc, subcutaneous; iv, intravenous; $t_{1/2}$ drug half-life.

Other Drugs That Reduce Thrombin Generation in HIT

Argatroban is a small-molecule thrombin inhibitor that inhibits clot-bound thrombin (Lunven et al., 1996). Anecdotal reports suggest that HIT patients can benefit from this drug (Matsuo et al., 1992; Lewis et al., 1996, 1997). A prospective cohort treatment study with historical controls suggested that the drug decreases thrombotic events in patients with clinically suspected HIT (see Table 2). However, a higher mortality rate was observed in the argatroban-treated patients (Lewis, 1997). A possible explanation for this finding is that patients who received argatroban may have had greater disease severity, or even other life-threatening explanations for their thrombocytopenia, as many patients tested negative for HIT antibodies in this trial (Walenga et al., 1999). Argatroban is undergoing reevaluation by the U.S. Food and Drug Administration (FDA; application resubmitted, December 1998), following its initial failure to receive approval as a treatment of HIT.

Other drugs with antithrombin activity described anecdotally as treatment for HIT include Hirulog (bivalirudin) (Chamberlin et al., 1995; Nand, 1993; Reid and Alving, 1994) and the glycosaminoglycan agent, dermatan sulfate (Agnelli et al., 1994). Theoretically, the heparin-binding pentasaccharide should not cause HIT or cross-react with HIT antibodies (Elalamy et al., 1995; Greinacher et al., 1995; Amiral et al., 1997), but there is no reported experience with this agent for HIT.

D. Anticoagulation of the HIT Patient Without Thrombosis

Approximately 50% of patients with HIT do not have a new HIT-associated thrombosis at the time HIT is first clinically suspected on the basis of thrombocytopenia alone (Warkentin and Kelton, 1996; Greinacher et al., 1999a,b). In a retrospective cohort study of 62 such patients with "isolated thrombocytopenia," the subsequent 30-day cumulative thrombotic event rate was high (52.8%; see Fig. 2 in Chap. 4). The rate of thrombosis was similar in the two largest patient subgroups: patients treated with discontinuation of heparin therapy alone (20/36, 56%), and patients treated with substitution of warfarin for heparin (10/21, 48%). Overall, 6 of the 62 patients developed pulmonary embolism (2 fatal); another patient who died suddenly may also have had a fatal pulmonary embolism. The early thrombotic event rates, approximately 10 and 18% at 1- and 2-days follow-up, respectively, mirrored the experience of the prospective treatment cohort studies (Greinacher et al., 1999a,b).

A small patient series by Boon et al. (1994) made similar observations: two of three patients with HIT developed thrombosis, despite stopping heparin administration (deep vein thrombosis [DVT], day 1; pulmonary embolism, day 2). Warkentin et al. (1995) identified four patients in a clinical trial that met the clinical criteria for isolated HIT following orthopedic surgery: three of four subsequently developed thrombosis (two patients with DVT on day 2; one patient with DVT on day 1 and pulmonary embolism on day 7).

The very high initial thrombotic event rates (5–10%/day over the first 1–2 days) observed in these prospective and retrospective studies suggest that many patients may have had subclinical DVT at the time that HIT was first suspected. The data support the recommendation that antithrombotic treatment for HIT be started before serological confirmation is received, even in patients without clinical evidence of thrombosis.

We generally prescribe an alternative anticoagulant in therapeutic doses in this situation. Prophylactic-dose anticoagulation is a reasonable option in HIT patients judged to be at higher risk for bleeding complications, as is regular screening for venous thrombosis without anticoagulation in a patient at very high bleeding risk. Thrombocytopenia itself should not be considered a contraindication to anticoagulation in patients with HIT, as petechiae and other spontaneous hemorrhagic manifestations are not usually seen in these patients (see Chap. 3). However, if the platelet count is fewer than 20×10^9/L and bleeding signs, but not thrombosis, are observed, then alternative diagnoses such as posttransfusion purpura or other drug-dependent immune thrombocytopenic disorders should be considered (see Chap. 2).

> *Recommendation.* Alternative anticoagulation with an appropriate anticoagulant, such as danaparoid or lepirudin, should be considered in patients with clinically suspected HIT even in the absence of symptomatic thrombosis. Anticoagulation should be continued at least until recovery of the platelet counts to a stable plateau. Patients should be assessed carefully for lower limb DVT, especially those at highest risk for venous thromboembolism, such as postoperative patients (grade C-2).

E. Longer-Term Anticoagulant Management of the HIT Patient with Thrombosis

Acute HIT by itself is not an indication for longer-term anticoagulation (i.e., 3–6 months). However, HIT-associated thrombosis, or the underlying disease itself, often is. For long-term control of thrombosis, oral anticoagulants of the coumarin class (e.g., warfarin or phenprocoumon) are the treatment of choice. Generally, it takes at least 5 days of oral anticoagulant therapy before therapeutic functional hypoprothrombinemia is achieved (Harrison et al., 1997). It is important that thrombin generation be controlled in patients with acute HIT before initiation of coumarin treatment, particularly in patients with severe HIT-associated DVT, because coumarin-induced venous limb gangrene is a potential outcome (Warkentin et al., 1997; see Chap. 3). It is our practice to postpone starting administration of coumarin anticoagulants until therapeutic anticoagulation is achieved with danaparoid or lepirudin, and substantial platelet count recovery has occurred (generally, $\geq 100 \times 10^9$/L).

Recommendation. The drug of choice for longer-term anticoagulation of HIT patients is an oral anticoagulant of the coumarin class (e.g., warfarin or phenprocoumon). However, in a patient with acute HIT, oral anticoagulant therapy should be delayed until the patient is adequately anticoagulated with a rapidly acting parenteral anticoagulant, and ideally not until there has been substantial platelet count recovery (grade C-1).

In case of coumarin overdose and severe bleeding during the first 3 months after an episode of HIT, prothrombin complex concentrates should only be used with extreme caution to ''reverse'' coumarin anticoagulation. This is because these concentrates contain heparin, and have caused recurrent thrombocytopenia and thrombosis in patients with circulating HIT antibodies (Greinacher et al., 1992).

Recommendation. Prothrombin complex concentrates should not be used to reverse coumarin anticoagulation in a patient with acute or recent HIT unless bleeding is otherwise unmanageable (grade C-2).

F. Reexposure of the HIT Patient to Heparin

Heparin Reexposure of the Patient with Acute or Recent HIT

Deliberate or accidental readministration of heparin to a patient with acute or recent HIT can cause an abrupt platelet count fall, sometimes complicated by thrombosis or acute systemic reactions (see Chap. 3). Accordingly, deliberate heparin rechallenge for diagnostic purposes is not recommended, especially because sensitive assays for HIT antibodies are available. It is, however, important to test acute serum or plasma, because HIT antibodies are transient and usually become undetectable within a few weeks after an episode of HIT. This is a grade A recommendation because the diagnostic usefulness of laboratory assays for HIT has been established in controlled studies (see Chap. 11).

Recommendation. Deliberate reexposure to heparin of a patient with acute or recent HIT for diagnostic purposes is not recommended. Rather, the diagnosis should be confirmed by testing acute patient serum or plasma for HIT antibodies using a sensitive activation or antigen assay (grade A-1).

Heparin Reexposure of the Patient with a History of Remote HIT

The HIT antibodies are usually not detectable 3 months after an episode of HIT (Warkentin and Kelton, 1998). There are few data describing the clinical and serological outcomes of patients with previously documented HIT in the remote past (arbitrarily, > 3 months ago, or sooner, if HIT antibodies have disappeared). One patient who developed fatal HIT on day 15 of UFH treatment had a history of HIT complicated by thrombosis 6 years earlier (Gruel et al., 1990). However, several patients with previous remote HIT have been observed in whom repeat heparin use caused neither HIT nor HIT antibody formation (Warkentin and Kelton, 1998).

Because there are acceptable alternative anticoagulant options for most prophylactic and therapeutic indications, it is prudent to avoid both UFH and LMWH completely in patients with a previous history of HIT. Indeed, to minimize the risk for accidental future use of heparin, it can be helpful to give the patient a permanent record of the HIT incident (Table 5). As discussed in the following section, however, there are special circumstances, such as cardiac or vascular surgery, during which it is reasonable to use heparin for a patient with a previous history of HIT, provided certain precautions are taken.

Table 5 Patient Drug Sensitivity Record

Patient Drug Sensitivity Record

Patients name ____________________; birth date ____________________

developed heparin-induced thrombocytopenia (HIT) on ____________________ (date) during

treatment with ____________________ (heparin name); ____________________ (dosage)

The clinical diagnosis was verified by a laboratory asssay:

yes/no ________

Type of assay ____________________

Laboratory address ____________________

The patient should not receive heparin again.[a] If future parenteral anticoagulation is required, hirudin (Refludan, Revasc) or danaparoid sodium (Orgaran) can be used.

Name of the physician and address ____________________

Place, date, and signature ____________________

[a] Under special circumstances, brief (<48 h) reexposure to heparin may be safe (e.g., for cardiac surgery, provided that HIT antibodies are no longer detectable). Please consult with a specialized center if such an approach is considered.

Recommendation. Heparin should not be used for antithrombotic prophylaxis or therapy in a patient with a previous history of HIT, except under special circumstances (e.g., cardiac or vascular surgery) (grade C-2).

IV. HIT IN SPECIAL CLINICAL SITUATIONS

A. Cardiopulmonary Bypass or Vascular Surgery

Management of the Patient with Acute or Recent HIT

For patients with acute HIT who require heart surgery, or with recent HIT and persistence of circulating HIT antibodies, it is possible to use an alternative anticoagulant during cardiopulmonary bypass (CPB). Two anticoagulant options for these patients are danaparoid and lepirudin. Unfortunately, the lack of a specific antidote, and the need for special intraoperative monitoring (anti-Xa levels and ecarin-clotting time for danaparoid and lepirudin, respectively), mean that neither drug is ideal for managing CPB. This topic is discussed in detail in Chap. 17. Danaparoid and lepirudin have also been used to flush blood vessels during vascular surgery in patients with acute HIT (see pp. 277, 329).

Recommendation. Heparin should not be used for heart or vascular surgery in a patient with acute or recent HIT with detectable HIT antibodies. Either danaparoid or lepirudin are appropriate alternatives for intraoperative anticoagulation, provided that rapid-turnaround laboratory monitoring and blood product support to manage potentially severe bleeding complications are available (grade C-2).

Management of the Patient Following Disappearance of HIT Antibodies

The drawbacks of danaparoid and lepirudin for CPB provide a rationale for the use of heparin in two groups of patients with a previous history of HIT: (1) a patient with a history of HIT, but who no longer has circulating HIT antibodies detected by sensitive laboratory assay; and (2) a patient with acute or recent HIT who requires elective heart surgery. In the latter situation, it is reasonable to delay cardiac surgery until HIT antibodies become undetectable, which usually occurs in a few weeks (median, 50 days) (Warkentin and Kelton, 1998).

It is feasible to give UFH for cardiac or vascular surgery in a patient with a previous history of HIT, provided that HIT antibodies are not detectable at the time of surgery (Olinger et al., 1984; Smith et al., 1985; Makhoul et al., 1987; Warkentin and Kelton, 1998). We recommend that heparin be avoided completely both before surgery (to prevent restimulation of HIT antibodies) and after surgery (thus making HIT unlikely even if HIT antibodies are reformed). Current evidence suggests that there is a minimum time to formation of clinically significant

HIT antibodies of 5 days even in patients who have a previous history of HIT (Cadroy et al., 1994; Warkentin and Kelton, 1998). The patient should receive routine doses of UFH for the surgical procedure itself. Preoperative anticoagulation (e.g., for heart catheterization) and postoperative antithrombotic prophylaxis can be achieved with an agent such as danaparoid (see Chap. 14).

Recommendation. In a patient with a previous history of HIT, heart or vascular surgery can be performed using heparin, provided that HIT antibodies are absent (by sensitive assay), and heparin use is restricted to the surgical procedure itself (grade C-1).

B. HIT During Pregnancy

There are a few reports describing HIT during pregnancy (Meytes et al., 1986; Henny et al., 1986; Copplestone and Oscier, 1987; Calhoun and Hesser 1987; van Besien et al., 1991; Greinacher et al., 1993a). Danaparoid has been used without adverse incident in at least 13 pregnant women using dosing schedules similar to those in nonpregnant patients. Danaparoid does not cross the placenta, based on cord blood assessment (see Chap. 14).

Only one report describes the use of lepirudin during pregnancy (Huhle et al., 1999). In preclinical experiments, lepirudin in very high doses induced increased mortality in pregnant animals (information provided by the manufacturer).

Recommendation. Danaparoid is preferred for parenteral anticoagulation of pregnant patients with HIT, or in those who have a previous history of HIT (grade C-2).

C. Treatment of HIT in Children

There are only a few reports describing the management of HIT in children (Potter et al., 1992; Klement et al., 1996; Murdoch et al., 1993; Oriot et al., 1990; Schiffmann et al., 1997); therefore, no clear treatment recommendations can be made. Single cases suggest that lepirudin and danaparoid can be used successfully in these children. The dosing schedules for adults (appropriately weight-adjusted for the child) can be used as a guideline, but careful monitoring is recommended.

V. ADJUNCTIVE THERAPIES

A. Medical Thrombolysis

Thrombocytopenia is not a contraindication to thrombolytic therapy in patients with HIT. Streptokinase (Fiessinger et al., 1984; Cohen et al., 1985; Bounameaux et al., 1986; Cummings et al., 1986; Mehta et al., 1991), urokinase (Leroy et al.,

1985; Krueger et al., 1985; Clifton and Smith, 1986), and tissue plasminogen activator (t-PA) (Schiffmann et al., 1997; Dieck et al., 1990) have been used both systemically and by local infusion (Quinones-Baldrich et al., 1989). In patients at high bleeding risk, an ultra–low-dose t-PA (2 mg/h over 12 h) was successfully applied without bleeding complications (Olbrich et al., 1998). As thrombin generation is not inhibited by thrombolysis, concomitant danaparoid or lepirudin should be given, in reduced dose, until the fibrinolytic effects have waned.

Recommendation. Regional or systemic pharmacological thrombolysis should be considered as a treatment adjunct in selected patients with limb-threatening thrombosis or pulmonary embolism with severe cardiovascular compromise (grade C-2).

B. Surgical Thromboembolectomy

Vascular surgery is often needed to salvage an ischemic limb threatened by HIT-associated acute arterial thromboembolism involving large arteries (Sobel et al., 1988). Either danaparoid or lepirudin can provide intraoperative anticoagulation. One author (AG) uses one of the following solutions to flush the vessel postembolectomy: (1) lepirudin, 0.1 mg/mL saline (one 50-mg ampule in 500 mL saline), using up to 250 mL in a normal-weight patient, and assessing the aPTT before giving more lepirudin to avoid overdosage (the lepirudin flushes thus can achieve therapeutic intraoperative anticoagulation; see p. 329); (2) danaparoid, 3 anti-Xa U/mL (one 750 U ampule in 250 mL saline), using up to 50 mL in a normal-weight patient (this small flush dose is used because systemic anticoagulation is achieved by giving a 2250 U bolus of danaparoid preoperatively (see p. 296).

Recommendation. Surgical thromboembolectomy is an appropriate adjunctive treatment for selected patients with limb-threatening large-vessel arterial thromboembolism. Thrombocytopenia is not a contraindication to surgery. An alternative anticoagulant to heparin should be used for intraoperative anticoagulation (grade C-1).

C. Intravenous Gammaglobulin

In vitro, both intact IgG as well as its Fc fragments inhibit HIT antibody-induced platelet activation, an effect that depends somewhat on the method of immunoglobulin preparation (Greinacher et al., 1994a; see Chap. 9). Case reports describe rapid increase in the platelet counts after high-dose intravenous (iv) IgG (Prull et al., 1992; Frame et al., 1989; Vender et al., 1986; Nurden et al., 1991; Grau et al., 1992; Warkentin and Kelton, 1994). The possibility that ivIgG treatment interrupts platelet activation by HIT antibodies provides a rationale for its use as an adjunct to anticoagulant therapy in certain life- or limb-threatening situations. The dose should be 1 g/kg body weight per day for 2 consecutive days.

Recommendation. ivIgG is a possible adjunctive treatment in selected patients requiring rapid blockade of the Fc receptor-dependent platelet-activating effects of HIT antibodies (e.g., management of patients with sinus vein thrombosis, severe limb ischemia, or very severe thrombocytopenia) (grade C-2).

D. Plasmapheresis

Plasmapheresis has been associated with successful treatment outcomes in uncontrolled studies of patients with severe HIT (Vender et al., 1986; Bouvier et al., 1988; Nand and Robinson 1988; Thorp et al., 1990; Manzano et al., 1990; Brady et al., 1991; Poullin et al., 1998). Whether this is due to removal of HIT antibodies or pathogenic immune complexes, or even correction of acquired natural anticoagulant deficiencies by normal plasma replacement, is unresolved. For example, a patient with warfarin-induced acquired protein C deficiency and severe venous limb ischemia may have benefited from correction of the protein C deficiency with apheresis using plasma replacement (Warkentin et al., 1997).

Recommendation. Plasmapheresis, using plasma as replacement fluid, may be a useful adjunctive therapy in selected patients with acute HIT and life- or limb-threatening thrombosis suspected or proved to have acquired deficiency of one or more natural anticoagulant proteins (grade C-2).

E. Antiplatelet Agents

Dextran

Dextran in high concentrations inhibits platelet function and fibrinogen polymerization. It also inhibits HIT antibody-mediated platelet aggregation (Sobel et al., 1986). However, a prospective randomized trial (Chong, 1996; see Chap. 14) showed that in patients with severe HIT-associated thrombosis, dextran was less effective therapy than danaparoid. It is unknown whether dextran would provide additional clinical benefit if combined with another anticoagulant. Neither of us uses dextran for the management of HIT.

Recommendation. Dextran should not be used as primary therapy for acute HIT complicated by thrombosis (grade C-1).

Acetylsalicylic Acid and Dipyridamole

Both acetylsalicylic acid (aspirin, ASA) and dipyridamole have been used in HIT patients with variable success (Makhoul et al., 1986; Laster et al., 1989; Matsuo et al., 1989; Hall et al., 1992; Janson et al., 1983; Kappa et al., 1987, 1989; Gruel et al., 1991; Almeida et al., 1998). Sometimes, the platelet count appeared to rise promptly with the application of antiplatelet therapy (Warkentin, 1997). However, HIT antibodies are potent platelet activators, and their effect cannot always be blocked in vitro by ASA or dipyridamole. These antiplatelet agents may be used as adjunctive therapy, but one should note that they can cause prolonged platelet inhibition. Because there is little information on the interactions of danaparoid or lepirudin with antiplatelet agents, combined use should probably be restricted to patients judged to be at high risk for arterial thromboembolism.

> *Recommendation.* Antiplatelet agents, such as aspirin, may be used as adjuncts to anticoagulant therapy of HIT, particularly in selected patients at high risk for arterial thromboembolism. The possible benefit in preventing arterial thrombosis should be weighed against the potential for increased bleeding (grade C-2).

Platelet Glycoprotein IIb/IIIa Inhibitors

Several platelet glycoprotein (GP) IIb/IIIa inhibitors are now available that potently block fibrinogen binding to platelets. They also can reduce thrombin generation by inhibiting the exposure of procoagulant phospholipid surfaces on platelets (Pedicord et al., 1998; Keularts et al., 1998, Hérault et al., 1998). In vitro, GP IIb/IIIa antagonists inhibit platelet aggregation (Hérault et al., 1997), endothelial cell activation (Herbert et al., 1998), and platelet microparticle generation (Mak et al., 1998) by HIT antibodies. However, Fc receptor-dependent platelet activation by HIT antibodies is independent of the GP IIb/IIIa complex (Greinacher et al., 1994a); therefore, GP IIb/IIIa inhibitors do not inhibit platelet granule release (Tsao et al., 1997; Polgár et al., 1998). As these agents do not have a direct anticoagulant effect, they probably need to be combined with an anticoagulant (danaparoid or lepirudin) to treat HIT. Because there are no data available on the interaction of these newer anticoagulants with the GP IIb/IIIa inhibitors, and because a synergistic effect on bleeding is likely, combined use for the management of HIT should be considered experimental. Theoretically, synthetic GP IIb/IIIa inhibitors with a short half-life could be safer than agents with a long half-life (e.g., abciximab)

> *Recommendation.* GP IIb/IIIa inhibitors should be considered experimental treatment in HIT and used with extreme caution if combined with anticoagulant drugs (grade C-2).

VI. CAVEATS FOR THE TREATMENT OF HIT

A. Low Molecular Weight Heparin

Low molecular weight heparin is less likely than UFH to cause HIT antibody formation as well as clinical HIT (Warkentin et al., 1995). Furthermore LMWH binds less avidly to platelets than does UFH (Greinacher et al., 1993b). With functional assays employing platelet-rich plasma, several investigators reported a reduced cross-reactivity of HIT antibodies with LMWH compared with UFH (Ramakrishna et al., 1995; Slocum et al., 1996; Vun et al., 1996); however, with sensitive washed platelet functional assays, the cross-reactivity rate of LMWH is nearly 100% (Greinacher et al., 1992; Warkentin et al., 1995; see Chap. 11).

Owing to the unavailability of other anticoagulant options during the 1980s, LMWH preparations were often used in Europe for further parenteral anticoagulation of HIT patients. No prospective cohort studies are available, but case reports (Roussi et al., 1984; Leroy et al., 1985; Vitoux et al., 1986; Gouault-Heilmann et al., 1987; Bauriedel et al., 1988; Kirchmeier and Bender, 1988) and a review (Reuter, 1987) suggest that LMWH may benefit some patients. Other case series, however, clearly show that LMWH is associated with disastrous complications in HIT patients (Horellou et al., 1984; Leroy et al., 1985; Gouault-Heilmann et al., 1987; Greinacher et al., 1992; Kleinschmidt et al., 1993). Unfortunately, no laboratory assay reliably predicts these differing treatment responses.

In our experience, treatment of HIT with LMWH is frequently unsuccessful. Of eight consecutive HIT patients who received LMWH, thrombocytopenia persisted in all, and new thromboembolic events occurred in two patients (Greinacher et al., 1992). After LMWH became available in North America, a similar experience was observed in seven HIT patients treated with LMWH (Warkentin, 1997).

Recommendation. LMWH should not be used to treat patients with acute HIT (grade C-1).

B. Oral Anticoagulants (Vitamin K Antagonists)

Although oral anticoagulants, such as warfarin, phenprocoumon, and other coumarin agents, are an important part of the longer-term management of patients with HIT-associated thrombosis, they are ineffective, and potentially dangerous, when given as single therapy, or in combination with ancrod, in patients with acute HIT (Warkentin et al., 1997; see Chap. 3). In patients with active DVT, oral anticoagulants may cause thrombosis to progress to involve even the microvasculature, leading to coumarin-induced venous limb gangrene. This syndrome appears to result from a transient disturbance in procoagulant–anticoagulant balance: increased thrombin generation associated with HIT remains high during early warfarin treatment, while simultaneously, there is severe, acquired deficiency in the natural anticoagulant, protein C. Although high doses of oral anticoagulants may be more likely to cause this syndrome, even relatively low doses that produce a rise in the INR to higher than 4.0 can cause limb gangrene in some patients. Thus, warfarin and phenprocoumon should always be given in combination with an agent that reduces thrombin generation in patients with acute HIT. Furthermore, it is prudent to delay coumarin anticoagulation until the HIT is adequately controlled by the parenteral anticoagulant, as judged by improved or stabilized thrombotic signs and partial or complete platelet count recovery.

Recommendation. Oral anticoagulants are contraindicated in patients with acute HIT, unless combined with an agent that reduces thrombin generation (grade C-1).

C. Ancrod

Ancrod is a defibrinogenating enzyme obtained from the venom of the Malayan pit viper. The thrombin-like enzyme cleaves fibrinopeptide A from fibrinogen but, in contrast with thrombin, does not proteolyze fibrinopeptide B (Bell, 1997). On the basis of uncontrolled studies, ancrod has been used successfully to treat several patients with HIT, primarily in Canada (Demers et al., 1991; Cole et al., 1990; Teasdale et al., 1989).

However, ancrod does not inhibit thrombin generation, and in HIT patients it even appears to increase thrombin generation initially (Warkentin, 1998). Animal models indicate that under special clinical circumstances, such as septicemia, ancrod contributes to enhanced fibrin deposition (Krishnamurti et al., 1993). These data could help explain why some patients have developed venous limb gangrene during combined treatment with ancrod and warfarin (Warkentin et al., 1997; Gupta et al., 1998) (i.e., increased thrombin generation during ancrod treatment could contribute to the disturbance in procoagulant–anticoagulant balance during warfarin therapy that has been hypothesized to explain venous limb gangrene; Warkentin et al., 1997). In a retrospective nonblinded comparison, ancrod appeared to be less effective than danaparoid in one medical community (Warkentin, 1996).

Another disadvantage of ancrod is that it cannot effect rapid anticoagulation, as the drug must be given over at least 12–24 h to avoid causing intravascular fibrin deposition by overwhelming the capacity of the fibrinolytic mechanisms. Also, it is difficult to predict the level of hypofibrinogenemia that is produced by a given dose of the drug. Long-term ancrod administration has also been complicated by formation of neutralizing antiancrod antibodies (Sapru et al., 1975; Thomson et al., 1976).

Recommendation. Ancrod should not be used to treat patients with HIT (grade C-1).

D. Platelet Transfusions

Usually there is no need to treat thrombocytopenia with platelet transfusions, as patients with HIT rarely bleed spontaneously. Indeed, platelet transfusions should be avoided because the transfused platelets can be activated by the same immune mechanisms as the patient's own platelets. Anecdotal experience describes thrombotic events soon after platelet transfusions given to patients with acute HIT (Babcock et al., 1976; Cimo et al., 1979). A consensus conference (Contreras, 1998) stated that thrombotic thrombocytopenic purpura (TTP) and HIT are two disorders in which prophylactic platelet transfusions are not recommended because of the risk of precipitating thrombosis.

Recommendation. Prophylactic platelet transfusions are contraindicated in patients with HIT (grade C-2).

Therapeutic platelet transfusions are appropriate for patients with HIT who develop severe hemorrhage, particularly if the heparin administration has been discontinued for more than a day.

E. Vena Cava Filters

Vena cava (Greenfield) filters are sometimes used to manage patients judged to be at high risk for life-threatening pulmonary embolism. However, their use can be complicated by massive vena cava thrombosis, including the renal veins, and other serious progression of venous thromboembolism, especially if pharmacological anticoagulation is not given (Sobel et al., 1988; Jouanny et al., 1993). In our opinion, these devices should rarely be used in patients with acute HIT.

REFERENCES

Agnelli G, Iorio A, De Angelis V, Nenci GG. Dermatan sulphate in heparin-induced thrombocytopenia [letter]. Lancet 344:1295–1296, 1994.

Almeida JI, Coats R, Liem TK, Silver D. Reduced morbidity and mortality rates of the heparin-induced thrombocytopenia syndrome. J Vasc Surg 27:309–316, 1998.

Amiral J, Lormeau JC, Marfaing-Koka A, Vissac AM, Wolf M, Boyer-Neumann C, Tardy B, Herbert JM, Meyer D. Absence of cross-reactivity of SR90107A/ORG31540 pentasaccharide with antibodies to heparin–PF4 complexes developed in heparin-induced thrombocytopenia. Blood Coagul Fibrinolysis 8:114–117, 1997.

Babcock RB, Dumper CW, Scharfman WB. Heparin-induced thrombocytopenia. N Engl J Med 295:237–241, 1976.

Bauriedel G, Gerbig H, Riess H, Samtleben W, Steinbeck G. Heparin-induzierte Thrombozytopenie. Weiterbehandlung mit niedermolekularem Heparin. Munch Med Wochenschr 8:133–134, 1988.

Bell WR Jr. Defibrinogenating enzymes. Drugs 54(suppl 3):18–31, 1997.

Boon DMS, Michiels JJ, Stibbe J, van Vliet HHDM, Kappers-Klunne MC. Heparin-induced thrombocytopenia and antithrombotic therapy [letter]. Lancet 344:1296, 1994.

Bounameaux H, de Moerloose P, Schneider PA, Leuenberger A, Krähenbühl B, Bouvier CA. Thrombose arterielle femorale associee a une thrombopenie induit par l'hcparin. Schweiz Med Wochenschr 116:1576–1579, 1986.

Bouvier JL, Lefevre P, Villain P, Elias A, Durand JM, Juhan I, Serradimigni A. Treatment of serious heparin-induced thrombocytopenia by plasma exchange: report on 4 cases. Thromb Res 51:335–336, 1988.

Brace LD, Fareed J. Heparin-induced platelet aggregation. II. Dose/response relationships for two low molecular weight heparin fractions (CY 216 and CY 222). Thromb Res 59:1–14, 1990.

Brady J, Riccio JA, Yumen OH, Makary AZ, Greenwood SM. Plasmapheresis: a therapeutic option in the management of heparin-associated thrombocytopenia with thrombosis. Am J Clin Pathol 96:394–397, 1991.

Burgess JK, Chong BH. The platelet proaggregating and potentiating effects of unfractionated heparin, low molecular weight heparin and heparinoid in intensive care patients and healthy controls. Eur J Haematol 58:279–285, 1997.

Cadroy Y, Amiral J, Raynaud H, Brunel P, Mazaleyrat A, Sauer M, Sie P. Evolution of antibodies anti-PF4/heparin in a patient with a history of heparin-induced thrombocytopenia reexposed to heparin (letter). Thromb Haemost 72:783–784, 1994.

Calhoun BC, Hesser JW. Heparin-associated antibody with pregnancy: discussion of two cases. Am J Obstet Gynecol 156:964–966, 1987.

Chamberlin JR, Lewis B, Leya F, Wallis D, Messmore H, Hoppensteadt D, Walenga JM, Moran S, Fareed J, McKiernan T. Successful treatment of heparin-associated thrombocytopenia and thrombosis using Hirulog. Can J Cardiol 11:511–514, 1995.

Chong BH. Low molecular weight heparinoid and heparin-induced thrombocytopenia [abstr]. Aust NZ J Med 26:331, 1996.

Chong BH, Murray B, Berndt MC, Dunlop LC, Brighton T, Chesterman CN. Plasma P-selectin is increased in thrombotic consumptive platelet disorders. Blood 83:1535–1541, 1994.

Chong BH. Low molecular weight heparinoid and heparin-induced thrombocytopenia [abstr]. Aust NZ J Med 26:331, 1996.

Cimo PL, Moake JL, Weinger RS, Ben-Menachem Y, Khalil KG. Heparin-induced thrombocytopenia: association with a platelet aggregating factor and arterial thromboses. Am J Hematol 6:125–133, 1979.

Cines DB, Tomaski A, Tannenbaum S. Immune endothelial-cell injury in heparin-associated thrombocytopenia. N Engl J Med 316:581–589, 1987.

Clifton GD, Smith MD. Thrombolytic therapy in heparin-associated thrombocytopenia with thrombosis. Clin Pharm 5:597–601, 1986.

Cole CW, Fournier LM, Bormanis J. Heparin-associated thrombocytopenia and thrombosis: optimal therapy with ancrod. Can J Surg 33:207–210, 1990.

Cohen JI, Cooper MR, Greenberg CS. Streptokinase therapy of pulmonary emboli with heparin-associated thrombocytopeia. Arch Intern Med 145:1725–1726, 1985.

Contreras M. The appropriate use of platelets: an update from the Edinburgh Consensus Conference. Br J Haematol 101(suppl 1):10–12, 1998.

Cook DJ, Guyatt GH, Laupacis A, Sackett DL, Goldberg RJ. Clinical recommendations using levels of evidence for antithrombotic agents. Chest 108(suppl):227S–230S, 1995.

Copplestone A, Oscier DG. Heparin-induced thrombocytopenia in pregnancy. Br J Haematol 65:248, 1987.

Cummings JM, Mason TJ, Chomka EV, Pouget JM. Fibrinolytic therapy of acute myocardial infarction in the heparin thrombosis syndrome. Am Heart J 112:407–409, 1986.

Danhof M, de Boer A, Magnani HN, Stiekema JCJ. Pharmacokinetic considerations on Orgaran (Org 10172) therapy. Hemostasis 22:73–84, 1992.

Demers C, Ginsberg JS, Brill-Edwards P, Panju A, Warkentin TE, Anderson DR, Turner C, Kelton JG. Rapid anticoagulation using ancrod for heparin-induced thrombocytopenia. Blood 78:2194–2197, 1991.

Dieck JA, Rizo-Patron C, Unisa A, Mathur V, Massumi GA. A new manifestation and treatment alternative for heparin-induced thrombosis. Chest 98:1524–1526, 1990.

Elalamy I, Lecrubier C, Potevin F, Abdelouahed M, Bara L, Marie JP, Samama M. Absence of in vitro cross-reaction of pentasaccharide with the plasma heparin-dependent factor of twenty-five patients with heparin-associated thrombocytopenia. Thromb Haemost 74:1384–1385, 1995.

Fiessinger JN, Aiach M, Rocanto M, Debure C, Gaux JC. Critical ischemia during heparin-induced thrombocytopenia. Treatment by intra-arterial streptokinase. Thromb Res 33:235–238, 1984.

Frame JN, Mulvey KP, Phares JC, Anderson MJ. Correction of severe heparin-associated thrombocytopenia with intravenous immunoglobulin. Ann Intern Med 111:946–947, 1989.

Gouault-Heilmann M, Huet Y, Adnot S, Contant G, Bonnet F, Intrator L, Payen D, Levent M. Low molecular weight heparin fractions as an alternative therapy in heparin-induced thrombocytopenia. Haemostasis 17:134–140, 1987.

Grau E, Linares M, Olaso MA, Ruvira J, Sanchis J. Heparin-induced thrombocytopenia—response to intravenous immunoglobulin in vivo and in vitro. Am J Hematol 39: 312–312, 1992.

Greinacher A. Antigen generation in heparin-associated thrombocytopenia: the nonimmunologic type and the immunologic type are closely linked in their pathogenesis. Semin Thromb Hemost 21:106–116, 1995.

Greinacher A, Michels I, Mueller-Eckhardt C. Heparin-associated thrombocytopenia: the antibody is not heparin-specific. Thromb Haemost 67:545–549, 1992.

Greinacher A, Eckhardt T, Mussmann J, Mueller-Eckhardt C. Pregnancy complicated by heparin-associated thrombocytopenia: management by a prospectively in vitro selected heparinoid (Org 10172). Thromb Res 71:123–126, 1993a.

Greinacher A, Michels I, Liebenhoff U, Presek P, Mueller-Eckhardt C. Heparin-associated thrombocytopenia: immune complexes are attached to the platelet membrane by the negative charge of highly sulfated oligosaccharides. Br J Haematol 84:711–716, 1993b.

Greinacher A, Liebenhoff U, Kiefel V, Presek P, Mueller-Eckhardt C. Heparin-associated thrombocytopenia: the effects of various intravenous IgG preparations on antibody mediated platelet activation—a possible new indication for high dose i.v. IgG. Thromb Haemost 71:641–45, 1994a.

Greinacher A, Poetzsch B, Amiral J, Dummel V, Eichner A, Mueller-Eckhard C. Heparin-associated thrombocytopenia: isolation of the antibody and characterization of a multimolecular PF4–heparin complex as the major antigen. Thromb Haemost 71: 247–251, 1994b.

Greinacher A, Alban S, Dummel V, Franz G, Mueller-Eckhardt C. Characterization of the structural requirements for a carbohydrate based anticoagulant with a reduced risk of inducing the immunological type of heparin-associated thrombocytopenia. Thromb Haemost 74:886–892, 1995.

Greinacher A, Völpel H, Janssens U, Hach-Wunderle V, Kemkes-Matthes B, Eichler P, Mueller-Velten HG, Pötzsch B. Recombinant hirudin (lepirudin) provides safe and effective anticoagulation in patients with the immunologic type of heparin-induced thrombocytopenia: a prospective study. Circulation 99:73–80, 1999a.

Greinacher A, Janssens U, Berg G, Böck M, Kwasny H, Kemkes-Matthes B, Eichler P, Völpel H, Pötzsch B, Luz M. Lepirudin (recombinant hirudin) for parenteral anticoagulation in patients with heparin-induced thrombocytopenia. Circulation 100:587–593, 1999b.

Gruel Y, Lang M, Darnige L, Pacouret G, Dreyfus X, Leroy J, Charbonnier B. Fatal effect of re-exposure to heparin after previous heparin-associated thrombocytopenia and thrombosis. Lancet 336:1077–1078, 1990.

Gruel Y, Lermusiaux P, Lang M, Darnige L, Rupin A, Delahousse B, Guilmot JL, Leroy J. Usefulness of antiplatelet drugs in the management of heparin-associated thrombocytopenia and thrombosis. Ann Vasc Surg 5:552–555, 1991.

Gupta AK, Kovacs MJ, Sauder DN. Heparin-induced thrombocytopenia. Ann Pharmacother 32:55–59, 1998.

Guyatt GH, Cook DJ, Sackett DL, Eckman M, Pauker S. Grades of recommendation for antithrombotic agents. Chest 114(suppl):441S–444S, 1998.

Hall AV, Clark WF, Parbtani A. Heparin-induced thrombocytopenia in renal failure. Clin Nephrol 38:86–89, 1992.

Harrison L, Johnston M, Massicotte MP, Crowther M, Moffat K, Hirsh J. Comparison of 5-mg and 10-mg loading doses in initiation of warfarin therapy. Ann Intern Med 126:133–136, 1997.

Henny CHP, ten Cate H, ten Cate JW, Prummel MF, Peters M, Büller HR. Thrombosis prophylaxis in an AT III deficient pregnant women: application of a low molecular weight heparinoid. Thromb Haemost 55:301, 1986.

Hérault JP, Lalé A, Savi P, Pflieger AM, Herbert JM. In vitro inhibition of heparin-induced platelet aggregation in plasma from patients with HIT by SR 121566, a newly developed Gp IIb/IIIa antagonist. Blood Coagul Fibrinolysis 8:206–207, 1997.

Hérault JP, Peyrou V, Savi P, Bernat A, Herbert JM. Effect of SR121566A, a potent GP IIb–IIIa antagonist on platelet-mediated thrombin generation in vitro and in vivo. Thromb Haemost 79:383–388, 1998.

Herbert JM, Savi P, Jeske WP, Walenga JM. Effect of SR 121566A, a potent GP IIb–IIIa antagonist, on the HIT serum/heparin-induced platelet mediated activation of human endothelial cells. Thromb Haemost 80:326–331, 1998.

Hirsh J, Warkentin TE, Raschke R, Granger C, Ohman EM, Dalen JE. Heparin and low-molecular-weight heparin. Mechanisms of action, pharmacokinetics, dosing considerations, monitoring, efficacy, and safety. Chest 114:489S–510S, 1998.

Horellou MH, Conard J, Lecrubier C, Samama M, Roque-D'Orbcastel O, de Fenoyl O, Di

Maria G, Bernadou A. Persistent heparin-induced thrombocytopenia despite therapy with low molecular weight heparin. Thromb Haemost 51:134, 1984.

Huhle G, Geberth M, Hoffmann U, Harenberg J, Heene DL. Management of heparin-associated thrombocytopenia in pregnancy with subcutaneous r-hirudin. Br J Obstet Gynaecol 1999. In press.

Janson PA, Moake JL, Garpinito C. Aspirin prevents heparin-induced platelet aggregation in vivo. Br J Haematol 53:166–168, 1983.

Jouanny P, Jeandel C, Laurain MC, Penin F, Cuny G. Thrombopénie a l'héparine et filtre cave. Difficultés du traitement. J Mal Vas. 18:320–322, 1993.

Kappa JR, Horn MK III, Fisher CA, Cottrell ED, Ellison A, Addonizio VP Jr. Efficacy of iloprost (ZK36374) versus aspirin in preventing heparin-induced platelet activation during cardiac operations. J Thorac Cardiovasc Surg 97:405–413, 1987.

Kappa JR, Fisher CA, Addonizio VP. Heparin-induced platelet activation: the role of thromboxane A_2 synthesis and the extent of granule release in two patients. J Vasc Surg 9:574–579, 1989.

Kelton JG, Sheridan D, Santos A, Smith J, Steeves K, Smith C, Brown C, Murphy WG. Heparin-induced thrombocytopenia: laboratory studies. Blood 72:925–930, 1988.

Keularts IMLW, Béguin S, de Zwaan C, Hemker HC. Treatment with a GPIIb/III antagonist inhibits thrombin generation in platelet rich plasma from patients. Thromb Haemost 80:370–371, 1998.

Kirchmaier CM, Bender N. Heparin-induzierte Thrombozytopenie mit arterieller und venöser Thrombose. Inn Med 15:174–178, 1988.

Kleinschmidt S, Ziegenfuss T, Seyfert UT, Greinacher A. Septisch toxisches Herz Kreislauf Versagen als Folge einer Heparin-induzierten Thrombozytopenie mit ''White Clot Syndrome.'' Anaesthesiol Intensivmed Notfallmed Schmerzther 28:58–60, 1993.

Klement D, Rammos S, von Kries R, Kirschke W, Kniemeyer HW, Greinacher A. Heparin as a cause of thrombus progression. Heparin-associated thrombocytopenia is an important differential diagnosis in paediatric patients even with normal platelet counts. Eur J Pediatr 155:11–14, 1996.

Krishnamurti C, Bolan C, Colleton CA, Reilly TM, Alving BM. Role of plasminogen activator inhibitor-1 in promoting fibrin deposition in rabbits infused with ancrod or thrombin. Blood 82:3631–3636, 1993.

Krueger SK, Andreas E, Weinand E. Thrombolysis in heparin-induced thrombocytopenia with thrombosis. Ann Intern Med 103:159, 1985.

Laster JL, Elfrink R, Silver D. Reexposure to heparin of patients with heparin-associated antibodies. J Vasc Surg 9:677–681, 1989.

Leroy J, Leclerc MH, Delahousse B, Guerois C, Foloppe P, Gruel Y, Toulemonde F. Treatment of heparin-associated thrombocytopenia and thrombosis with low molecular weight heparin (CY 216). Semin Thromb Hemost 11:326–329, 1985.

Lewis BE. Preliminary results of a prospective randomized controlled trial of argatroban versus conventional therapy for heparin-induced thrombocytopenia. XVIth International Congress of the International Society on Thrombosis and Haemostasis, Florence, Italy, June 12, 1997.

Lewis BE, Iaffaldano R, McKiernan TL, et al. Report of successful use of argatroban as an alternative anticoagulant during coronary stent implantation in a patient with heparin-induced thrombocytopenia and thrombosis syndrome. Cathet Cardiovasc Diagn 38:206–209, 1996.

Lewis BE, Walenga JM, Wallis DE. Anticoagulation with Novastan (argatroban) in patients with heparin-induced thrombocytopenia and heparin-induced thrombocytopenia and thrombosis syndrome. Semin Thromb Hemost 23:197–202, 1997.

Lunven C, Gauffeny C, Lecoffre C, O'Brienc DP, Roome NO, Berry CN. Inhibition by argatroban, a specific thrombin inhibitor, of platelet activation by fibrin clot-associated thrombin. Thromb Haemost 75:154–160, 1996.

Magnani HN. Heparin-induced thrombocytopenia (HIT): an overview of 230 patients treated with Orgaran (Org 10172). Thromb Haemost 70:554–561, 1993.

Magnani HN. Orgaran (danaparoid sodium) use in the syndrome of heparin-induced thrombocytopenia. Platelets 8:74–81, 1997.

Mak KH, Kottke-Marchant K, Brooks LM, Topol EJ. In vitro efficacy of platelet glycoprotein IIb/IIIa antagonist in blocking platelet function in plasma of patients with heparin-induced thrombocytopenia. Thromb Haemost 80:989–993, 1998.

Makhoul RG, Greenberg CS, McCann RL. Heparin-associated thrombocytopenia and thrombosis: a serious clinical problem and potential solution. J Vasc Surg 4:522–528, 1986.

Makhoul RG, McCann RL, Austin EH, Greenberg CS, Lowe JE. Management of patients with heparin-associated thrombocytopenia and thrombosis requiring cardiac surgery. Ann Thorac Surg 43:617–621, 1987.

Manzano L, Yebra M, Vargas JA, Barbolla L, Alvarez-Mon M. Plasmapheresis in heparin-induced thrombocytopenia and thrombosis [letter]. Stroke 21:1236, 1990.

Matsuo T, Yamada T, Chikahira Y, Kadowaki S. Effect of aspirin on heparin-induced thrombocytopenia (HIT) in a patient requiring hemodialysis. Blut 59:393–395, 1989.

Matsuo T, Kario K, Chikahira Y, Nakao K, Yamada T. Treatment of heparin-induced thrombocytopenia by use of argatroban, a synthetic thrombin inhibitor. Br J Haematol 82:627–629, 1992.

McIntyre KM. Medicolegal implications of the consensus conference, with special attention to the Fifth Antithrombotic Therapy Consensus Conference. Chest 114:742S–747S, 1998.

Mehta DP, Yoder EL, Appel J, Bergsman KL. Heparin-induced thrombocytopenia and thrombosis: reversal with streptokinase. A case report and review of literature. Am J Hematol 36:275–279, 1991.

Meytes D, Ayalon H, Virag I, Weisbort Y, Zakut H. Heparin-induced thrombocytopenia and recurrent thrombosis in pregnancy. A case report. J Reprod Med 31:993–996, 1986.

Murdoch IA, Beattie RM, Silver DM. Heparin-induced thrombocytopenia in children. Acta Paediatr 82:495–497, 1993.

Nand S, Robinson JA. Plasmapheresis in the management of heparin-associated thrombocytopenia with thrombosis. Am J Hematol 28:204–206, 1988.

Nand S. Hirudin therapy for heparin-associated thrombocytopenia and deep venous thrombosis. Am J Hematol 43:310–311, 1993.

Nurden AT, Laroche-Traineau J, Jallu V, Broult J, Durrieu C, Besse P, Brossel C, Hourdillé P. Heparin-induced thrombocytopenia: observation of the nature of the antibody activities and on the use of gammaglobulin concentrates in a patient with thrombotic complications. [abstr]. Thromb Haemost 65:796, 1991.

Olbrich K, Wiersbitzky M, Wacke W, Eichler P, Zinke H, Schwock M, Möx B, Kraatz G, Motz W, Greinacher A. Atypical heparin-induced thrombocytopenia complicated by intracardiac thrombus, effectively treated with ultra-low-dose rt-PA lysis and recombinant hirudin (lepirudin). Blood Coagul Fibrinolysis 9:273–277, 1998.

Olinger GN, Hussey CV, Olive JA, Malik MI. Cardiopulmonary bypass for patients with previously documented heparin-induced platelet aggregation. J Thorac Cardiovasc Surg 87:673–677, 1984.

Oriot D, Wolf M, Wood C, Brun P, Sidi D, Devictor D, Tchernia G, Huault G. Thrombopénie sévère induite par l'héparine chez un nourrisson porteur d'une myocardite aiguë. Arch Fr Pediatr 47:357–359, 1990.

Ortel TL, Chong BH. New treatment options for heparin-induced thrombocytopenia. Semin Hematol 35:26–34, 1998.

Pedicord DL, Thomas BE, Mousa SA, Dicker IB. Glycoprotein IIb/IIIa receptor antagonists inhibit the development of platelet procoagulant activity. Thromb Res 90:247–258, 1998.

Polgár J, Eichler P, Greinacher A, Clemetson KJ. Adenosine diphosphate (ADP) and ADP receptor play a major role in platelet activation/aggregation induced by sera from heparin-induced thrombocytopenia patients. Blood 91:549–554, 1998.

Potter C, Gill JC, Scott JP, McFarland JG. Heparin-induced thrombocytopenia in a child. J Pediatr 121:135–138, 1992.

Poullin P, Pietri P, Lefevre P. Heparin-induced thrombocytopenia with thrombosis: successful treatment with plasma exchange [letter]. Br J Haematol 102:630–631, 1998.

Prull A, Nechwatal R, Riedel H, Mäurer W. Therapie des Heparin-induzierten Thrombose–Thrombozytopenie Syndroms mit Immunglobulinen. Dtsch Med Wochenschr 117:1838–1842, 1992.

Quinones-Baldrich WJ, Baker JD, Busuttil RW, Machleder HI, Moore WS. Intraoperative infusion of lytic drug for thrombotic complications of revascularisation. J Vasc Surg 10:408–417, 1989.

Ramakrishna R, Manoharan A, Kwan YL, Kyle PW. Heparin-induced thrombocytopenia: cross-reactivity between standard heparin, low molecular weight heparin, dalteparin (Fragmin) and heparinoid, danaparoid (Orgaran). Br J Haematol 91:736–738, 1995.

Reid T III, Alving BM. Hirulog therapy for heparin-associated thrombocytopenia and deep venous thrombosis. Am J Hematol 45:352–353, 1994.

Reininger CB, Greinacher A, Graf J, Lasser R, Steckmeier B, Schweiberer L. Platelets of patients with peripheral arterial disease are hypersensitive to heparin. Thromb Res 81:641–649, 1996.

Reuter HD. Niedermolekulares Heparin in der Therapie der Heparininduzierten Thrombozytopenie. Med Klin 82:115–118, 1987.

Roussi JH, Houboyan LL, Goguel AF. Use of low-molecular-weight heparin in heparin-induced thrombocytopenia with thrombotic complications. Lancet 1:1183, 1984.

Salzman EW, Rosenberg RD, Smith MH, Lindon JN, Favreau L. Effect of heparin and heparin fractions on platelet aggregation. J Clin Invest 65:64–73, 1980.

Sapru RP, Moza AK, Kumar M, Ganguly NK. Antibodies to Arvin following prolonged intravenous therapy. Thromb Res 7:635–641, 1975.

Schiffmann H, Unterhalt M, Harms K, Figulla HR, Völpel H, Greinacher A. Erfolgreiche Behandlung einer Heparin-induzierten Thrombozytopenie Typ II im Kindesalter mit rekombinantem Hirudin. Monat Kinderheilkd 145:606–612, 1997.

Slocum MM, Adams JG Jr, Teel R, Spadone DP, Silver D. Use of enoxaparin in patients with heparin-induced thrombocytopenia syndrome. J Vasc Surg 23:839–849, 1996.

Smith JP, Walls JT, Muscato MS, McCord ES, Worth ER, Curtis JJ, Silver D. Extracorporeal circulation in a patient with heparin-induced thrombocytopenia. Anaesthesiology 62:363–365, 1985.

Sobel M, Adelman B, Greenfield LJ. Dextran 40 reduces heparin-mediated platelet aggregation. J Surg Res 40:382–387, 1986.

Sobel M, Adelman B, Szentpeterey S, Hofmann M, Posner MP, Jenvey W. Surgical management of heparin-associated thrombocytopenia. Strategies in the treatment of venous and arterial thromboembolism. J Vasc Surg 8:395–401, 1988.

Teasdale SJ, Zulys VJ, Mycyk T, Baird RJ, Glynn MF. Ancrod anticoagulation for cardiopulmonary bypass in heparin-induced thrombocytopenia and thrombosis. Ann Thorac Surg 48:712–713, 1989.

Thomson NC, Hutcheon AW, Dagg JH. Acquired resistance to prolonged treatment with intravenous ''Arvin'' (ancrod). Br J Clin Pract 30:232–233, 1976.

Thorp D, Canty A, Whiting J, Dart G, Lloyd JV, Duncan E, Gallus A. Plasma exchange and heparin-induced thrombocytopenia. Prog Clin Biol Res 337:521–522, 1990.

Tsao PW, Forsythe MS, Mousa SA. Dissociation between the anti-aggregatory and anti-secretory effects of platelet integrin $\alpha IIb\beta_2$ (GPIIb/IIIa) antagonists, c7E3 and DMP728. Thromb Res 89:137–146, 1997.

Van Besien K, Hoffman R, Golichowski A. Pregnancy associated with lupus anticoagulant and heparin-induced thrombocytopenia: management with a low molecular weight heparinoid. Thromb Res 62:23–29, 1991.

Vender JS, Matthew EB, Silverman IM, Konowitz H, Dau PC. Heparin-associated thrombocytopenia: alternative managements. Anesth Analg 65:520–522, 1986.

Visentin GP, Ford SE, Scott PJ, Aster RH. Antibodies from patients with heparin-induced thrombocytopenia/thrombosis are specific for platelet factor 4 complexed with heparin or bound to endothelial cells. J Clin Invest 93:81–88, 1994.

Vitoux JF, Mathieu JF, Roncato M, Fiessinger JN, Aiach M. Heparin-associated thrombocytopenia treatment with low-molecular weight heparin. Thromb Haemost 55:37–39, 1986.

Vun CM, Evans S, Chong BH. Cross-reactivity study of low molecular weight heparins and heparinoid in heparin-induced thrombocytopenia. Thromb Res 81:525–532, 1996.

Walenga JM, Jeske WP, Wood JJ, Ahmad S, Lewis BE, Bakhos M. Laboratory tests for heparin-induced thrombocytopenia: a multicenter study. Semin Hematol 36(suppl 1):22–28, 1999.

Warkentin TE. Danaparoid (Orgaran) for the treatment of heparin-induced thrombocytopenia (HIT) and thrombosis: effects on in vivo thrombin and cross-linked fibrin generation, and evaluation of the clinical significance of in vitro cross-reactivity (XR) of danaparoid for HIT–IgG [abstr]. Blood 88(suppl 1):626a, 1996.

Warkentin TE. Heparin-induced thrombocytopenia. Pathogenesis, frequency, avoidance and management. Drug Safety 17:325–341, 1997.

Warkentin TE. Limitations of conventional treatment options for heparin-induced thrombocytopenia. Semin Hematol 35(suppl 5):17–25, 1998.

Warkentin TE, Kelton JG. Interaction of heparin with platelets, including heparin-induced thrombocytopenia. In: Bounameaux H, ed. Low-Molecular-Weight Heparins in Prophylaxis and Therapy of Thromboembolic Diseases. New York: Marcel Dekker, 1994:75–127.

Warkentin TE, Kelton JG. A 14-year study of heparin-induced thrombocytopenia. Am J Med 101:502–507, 1996.

Warkentin TE, Kelton JG. Timing of heparin-induced thrombocytopenia (HIT) in relation to previous heparin use: absence of an anamnestic immune response, and implications for repeat heparin use in patients with a history of HIT [abstr]. Blood 92(suppl 1):182a, 1998.

Warkentin TE, Hayward CPM, Boshkov LK, Santos AV, Sheppard JI, Bode AP, Kelton JG. Sera from patients with heparin-induced thrombocytopenia generate platelet-derived microparticles with procoagulant activity: an explanation for the thrombotic complications of heparin-induced thrombocytopenia. Blood 84:3691–3699, 1994.

Warkentin TE, Levine MN, Hirsh J, Horsewood P, Roberts RS, Gent M, Kelton JG. Heparin-induced thrombocytopenia in patients treated with low-molecular-weight heparin or unfractionated heparin. N Engl J Med 332:1330–1335, 1995.

Warkentin TE, Elavathil LJ, Hayward CPM, Johnston MA, Russett JI, Kelton JG. The pathogenesis of venous limb gangrene associated with heparin-induced thrombocytopenia. Ann Intern Med 127:804–812, 1997.

Warkentin TE, Chong BH, Greinacher A. Heparin-induced thrombocytopenia: towards consensus. Thromb Haemost 79:1–7, 1998.

14

Danaparoid for the Treatment of Heparin-Induced Thrombocytopenia

Beng Hock Chong
University of New South Wales and Prince of Wales Hospital, Sydney, New South Wales, Australia

I. INTRODUCTION

In patients with heparin-induced thrombocytopenia (HIT), cessation of heparin is mandatory. Thereafter, an alternative anticoagulant is often needed for the treatment of venous or arterial thrombosis, or for other indications (Chong, 1995). Currently, two antithrombotic agents, danaparoid sodium and recombinant hirudin (r-hirudin), have been approved in various countries for the treatment of patients with HIT (Warkentin et al., 1998). The clinical use of danaparoid in HIT patients will be reviewed in this chapter, and r-hirudin is discussed in Chap. 15. Danaparoid (Orgaran, Organon NV, The Netherlands; formerly known as Org 10172 and Lomoparan) has been used extensively to treat HIT patients. Worldwide, many hundreds of patients have been successfully treated with this drug (Ortel and Chong, 1998).

A. Chemistry, Pharmacology, Pharmacodynamics, and Pharmacokinetics

Chemistry

Although danaparoid is often referred to as a low molecular weight (LMW) heparinoid (implying that it has heparin-like activity), there are, in fact, substantial differences in the chemistry, pharmacology, and pharmacokinetics between danaparoid and both unfractionated heparin (UFH) and low molecular weight heparin (LMWH).

Danaparoid consists of a mixture of LMW glycosaminoglycans; namely, heparan sulfate (84%), dermatan sulfate (12%), and chondroitin sulfate (4%) (Meuleman, 1992). A small proportion of the heparan sulfate molecules have high affinity for antithrombin (AT, formerly known as antithrombin III) (Meuleman, 1992; Ofosu, 1992). Danaparoid has an average molecular mass of approximately 6000 Da. It does not contain heparin or heparin fragments, and differs in chemical composition from heparin in that the repeating disaccharide subunits in heparan sulfate, its principal constituent, are predominantly glucuronic acid and *N*-acetyl-glucosamine, whereas in heparin, they are mostly iduronic acid and glucosamine-*N*-sulfate (Gordon et al., 1990) (Fig. 1). Compared with LMWH, danaparoid has a lower degree of sulfation and a lower charge density. These two factors play an important role in its binding (or more precisely, its lack of binding) to plasma proteins and platelets, which is particularly relevant for the pharmacological profile of the drug (Casu, 1991; see Chap. 8).

Pharmacology

Danaparoid exerts its antithrombotic effects predominantly by inhibition of factor Xa; it has only minimal antifactor IIa (antithrombin) activity. Its ratio of antifactor Xa (anti-Xa) to antithrombin (anti-IIa) is 22:1 or higher, which is considerably greater than that of LMWH (2:1–4:1) and UFH (1:1) (Meuleman et al., 1982;

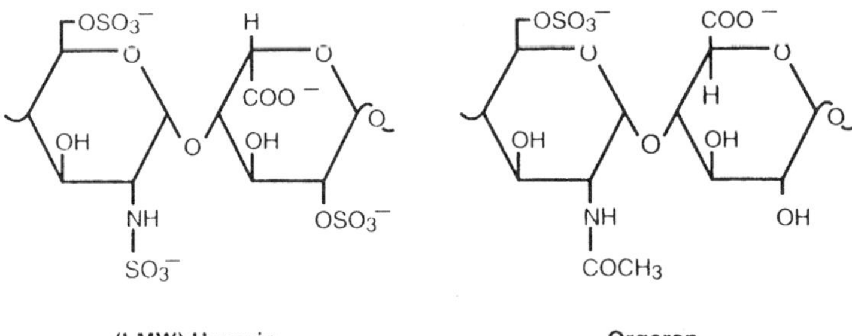

Figure 1 Comparison of predominant disaccharide structure of heparin with danaparoid. The low molecular weight (LMW) heparin disaccharide is mostly (left) glucosamine-*N*-sulfate and (right) iduronic acid, whereas danaparoid's principal constituent, heparan sulfate, is predominantly (left) *N*-acetyl-glucosamine and (right) glucuronic acid. The degree of sulfation (sulfate groups per disaccharide unit) for heparin and danaparoid are approximately 2.0–2.5 and 1.0–1.5, respectively (see Chap. 8).

Gordon et al., 1990; Meuleman, 1992). Its inhibition of factor Xa is mediated by AT, and its minor effect on thrombin by both AT and heparin cofactor II. Its highly selective inhibition of factor Xa confers on this drug the advantage of a linear inhibitory effect on thrombin generation and fibrin formation. Another advantage is that danaparoid does not interfere with normal platelet function (Meuleman et al., 1982; Mikhailidis et al., 1984, 1987; Meuleman, 1987). Thus, unlike UFH, danaparoid does not interfere with platelet accretion to experimental thrombi, although thrombus growth is markedly reduced by its prevention of fibrin accretion. Similarly, danaparoid has minimal effects on formation of the platelet-dependent hemostatic plug (Meuleman, 1992). These beneficial characteristics of danaparoid contribute to the high therapeutic index (i.e., favorable benefit/risk ratio) of this drug.

Pharmacodynamics and Pharmacokinetics

Danaparoid has a pharmacokinetic profile different from that of UFH or LMWH. It is well-absorbed after subcutaneous administration in humans, with its bioavailability approaching 100% (Stiekema et al., 1989; Danhof et al., 1992). In comparison, the bioavailability of LMWH is 87–92%, and that of UFH only 15–20% (Skoutakis, 1997). Danaparoid's plasma anti-Xa levels peak 4–5 h following subcutaneous injection (Danhof et al., 1992). Unlike UFH, it is not neutralized by plasma proteins, such as platelet factor 4 (PF4) and histidine-rich glycoprotein; hence, after subcutaneous or intravenous administration, more predictable plasma levels of the drug are obtained.

Danaparoid is eliminated mainly by the kidneys. It has a relatively long plasma anti-Xa half-life ($t_{1/2}$) of about 25 h. Plasma $t_{1/2}$ values of anti-IIa activity and thrombin generation-inhibiting activity are much shorter, ranging from 2 to 4 h and 3 to 7 h, respectively (Bradbrook et al., 1987; Stiekema et al., 1989; Danhof et al., 1992). In patients with impaired renal function, the drug has a tendency to accumulate, and the dose should be reduced accordingly.

Danaparoid's metabolism is not affected by hepatic cytochrome P-450, nor does it affect hepatic or renal handling of other drugs. It has no significant effect on the pharmacodynamics and pharmacokinetics of coumarin anticoagulants. Its pharmacokinetics are not modified by age or body weight; hence, dose adjustments are usually unnecessary in the elderly or in overweight patients (Stiekema et al., 1989; Danhof et al., 1992).

Similar to LMWH, protamine chloride only very minimally neutralizes the anticoagulant activity of danaparoid. There is no effective antidote for the drug (Stiekema et al., 1989), and in severe bleeding, the drug should be stopped and blood product replacement given, as indicated on clinical grounds. There is limited evidence that plasmapheresis can accelerate elimination of the drug (Schmahl et al., 1997), but this option may not be practical in an unstable patient.

II. CLINICAL USE OF DANAPAROID

A. Clinical Use of Danaparoid in Disorders Other Than HIT

Danaparoid has been studied for the prophylaxis and treatment of venous thromboembolism in several controlled clinical studies of routine (i.e., non-HIT) patients. These trials confirmed the efficacy of danaparoid as an antithrombotic agent and, in some trials, it was even more effective than other standard antithrombotic agents. Six prospective, randomized, controlled, and assessor-blind studies showed that danaparoid is more effective than warfarin, dextran, or low-dose UFH plus dihydroergotamine in preventing deep vein thrombosis (DVT) after total hip replacement or hip fracture surgery; and compared favorably with LMWH in patients undergoing total hip replacement surgery (Bergqvist et al., 1991; Gerhart et al., 1991; Hoek et al., 1992; Leyvraz et al., 1992; Organon report, 1994; Gent et al., 1996). In addition, there are also prospective controlled and uncontrolled studies, as well as case reports, demonstrating the efficacy of danaparoid in the treatment of DVT, acute thrombotic stroke, and disseminated intravascular coagulation complicating promyelocytic leukemia, as well as DVT prophylaxis and the prevention of fibrin deposition on the dialysis membrane during hemodialysis (Henny et al., 1983; Nieuwenhuis and Sixma, 1986; Cade et al., 1987; Biller et al., 1989; von Bonsdorff et al., 1990; Gallus et al., 1993; de Valk et al., 1995).

B. Clinical Use of Danaparoid in Patients with HIT

Danaparoid has been used extensively to treat patients with HIT (Chong and Magnani, 1992; Magnani, 1993, 1997). After the diagnosis of HIT, and discontinuation of heparin administration, patients often require an alternative anticoagulant for any one of the following indications: (1) treatment of a recent or new thrombosis; (2) prophylaxis of venous thromboembolism; (3) anticoagulation for cardiopulmonary bypass (CPB) surgery or peripheral arterial surgery; (4) anticoagulation of hemodialysis or hemofiltration; (5) cardiac catheterization or coronary angioplasty; or (6) maintenance of intravascular catheter patency. The rationale for the use of danaparoid to treat patients with HIT for these indications is that danaparoid is an effective antithrombotic–anticoagulant agent, as shown by the results of controlled trials (Skoutakis, 1997). Furthermore, it has a specific inhibitory effect on HIT antibody-induced platelet aggregation (Chong et al., 1989). Additionally, unlike LMWH, it has a low frequency of in vitro cross-reactivity with HIT antibodies (Makhoul et al., 1986; Chong et al., 1989; Greinacher et al., 1992; Kikta et al., 1993; Vun et al., 1996).

The largest clinical experience with the use of danaparoid in the treatment of patients with HIT is in the compassionate-use (named patient) program organized by the manufacturer (Organon NV, Oss, The Netherlands; Magnani, 1993, 1997). In a 15-year period from 1982, over 750 patients were treated under this program for the various foregoing indications (Ortel and Chong, 1998). The duration of treatment ranged from 1 day to 3.5 years. Interim, updated reports of this program have been published (Chong and Magnani, 1992; Magnani, 1993, 1997). The overall success rate, defined as platelet count recovery without new, progressive, or recurrent thrombosis during the danaparoid treatment period or thrombotic death during 3 months follow-up, and in the absence of any adverse effect necessitating treatment cessation, has been 91–94%, as judged by the local physician-investigators. However, as this definition does not include nonthrombotic death, the overall mortality observed in the program was 18%, including both the treatment and a 3-month posttreatment follow-up period. Most patients in this program received danaparoid for the treatment of acute thromboembolism, often in the setting of severe illness, such as renal or multisystem organ failure. Besides this compassionate-release program, one prospective, randomized clinical trial (Chong, 1996) has been performed showing danaparoid to be effective for the treatment of venous and arterial thrombosis in HIT patients (discussed subsequently).

Treatment of Venous and Arterial Thromboembolism

Patients with HIT frequently have one or more acute thromboses, which may have occurred before the development of HIT, as a complication of HIT itself, or both (Warkentin and Kelton, 1996). Venous thrombosis complicates HIT more often than does arterial occlusion. Indeed, in the compassionate-use program, the ratio of venous to arterial thrombosis was 2:1, with some patients having both types of thrombosis (Ortel and Chong, 1998). In HIT patients, nevertheless, after cessation of UFH administration, the acute thrombosis requires continuation of antithrombotic therapy. Currently, either danaparoid or r-hirudin are believed to be effective in this situation (Warkentin et al., 1998). These agents have in common the capacity to inhibit thrombin generation, either by inhibition of factor Xa (danaparoid) or by direct inhibition of thrombin (r-hirudin).

In the compassionate-use program, it was recommended that HIT patients with acute thrombosis receive intravenous danaparoid administered as a bolus of 2500 U, followed by an infusion of danaparoid at 400 U/h for 4 h, followed by 300 U/h for 4 h, and then 150–200 U/h for at least 5 days, aiming for a plasma anti-Xa level of 0.5–0.8 anti-Xa U/mL. Table 1 describes a similar protocol that takes into account the amount of danaparoid per marketed ampule (750 anti-Xa U/ampule), as well as certain initial bolus dose adjustments based on body weight. Danaparoid is also effective when administered subcutaneously (de Valk et al., 1995): in this situation, the equivalent 24-h actual or estimated intravenous dose is given in two to three divided doses by subcutaneous injection over a 24-h period. For example, 2250 U (3 ampules) every 12 h by subcutaneous injection is approximately equal to 190 U/h by intravenous infusion given over 24 h. In

Table 1 Danaparoid Dosing Schedules in HIT Patients

Clinical indication	Danaparoid dosing schedule
Venous thromboembolism	
Prophylaxis	750 U sc, b.i.d. or t.i.d.
Treatment	2250 U iv bolus[a] followed by 400 U/h for 4 h, 300 U/h for 4 h, then 150–200 U/h for ≥ 5 days, aiming for a plasma anti-Xa level of 0.5–0.8 U/mL *Subcutaneous administration schedule*: 1500–2250 U sc b.i.d. (bioavailability is almost 100% when given by sc injections; thus, 2250 U sc b.i.d. is approximately equal to an iv infusion rate of 200 U/h (4500 U/24 h vs. 4800 U/24 h, respectively)
Arterial thromboembolism: treatment	See venous thromboembolism treatment schedule
Embolectomy or other peripheral vascular surgery	*Preoperative*: 2250 U iv bolus[a]; *intraoperative flushes*: 750 U in 250 mL saline, using up to 50 mL (see p. 277); *postoperative*: 750 U sc t.i.d. (low-risk patients) or 150–200 U/h (high-risk patients) beginning at least 6 h after surgery
Hemodialysis (on alternate days)	3750 U iv before 1st and 2nd dialyses; 3000 U for 3rd dialysis; then 2250 U for subsequent dialyses, aiming for plasma anti-Xa level of < 0.3 U/mL before each dialysis and 0.5–0.8 U/mL during dialysis (see also Chap. 16).
Hemofiltration	2250 U iv bolus, followed by 600 U/h for 4 h, then 400 U/h for 4 h, then 200–400 U/h aiming for a plasma anti-Xa Level of 0.5–1.0 U/mL (see also Chap. 16).
Cardiopulmonary bypass surgery (CPB)	125 U/kg iv bolus after thoracotomy; 3 U/mL in priming fluid of apparatus; 7 U/kg/h iv infusion commencing after bypass hookup, and continued until 45 min before expectation of stopping bypass (see also Chap. 17)
Cardiac catheterization	*Preprocedure*: 2250 U iv bolus (3000 U if 75–90 kg and 3750 U if > 90 kg)
Percutaneous transluminal coronary angioplasty (PTCA) or intra-aortic balloon pump	*Preprocedure*: bolus as per foregoing; *post procedure*: 150–200 U/h for 1–2 days after PTCA (or until removal of balloon pump)
Catheter patency	750 U in 50 mL saline, then 5–10 mL per port, or as required
Pediatric dosage considerations	*Prophylaxis*: 10 U/kg sc b.i.d. *Treatment*: 30 U/kg b.w. iv bolus, then 1.2–2.0 U/kg b.w./h depending upon severity of thrombosis

Abbreviations: b.w., body weight; b.i.d., twice daily; iv, intravenous; t.i.d., three times daily.

[a] Adjust iv danaparoid bolus for body weight: < 60 kg, 1500 U; 60–75 kg, 2250 U; 75–90 kg, 3000 U; > 90 kg, 3750 U.

Compatibility with intravenous solutions: Danaparoid is compatible for dilution with any of the following solutions: saline, dextose, dextrose–saline, Ringer's, lactated Ringer's, 10% mannitol. Preparation of solution for infusion: There are several options. One approach I use is to add four ampules containing 3000 U (i.e., 750 anti-Xa U/0.6 mL ampule) of danaparoid to 300 mL of intravenous solution (i.e., a solution that comprises 10 U danaparoid per milliliter of intravenous solution; thus, an infusion rate of 40 mL/h corresponds to a dose of 400 U/h; 20 mL/h to an infusion rate of 200 U/h; and so on.

the compassionate-use program, 464 patients with acute thromboembolism were treated with danaparoid, with efficacy judged to be over 90% (Ortel and Chong, 1998).

Danaparoid treatment for HIT patients also proved efficacious in a prospective, randomized, controlled clinical study (Chong, 1996). In this trial, HIT patients with an acute thrombosis (venous, arterial, or both) were randomized to receive either danaparoid plus warfarin, or dextran 70 plus warfarin. Dextran is a glucose polymer, with an average molecular mass of 70 kDa. It is a weak antithrombotic agent that has been used to prevent DVT in postoperative patients (Aberg and Rausing, 1978; Bergqvist, 1980). It is known to block HIT antibody-induced platelet aggregation in vitro (Sobel et al., 1986), and it has been suggested as a potentially useful drug for the treatment of HIT. The reason for its use in the control group was that dextran 70 was the only rapidly acting antithrombotic drug available for the treatment of HIT-associated thrombosis in Australia at study commencement.

The danaparoid treatment regimen was slightly different from that of the compassionate-use program. Danaparoid was given as a bolus of 2400 U, followed by an infusion of 400 U/h for 2 h, 300 U/h for 2 h, and then 200 U/h for 5 days. In the dextran 70 arm, patients received dextran, 1 L on day 1, and then 500 mL/day from days 2 to 5. In both treatment arms, the patients also received warfarin, with doses adjusted to an INR of 2–4; the warfarin was continued for 3 months. Patients were also stratified at randomization, depending on the severity of their thrombosis, using predefined criteria.

Resolution of thrombocytopenia showed a nonsignificant trend in favor of danaparoid over dextran 70. Among the patients stratified as having ''mild'' thrombosis, a slightly higher percentage of patients treated with danaparoid (83%) improved compared with those who received dextran 70 (73%). In contrast, a substantial and significant difference in treatment outcome occurred in patients with ''serious'' thrombosis: 88% of danaparoid-treated patients recovered, compared with 44% of those treated with dextran 70. These data suggest that the use of an effective anticoagulant to treat thromboembolism associated with HIT is particularly important in those with more severe disease.

In the treatment of HIT patients, it is important to inhibit thrombin generation adequately with danaparoid until the acute thrombosis is well controlled. Furthermore, it generally takes at least 5 days of warfarin therapy before therapeutic functional hypoprothrombinemia is achieved (Harrison et al., 1997). Thus, even when oral anticoagulant therapy is begun soon after starting danaparoid, at least 5 days of danaparoid therapy are usually required. Many danaparoid-treated HIT patients also receive overlapping warfarin treatment, because oral anticoagulants are usually preferred when at least 3–6 months of further anticoagulation is indicated because of venous or arterial thromboembolism. Warfarin administration can be started safely together with danaparoid in patients who do not have severe HIT-associated thrombosis (Chong, 1996). However, in HIT patients with severe or extensive thrombosis, it is prudent to delay administration of warfarin until the thrombotic process is controlled and substantial resolution of the thrombocytopenia has occurred. This caveat is based on the observation that warfarin may aggravate the thrombotic process during the first few days of its administration, by reducing levels of the natural anticoagulant protein C, particularly when there is uncontrolled thrombin generation (Warkentin, 1996; Warkentin et al., 1997; Poetzsch et al., 1996; see Chaps. 3 and 12). Warfarin does not neutralize activated coagulation factors, and thus sufficient time must pass before its antithrombotic effects are achieved through reduction in the vitamin K-dependent procoagulant factors, particularly prothrombin. Danaparoid therapy usually is discontinued when the INR is at, or near, the target therapeutic range, and provided the acute thrombosis appears controlled on clinical grounds. Danaparoid does not interfere with INR measurements during oral anticoagulant therapy.

Prophylaxis of Venous Thromboembolism

Patients with a previous history of HIT may require an alternative anticoagulant to prevent venous thromboembolism if they are in a high-risk situation, such as following surgery. UFH cannot be used, particularly during the first 1 or 2 months after the onset of HIT when HIT antibodies still circulate. Thereafter, although HIT antibodies are usually undetectable, and the risk of HIT is possibly relatively low (Warkentin and Kelton, 1998), most physicians are understandably reluctant to readminister heparin in this situation.

Danaparoid is an effective and convenient drug for the prevention of venous thromboembolism in patients with prior HIT. In the compassionate-use program, 390 patients received danaparoid, 750 U by subcutaneous injection, usually twice daily for DVT prophylaxis for many postoperative settings, including following general, gynecological, neurological, cancer, and organ transplant surgery. A high rate of success was observed (Magnani, 1997; Ortel and Chong, 1998).

Prophylaxis of Arterial Thromboembolism

Danaparoid has been used to prevent arterial thromboembolism in patients undergoing various vascular operations, including peripheral artery bypass graft surgery, embolectomy, and endarterectomy. In these patients, it was given as a preoperative intravenous bolus of 2500 U and, in some, it was also administered postoperatively. Given as an intravenous bolus of 2500 U, immediately before the procedure, danaparoid has also been used to provide antithrombotic cover for percutaneous coronary angioplasty, with or without stenting, and for insertion of inferior vena cava filters and intra-aortic balloon devices.

Anticoagulation for Cardiopulmonary Bypass Surgery

Patients with acute HIT, or recent previous HIT with persisting HIT antibodies, may need to undergo cardiac surgery. UFH is contraindicated for these patients, necessitating an alternative anticoagulant for use during cardiopulmonary bypass surgery (CPB). After successful experiments in dogs, danaparoid has been used since 1985 for CPB in these patients (Henney et al., 1985; Magnani, 1993; Wilhelm et al., 1996; Christiansen et al., 1998). A recent report summarizes the experience of 47 evaluable patients who underwent CPB using danaparoid (Magnani et al., 1997).

The initial recommended dosing schedule consisted of 8750 U by intravenous bolus postthoracotomy (with the bolus dose changed to 5,000 and 10,000 U for patients weighing < 60 and > 90 kg, respectively) plus 7500 U danaparoid given in the priming fluid of the CPB machine. Further intraoperative booster injections were recommended up to an hourly basis, if necessary, because of fibrin clot formation. In the 47 reported patients who received danaparoid for CPB under the compassionate-use program, the recommended dosing schedule was not strictly followed in all patients. Some received inappropriate or wrongly timed booster doses (too near to surgical closure) and others received substantially higher doses in erroneous attempts to obtain the same activated-clotting time (ACT) prolongation as with UFH, even though anticoagulant-effective danaparoid doses do not prolong the ACT (Gitlin et al., 1998).

Despite suboptimal dosing in some patients, cardiac surgery nevertheless could be successfully completed in 45 of the 47 patients (Magnani et al., 1997). In two patients, the operations had to be abandoned because of formation of "clots" in the operative field or in the CPB circuit. In another 16 patients, intraoperative clots were seen, but dissolved on booster doses of danaparoid. No patients in this series had detectable in vitro cross-reactivity; thus, intraoperative clot formation is unlikely to be attributable to a manifestation of in vivo cross-reactivity. Intraoperative clot formation did not result in clinically evident thrombosis in any of the patients.

Increased postoperative bleeding was a significant problem with the use of danaparoid for CPB (Magnani et al., 1997). Eleven (22%) of the patients suffered severe postoperative blood loss, and another 33% had mild-to-moderate bleeding. Possible reasons for the excessive bleeding included (1) excessive danaparoid dosing owing to ad hoc protocol modifications; (2) administration of danaparoid booster doses too close to the end of surgery; (3) use of blood salvage techniques that returned anticoagulant-containing blood to the patient; and (4) the long plasma half-life of danaparoid and lack of an antidote to neutralize its anticoagulant effect (Skoutakis, 1997). It is also theoretically possible that suboptimal anticoagulation during CPB would paradoxically be associated with greater postoperative bleeding, as greater in vivo thrombin generation during CPB might lead to greater postoperative blood loss from secondary hyperfibrinolysis. This issue is raised because the empirically modified protocol subsequently described may, therefore, not necessarily be associated with reduction in bleeding outcomes.

On review of this experience, it was hypothesized that unnecessarily high drug doses contributed to postoperative bleeding. Supporting evidence included the observation that no severe bleeding was observed in patients who received a total dose of danaparoid of 16,250 U or less (i.e., ≤ 250 U/kg) (Magnani et al, 1997). Therefore, a new dosing regimen (see Table 1) was developed that delivers no more than 232 U/kg of the drug). Continuous intraoperative danaparoid infusion is also recommended, which may reduce the need for a further drug bolus shortly before wound closure, as well as provide therapeutic drug levels throughout CPB. Only a few patients have undergone cardiac surgery using the revised protocol, and it is too early to know whether the outcomes will be improved.

In view of these disadvantages with using danaparoid for CPB (Westphal et al., 1997), other therapeutic options should be considered. One approach reported to be successful in elective cardiac surgical settings is to await the disappearance of HIT antibodies, and then to use UFH for the period of CPB only, with or without antiplatelet agents (Makhoul et al., 1987; Addonizio et al., 1987; Laster et al., 1989; Kappa et al., 1990; Warkentin and Kelton, 1998). It appears that HIT antibodies do not recur rapidly in this setting, thus providing a rationale for this treatment approach (Warkentin and Kelton, 1998). For patients who need urgent cardiac surgery and who still have circulating HIT antibodies, plasmapheresis has been used successfully to remove the antibody before surgery in a few patients (Nand and Robinson, 1988; Thorp et al., 1990). These approaches, as well as the use of r-hirudin, are discussed further in Chaps. 13 and 17.

Hemodialysis and Hemofiltration

Danaparoid has been used to anticoagulate patients with HIT requiring hemodialysis or hemofiltration, in one of several clinical settings. First, patients with chronic or acute renal failure undergoing regular hemodialysis with UFH occasionally develop HIT, thus necessitating use of an alternative anticoagulant for subsequent dialyses. Second, very ill patients in intensive care settings who develop HIT not uncommonly have a need for anticoagulation during hemodialysis or hemofiltration. Third, danaparoid is useful for patients who experience difficulty in undergoing hemodialysis or hemofiltration with UFH because of repeated deposition of fibrin on the dialysis or hemofiltration membranes (Burgess and Chong, 1997). A change from UFH to danaparoid often allows continuation of hemodialysis or hemofiltration without further incident. This problem, which may be secondary to UFH-induced platelet aggregation and microthrombus formation, despite absence of HIT antibodies, may be a manifestation of nonimmune heparin-associated thrombocytopenia, although significant thrombocytopenia usually does not occur (Burgess and Chong, 1997).

Because danaparoid is cleared renally, the drug accumulates in the blood of patients with renal failure undergoing hemodialysis or hemofiltration with the heparinoid. A reduction in the dose of danaparoid generally is necessary for the second or third procedure after 2 or 3 days. For the first hemodialysis, an intravenous bolus of 3750 U (2500 U if the body weight is < 55 kg) is usually administered. A plasma anti-Xa level should be performed before the second and subsequent dialysis. The drug dose should be appropriately reduced (usually to 2250 or 3000 U), depending on whether hemodialysis is performed daily or every second day. The aim is to maintain a plasma anti-Xa level between 0.5 and 0.8 U/mL. For hemofiltration, the dosing regimen is the same as the intravenous infusion regimen used for the treatment of venous thrombosis (see Table 1). To avoid excessive accumulation of the drug in the blood, the infusion rate may be reduced on the second or subsequent day, according to the plasma anti-Xa levels.

Use in Children and Pregnant Women

Danaparoid has been used in only a very small number of pediatric and pregnant patients. Its major use in these patients has been for the treatment of HIT. Six children were treated with danaparoid for various indications, including maintenance of catheter patency, renal dialysis, and cardiac surgery. The treatment was successful in all except one patient in whom HIT occurred after a liver transplant complicated by graft rejection. In general, it was noted that children, particularly infants, often required higher doses of danaparoid than adults on a weight-adjusted basis.

Thirteen pregnant women with HIT were treated with danaparoid because of a past or recent venous thromboembolic event. About one-third started danaparoid in each trimester. The drug was discontinued in one patient because of possible cross-reactivity of the HIT antibodies with danaparoid in vitro and in vivo, in another because of persistent bleeding from placenta previa, and in a third because of onset of hemolysis–elevated liver enzymes–low platelets (HELLP) syndrome after 6 weeks of treatment. In the four neonates tested, the cord plasma showed no detectable anti-Xa activity, despite adequate levels in the mother, indicating that the drug does not cross the placenta. No increase in postpartum bleeding in danaparoid-treated pregnant mothers was reported. The doses of danaparoid used in these pregnant patients were the same as those used in nonpregnant women for the same clinical situations.

C. Laboratory Monitoring

Measurement of plasma anti-Xa levels using an amidolytic assay can be used for the laboratory monitoring of danaparoid's anticoagulant action. The heparinoid does not significantly prolong the activated partial thromboplastin time

(APTT), prothrombin time (INR), or activated-clotting time (ACT), except at very high doses. Hence, these assays cannot be used for laboratory monitoring of danaparoid. However, monitoring is not required in many clinical situations. The drug has a bioavailability of almost 100% after subcutaneous administration, and because of its lack of plasma protein interaction, predictable plasma levels are usually obtained with subcutaneous or intravenous use. However, laboratory monitoring is recommended in the following clinical settings: (1) patients with substantial renal impairment; (2) patients with unusually low or high body weight; (3) patients with life- or limb-threatening thrombosis; (4) patients with unexpected bleeding; and (5) critically ill or unstable patients.

It must be emphasized that for any assay of danaparoid-associated plasma anti-Xa activity, the standard calibration curve must be constructed using danaparoid, and not UFH or even LMWH (Laposata et al., 1998). Because of its lack of interaction with plasma heparin-binding proteins, danaparoid gives a dose-response relation different from these heparins, and plasma anti-Xa levels during danaparoid treatment will be overestimated if a LMWH standard curve is used. Indeed, there are differences in the stated therapeutic range among these various glycosaminoglycan anticoagulants (UFH, 0.2–0.4 U/mL by protamine titration; UFH, 0.3–0.7 anti-Xa U/mL; LMWH, 0.6–1.0 U/mL; danaparoid, 0.5–0.8 anti-Xa U/mL) (Hirsh et al., 1998; Laposata et al., 1998; Warkentin et al., 1998). In some clinical treatment settings using danaparoid, it might be advisable to aim for a lower anti-Xa level (e.g., about 0.3 U/mL for a patient judged to have a high risk of bleeding); sometimes, a higher target anti-Xa level should be sought (e.g., about 1.0 U/mL for a patient with life- or limb-threatening venous or arterial thrombosis).

Anti-Xa levels are determined using a chromogenic assay (i.e., a method similar to that performed for monitoring LMWH treatment). A standard reference curve must be constructed using various dilutions of danaparoid (e.g., 1.6, 1.0, 0.5, 0.3, and 0 U/mL danaparoid, diluted in pooled normal platelet-poor plasma). Control plasma samples are prepared by adding known quantities of danaparoid to normal pooled plasma aliquots (assuming 100% recovery of the known quantity of danaparoid added) in three different concentrations approximating treatment situations (e.g., 0.2, 0.7, and 1.25 U/mL, corresponding to low, mid, and high control danaparoid levels). Aliquots stored at −70°C are stable indefinitely if used only once, without refreezing and rethawing.

D. Cross-Reactivity of HIT Antibodies with Danaparoid

As danaparoid consists of a mixture of glycosaminoglycans (mainly heparan sulfate), it is not surprising that a small percentage of antibodies from HIT patients do cross-react with the drug. The cross-reactivity rate is low (mean, 9.6%) if aggregation studies using citrated platelet-rich plasma are performed (Makhoul et al., 1986; Kikta et al., 1993; Ramakrishna et al., 1995; Vun et al., 1996), but higher if more sensitive washed platelet activation (Warkentin, 1996) or a fluid-phase antigen assay (Newman et al., 1998) is used (see Chap. 11). Because activation HIT assays are highly dependent on the donor platelets used for testing, we have used highly reactive donor platelets under standardized conditions using platelet aggregation, to investigate the cross-reactivity of the HIT antibodies with danaparoid and LMWH. We found cross-reactivity rates of 7% with danaparoid and 83–89% with LMWH (Vun et al., 1996). However, with the sensitive fluid-phase antigen assay, we observed a higher cross-reactivity rate of 50% with danaparoid and again a much higher rate (88%) with LMWH (Newman et al., 1998; Fig. 2). Importantly, even when in vitro reactivity with danaparoid is observed, it is generally weak and quantitatively less than seen with LMWH.

The in vitro cross-reactivity of the HIT antibodies with danaparoid does not appear to be clinically significant. We have investigated the clinical significance of in vitro cross-reactivity in 21 patients treated with the LMW heparinoid (Newman et al., 1998). The 8 patients who tested positive with danaparoid by the fluid-phase enzyme immunoassay, but negative by the [^{14}C]serotonin-release washed platelet assay, recovered with resolution of their thrombocytopenia and thrombosis, in a fashion similar to the 11 patients who did not manifest in vitro cross-reactivity to danaparoid by both assays. Two patients tested positive by both activation and antigen assays: in 1 patient, both thrombocytopenia and pulmonary embolism resolved during danaparoid treatment. However, in the other patient, thrombocytopenia and extensive thrombosis persisted despite danaparoid therapy. It is unclear whether this unusual patient course represented a specific danaparoid treatment failure, as the patient's subsequent clinical course was characterized by consistent failure for all of the antithrombotic therapies used (Fig. 3).

Warkentin (1996) also evaluated the clinical significance of in vitro cross-reactivity with danaparoid in 29 HIT patients who had been treated with the heparinoid for HIT. This investigator found no difference in clinical outcomes, or in the time to platelet count recovery, between the two patient groups. However, there are isolated anecdotal reports of unfavorable clinical outcomes in HIT patients treated with danaparoid (Tandy/Poncet et al., 1995; Insler et al., 1997; Muhm et al., 1997). Cross-reactive antibodies were not always investigated in these studies. It remains possible that unrelated clinical factors might have caused the fall in the platelet count in these patients.

Overall, on the balance of current evidence, it would appear that in vitro cross-reactivity with danaparoid is not associated with adverse clinical outcomes in most patients. Accordingly, some investigators do not obtain cross-reactivity test results before instituting danaparoid therapy. This approach seems reasonable. It is based on several considerations: the overall low risk of in vivo cross-reactivity, the low predictivity of in vitro cross-reactivity testing, the lack of standardized test methods, and the potential for adverse clinical events during withholding of treatment pending the results of cross-reactivity testing. However, cross-reactivity testing should be performed in patients who develop new,

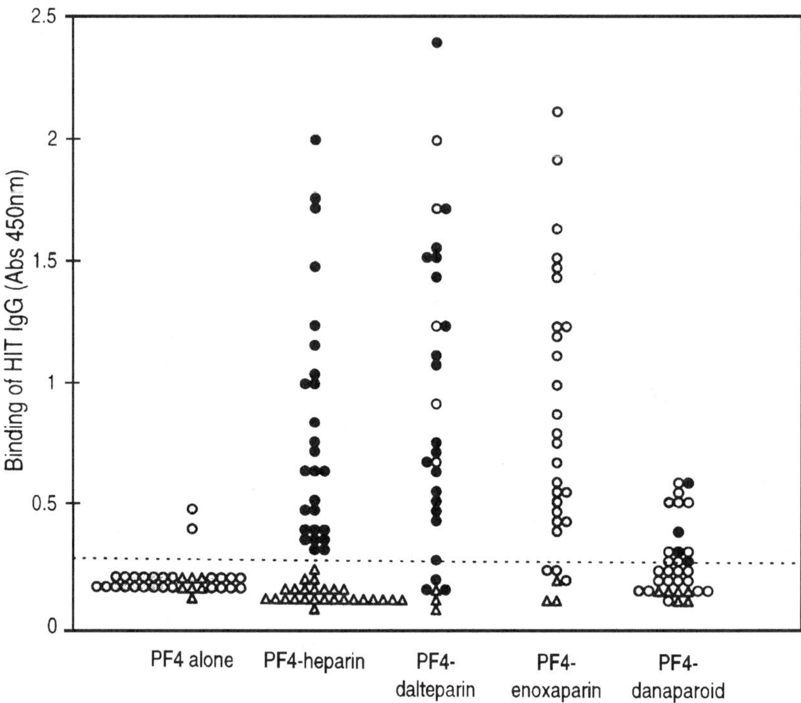

Figure 2 Cross-reactivity of HIT–IgG antibodies with PF4 complexed to heparin-like anticoagulants: The fluid-phase enzyme-linked immunoassay was used to assess the degree to which IgG present in HIT sera or plasma bound to PF4 alone, PF4–heparin, PF4–dalteparin (Fragmin), PF4–enoxaparin (Clexane), or PF4–danaparoid (Orgaran). The positive cutoff (dashed line) is 3 standard deviations above the mean (log transformed) absorbance of the normal samples using PF4–heparin. The binding of normal antibodies is indicated by triangles. Circles indicate HIT samples that have been positive (closed circle), negative (open circle), or not tested (speckled circle) in a functional assay with the corresponding drug. (From Newman et al., 1998.)

progressive, or recurrent thrombocytopenia or thrombosis during treatment with danaparoid.

E. Adverse Effects

Severe bleeding is the most serious adverse effect of danaparoid, but rarely occurs except in patients who are treated with very high doses of the drug, or who develop drug accumulation (renal failure), or who have additional hemostatic or

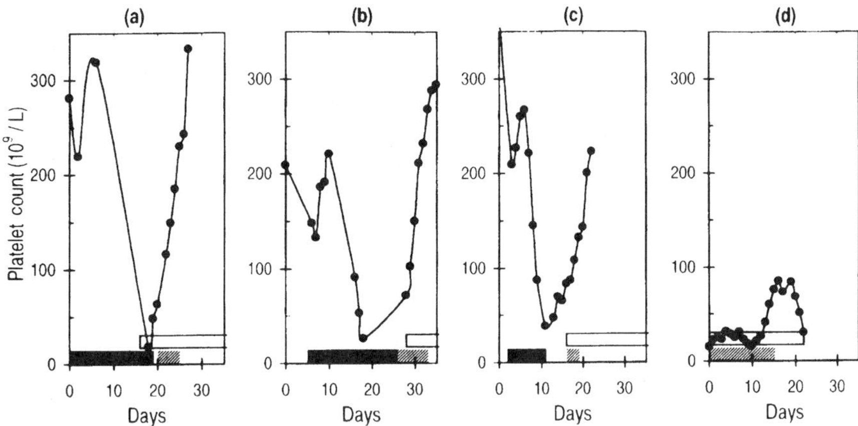

Figure 3 Serial platelet counts of representative HIT patients treated with danaparoid: Solid black bar shows duration of heparin administration, striped bar indicates danaparoid therapy, open bar shows warfarin therapy. (a) Typical profile of the 11 patients who were negative in both fluid-phase EIA and functional assay. (b) Typical profile of the 8 patients who were positive in the fluid-phase, but negative in a functional assay. (c) Profile of patient A, one of the two patients who were positive in both types of assay. She recovered during a short course of danaparoid. (d) Profile of patient B, the other patient positive in both assays. The profile indicates the course of HIT following transfer to a major hospital. Despite treatment with many antithrombotic agents, he eventually died following major thrombosis. (From Newman et al., 1998.)

vascular defects. However, serious bleeding occurred in a significant number of patients who had undergone CPB with danaparoid (Magnani et al., 1997; Westphal et al., 1997). In contrast, bleeding was not seen in the randomized trial in which HIT patients with venous or arterial thromboses received danaparoid (Chong, 1996). Compared with CPB patients, these patients underwent less intense anticoagulation, and did not suffer from the additional insults of CPB and chest incision.

Skin hypersensitivity reactions have been reported with danaparoid, but these are rare (Magnani, 1993). Elevated liver enzyme levels were observed in some patients, but osteoporosis (an important complication of prolonged UFH treatment) was not detected in any danaparoid-treated patients in the compassionate-use program, even in those treated for more than 3 months. Despite the issue of in vitro cross-reactivity with danaparoid, it is noteworthy that new-onset immune-mediated thrombocytopenia has never been reported with this agent.

F. Availability of Danaparoid

Table 2 lists the countries in which danaparoid has been approved for the treatment of HIT, either with or without associated thrombosis. Also listed are a number of countries, including the United States, Canada, France, the United Kingdom, and the Netherlands, where the drug has been approved for the prevention of DVT. In these countries, physicians have the legal option to prescribe danaparoid for HIT (i.e., for ''off-label'' use in a nonapproved indication; see Chap. 18).

Table 2 Countries in Which Danaparoid Is Approved for Clinical Use

	DVT prophylaxis		Heparin-induced thrombocytopenia	
Country	Postsurgery	Poststroke	Prophylaxis	Treatment
North America				
Canada	X	X		
United States	X[a]			
Europe				
Austria			X	X
Belgium	X		X	X
Denmark	X		X	X
Finland			X	X
France	X		X	
Germany			X	X
Great Britain	X			X
Greece	X			
Ireland	X			
Italy	X			
Luxembourg	X		X	X
Netherlands	X[b]	X[b]	X	X
Norway	X	X		
Portugal	X		X	X
Sweden	X	X		X
Switzerland	X[a]			
Australasia				
Australia	X			
Korea	X			
New Zealand	X	X	X	X

[a] Excluding prophylaxis in patients with stroke.

[b] Approval withdrawn to obtain approval for HIT.

III. CONCLUSION

Danaparoid is a safe and effective anticoagulant for the prevention or treatment of venous or arterial thrombosis in HIT patients, regardless of the presence of antibody cross-reactivity with the drug. It is also efficacious as an anticoagulant for hemodialysis–hemofiltration and cardiac surgery employing CPB. With the use of danaparoid for the cardiac surgery, serious postoperative bleeding can occur.

ACKNOWLEDGMENTS

I wish to thank Dr. H. Magnani for his helpful comments and critical review of the manuscript. Some of the studies described in this chapter were supported by a program grant from the National Health and Medical Research Council of Australia.

REFERENCES

Aberg M, Rausing A. The effect of dextran 70 on the structure of ex vivo thrombi. Thromb Res 12:1113–1122, 1978.

Addonizio VP Jr, Fisher CA, Kappa JR, Ellison N. Prevention of heparin-induced thrombocytopenia during open heart surgery with iloprost. Surgery 102:796–807, 1987.

Bergqvist D. Prevention of postoperative deep vein thrombosis in Sweden. Results of a survey. World J Surg 4:489–495, 1980.

Bergqvist D, Kettunen K, Fredin H, et al. Thromboprophylaxis in patients with hip fractures: a prospective, randomized, comparative study between Org 10172 and dextran 70. Surgery 109:617–622, 1991.

Biller J, Massey EW, Marler JR, et al. A dose escalation study of Org 10172 (low molecular weight heparinoid) in stroke. Neurology 39:262–265, 1989.

Bradbrook ID, Magnani HN, Moelker HCT, Morrison PJ, Robinson J, Rogers HJ, Spector RG, Van Dinther T, Wijnand H. Org 10172: a low molecular weight heparinoid anticoagulant with a long half-life in man. Br J Clin Pharmacol 23:667–675, 1987.

Burgess JK, Chong BH. The platelet proaggregating and potentiating effects of unfractionated heparin, low molecular weight heparin and heparinoid in intensive care patients and healthy controls. Eur J Haematol 58:279–285, 1997.

Cade JF, Wood M, Magnani HN, Westlake GW. Early clinical experience of a new heparinoid, Org 10172, in prevention of deep venous thrombosis. Thromb Res 45:497–503, 1987.

Casu B. Structural features of chondroitin sulphate, dermatan sulphate and heparan sulphate. Semin Thromb Haemost 17(suppl 1):9–14, 1991.

Chong BH. Heparin-induced thrombocytopenia. Br J Haematol 89:431–439, 1995.

Chong BH. Low molecular weight heparinoid and heparin-induced thrombocytopenia [abstr]. Aust NZ J Med 26:331, 1996.

Chong BH, Castaldi PA. Platelet proaggregating effect of heparin: possible mechanism for non-immune heparin-associated thrombocytopenia. Aust NZ J Med 16:715–716, 1986.

Chong BH, Ismail F. The mechanism of heparin-induced platelet aggregation. Eur J Haematol 43:245–251, 1989.

Chong BH, Magnani HN. Orgaran in heparin-induced thrombocytopenia. Haemostasis 22: 85–91, 1992.

Chong BH, Ismail F, Cade J, Gallus AS, Gordon S, Chesterman CN. Heparin-induced thrombocytopenia: studies with a new molecular weight heparinoid, Org 10172. Blood 73:1592–1596, 1989.

Danhof M, de Boer A, Magnani HN, Stiekema JCJ. Pharmacokinetic considerations on Orgaran (Org 10172). Hemostasis 22:73–84, 1992

de Valk HW, Banga JD, Wester JWJ, Brouwer CB, van Hessen MWJ, Meuwissen OJAT, Hart HC, Sixma JJ, Nieuwenhuis HK. Comparing subcutaneous danaparoid with intravenous unfractionated heparin for the treatment of venous thromboembolism. A randomized controlled trial. Ann Intern Med 123:1–9, 1995.

Gallus A, Cade J, Ockelford P, Hepburn S, Maas M, Magnani H, Bucknall T, Stevens J, Porteious F. Orgaran (Org 10172) or heparin for preventing venous thrombosis after elective surgery for malignant disease? A double-blind, randomised, multicentre comparison. Thromb Haemost 70:562–567, 1993.

Gent M, Hirsh J, Ginsberg JS, Powers PJ, Levine MN, Geerts WH, Jay RM, Leclerc J, Neemeh JA, Turpie AG. Low-molecular-weight heparinoid Orgaran is more effective than aspirin in the prevention of venous thromboembolism after surgery for hip fracture. Circulation 93:80–84, 1996.

Gerhart TN, Yett HS, Robertson LK, Lee MA, Smith M, Salzman EW. Low-molecular-weight heparinoid compared with warfarin for prophylaxis of deep-vein thrombosis in patients who are operated on for fracture of the hip. A prospective, randomized trial. J Bone Joint Surg 73A:494–502, 1991.

Getlin SD, Deeb GM, Yann C, Schmaier AH. Intraoperative monitoring of danaparoid sodium anticoagulation during cardiovascular operations. J Vasc Surg 27:568–575, 1998.

Gordon DL, Linhardt R, Adams HP. Low-molecular-weight heparins and heparinoids and their use in acute or progressing ischaemic stroke. Clin Neuropharmacol 13:522–543, 1990.

Greinacher A, Michels I, Muller-Eckhardt C. Heparin-associated thrombocytopenia: the antibody is not heparin specific. Thromb Haemost 67:545–549, 1992.

Harrison L, Johnston M, Massicotte MP, Crowther M, Moffat K, Hirsh J. Comparison of 5-mg and 10-mg loading doses in initiation of warfarin therapy. Ann Intern Med 126:133–136, 1997.

Henny CP, ten Cate H, ten Cate JW, Surachno S, van Bronswijk H, Wilmink JM, Ockelford PA. Use of a new heparinoid as anticoagulant during acute haemodialysis of patients with bleeding complications. Lancet 1:890–893, 1983.

Hirsh J, Warkentin TE, Raschke R, Granger C, Ohman EM, Dalen JE. Heparin and low-molecular-weight heparin. Mechanisms of action, pharmacokinetics, dosing considerations, monitoring, efficacy, and safety. Chest 114:489S–510S, 1998.

Hoek JA, Nurmohamed MT, Hamelynck KJ, Marti RK, Knipscheer HC, ten Cate H, Büller HR, Magnani HN, ten Cate JW. Prevention of deep vein thrombosis following total hip replacement by low molecular weight heparinoid. Thromb Haemost 67:28–32, 1992.

Insler SR, Kraenzler EJ, Bartholomew JR, Kottke-Marchant K, Lytle B, Starr NJ. Thrombosis during the use of the heparinoid Organon 10172 in a patient with heparin-induced thrombocytopenia. Anesthesiology 86:495–498, 1997.

Kappa JR, Fisher CA, Todd B, Stenach N, Bell P, Campbell F, Ellison N, Addonizio VP. Intraoperative management of patients with heparin-induced thrombocytopenia. Ann Thoracic Surg 49:714–722, 1990.

Kikta MJ, Keller MP, Humphrey PW, Silver D. Can low molecular weight heparins and heparinoids be safely given to patients with heparin-induced thrombocytopenia syndrome? Surgery 114:705–710, 1993.

Laposata M, Green D, Van Cott EM, Barrowcliffe TW, Goodnight SH, Sosolik RC. College of American Pathologists Conference Therapy. The clinical use and laboratory monitoring of low-molecular-weight heparin, danaparoid, hirudin and related compounds, and argatroban. Arch Pathol Lab Med 122:799–807, 1998.

Laster J, Elfrink R, Silver D. Re-exposure to heparin of patients with heparin-associated antibodies. Vasc Surg 9:677–681, 1989.

Leyvraz P, Bachmann F, Bohnet J, et al. Thromboembolic prophylaxis in total hip replacement: a comparison between the low molecular weight heparinoid Lomoparan and heparin-dihydroergotamine. Br J Surg 79:911–914, 1992.

Magnani HN. Heparin-induced thrombocytopenia (HIT): an overview of 230 patients treated with Orgaran (Org 10172). Thromb Haemost 70:554–561, 1993.

Magnani HN. Orgaran (danaparoid sodium) use in the syndrome of heparin-induced thrombocytopenia. Platelets 8:74–81, 1997.

Magnani HN, Beijering RJR, ten Cate JW, Chong BH. Orgaran anticoagulation for cardiopulmonary bypass in patients with heparin-induced thrombocytopenia. In: Pifarre R, ed. New Anticoagulants for the Cardiovascular Patient. Philadelphia: Hanley & Belfus, 1997:487–500.

Makhoul RG, Greenberg CS, McCann RL. Heparin-induced thrombocytopenia and thrombosis: a serious clinical problem and potential solution. J Vasc Surg 4:522–528, 1986.

Makhoul RG, McCann RL, Austin EH, Greenberg CS, Lowe JE. Management of patients with heparin-associated thrombocytopenia and thrombosis requiring cardiac surgery. Ann Thorac Surg 43:617–621, 1987.

Meuleman DG, Hobbelen PMJ, Van Dedem G, Moelker HCT. A novel anti-thrombotic heparinoid (Org 10172) devoid of bleeding inducing capacity: a survey of its pharmacological properties in experimental animal models. Thromb Res 27:353–63, 1982.

Meuleman DG. Synopsis of the anticoagulant and antithrombotic profile of the low molecular weight heparinoid Org 10172 in experimental models. Thromb Haemost 58: 376–80, 1987.

Meuleman DG. Orgaran (Org 10172): its pharmacological profile in experimental models. Haemostasis 22:58–65, 1992.

Mikhailidis DP, Barradas MA, Mikhailidis AM, Magnani H, Dandona P. Comparison of the effect of a conventional heparin and a low molecular weight heparinoid on platelet function. Br J Clin Pharmacol 17:43–48, 1984.

Mikhailidis DP, Fonseca VA, Barradas MA, Jeremy JY, Dandona P. Platelet activation following intravenous injection of a conventional heparin: absence of effect with a low molecular weight heparinoid (Org 10172). Br J Clin Pharmacol 24:415–424, 1987.

Muhm M, Claeys L, Huk I, Koppensteiner R, Kyrle PA, Minar E, Stumpflen A, Ehringer H, Polterauer P. Thromboembolic complications in a patient with heparin-induced thrombocytopenia (HIT) showing cross-reactivity to a low molecular weight heparin-treatment with Org 10172 (Lomoparan). Wien Klin Wochenschr 109:128–131, 1997.

Nand S, Robinson JA. Plasmapheresis in the management of heparin-associated thrombocytopenia with thrombosis. Am J Hematol 28:204–206, 1998.

Newman PM, Swanson RL, Chong BH. IgG binding to PF4–heparin complexes in the fluid phase and cross-reactivity with low molecular weight heparin and heparinoid. Thromb Haemost 80:292–297, 1998.

Nieuwenhuis HK, Sixma JJ. Treatment of disseminated intravascular coagulation in acute promyelocytic leukemia with low molecular weight heparinoid Org 10172. Cancer 58:761–764, 1986.

Ofosu FA. Anticoagulant mechanisms of Orgaran (Org 10172) and its fraction with high affinity to antithrombin III (Org 10849). Haemostasis 22:66–72, 1992.

Org 10172 hip joint replacement report, research protocol 004–023. West Orange, NJ: Organon Inc., 1994.

Ortel TL, Chong BH. New treatment options for heparin-induced thrombocytopenia. Semin Hematol 35(suppl 5):26–34, 1998.

Pötzsch B, Unrig C, Madlener K, Greinacher A, Müller-Berghaus G. APC resistance and early onset of oral anticoagulation are high thrombotic risk factors in patients with heparin-associated thrombocytopenia (HAT) [abstr]. Ann Hematol 72(suppl 1):A6, 1996.

Ramakrishna R, Manoharan A, Kwan YL, Kyle PW. Heparin-induced thrombocytopenia: cross-reactivity between standard heparin, low molecular weight heparin, dalteparin (Fragmin) and heparinoid (Orgaran). Br J Haematol 91:736–738, 1995.

Skoutakis VA. Danaparoid in the prevention of thrombo-embolic complications. Ann Pharmacother 31:876–887, 1997.

Sobel M, Adelman B, Greenfield LJ. Dextran 40 reduces heparin-mediated platelet aggregation. J Surg Res 40:382–387, 1986.

Stiekema JC, Wijnand HP, van Dinther TG, Moelker HCT, Dawes J, Vinchenzo A, Toeberich H. Safety and pharmacokinetics of the low molecular weight heparinoid Org 10172 administered to healthy elderly volunteers. Br J Clin Pharmacol 27:39–48, 1989.

Tardy/Poncet B, Mahul P, Beraud AM, Favre JP, Tardy B, Guyotat D. Failure of Orgaran therapy in a patient with a previous heparin-induced thrombocytopenia. Br J Haematol 90:69–70, 1995.

Thorp D, Canty A, Whiting J, Dart G, Lloyd JV, Duncan E, Gallus A. Plasma exchange and heparin-induced thrombocytopenia. Prog Clin Biol Res 337:521–522, 1990.

Von Bonsdorff M, Stiekema J, Harjanne A, Alapiessa U. A new low molecular weight heparinoid Org 10172 as anticoagulant in hemodialysis. Int J Artif Organs 13:103–108, 1990.

Vun CH, Evans S, Chong BH. Cross-reactivity study of low molecular weight heparins and heparinoid in heparin-induced thrombocytopenia. Thromb Res 81:525–532, 1996.

Warkentin TE. Heparin-induced thrombocytopenia: IgG-mediated platelet activation, platelet microparticle generation, and altered procoagulant/anticoagulant balance in the pathogenesis of thrombosis and venous limb gangrene complicating heparin-induced thrombocytopenia. Transf Med Rev 10:249–258, 1996.

Warkentin TE. Danaparoid (Orgaran) for the treatment of heparin-induced thrombocytopenia (HIT) and thrombosis: effects on in vivo thrombin and cross-linked fibrin generation, and evaluation of the clinical significance of in vitro cross-reactivity of danaparoid for HIT-IgG [abstr]. Blood 88:626a, 1996.

Warkentin TE, Kelton JG. A 14-year study of heparin-induced thrombocytopenia. Am J Med 101:502–507, 1996.

Warkentin TE, Kelton JG. Timing of heparin-induced thrombocytopenia (HIT) in relation to previous heparin use: absence of an anamnestic immune response, and implications for repeat heparin use in patients with a history of HIT [abstr]. Blood 92 (suppl 1):182a, 1998.

Warkentin TE, Elavathil LJ, Hayward CPM, Johnston MA, Russett JI, Kelton JG. The pathogenesis of venous limb gangrene associated with heparin-induced thrombocytopenia. Ann Intern Med 127:804–812, 1997.

Warkentin TE, Chong BH, Greinacher A. Heparin-induced thrombocytopenia: towards consensus. Thromb Haemost 79:1–7, 1998.

Westphal K, Martens S, Strouhal U, Matheis G. Heparin-induced thrombocytopenia type II: perioperative management using danaparoid in a coronary artery bypass patient with renal failure. Thorac Cardiovasc Surg 45:318–20, 1997.

15

Recombinant Hirudin for the Treatment of Heparin-Induced Thrombocytopenia

Andreas Greinacher
Ernst-Moritz-Arndt University, Greifswald, Germany

I. INTRODUCTION

Heparin-induced thrombocytopenia (HIT) is caused by immunological mechanisms. Usually, pathogenic antibodies are formed against complexes of sulfated oligosaccharides (e.g., heparin) and platelet factor 4 (PF4) (see Chaps. 6–8). Resulting immune complexes interact with platelet FcγIIa receptors, resulting in platelet activation and thrombocytopenia (Greinacher, 1995; Warkentin et al., 1998). HIT antibodies also activate endothelial cells. Together, platelet activation, platelet microparticle generation, and endothelial cell alteration promote thrombin generation, increasing the risk for thromboembolic complications (TECs) associated with HIT.

Immediate cessation of heparin administration is mandatory when HIT is clinically suspected. Despite stopping administration of heparin, increased thrombin generation persists for at least several days (Warkentin, 1998), and patients remain at high risk for thrombosis (Warkentin and Kelton, 1996; Greinacher et al., 1999a). Thus, many patients with HIT require further parenteral anticoagulation. Currently, two antithrombotic agents are approved in several countries for treatment or prophylaxis of thrombosis associated with HIT: danaparoid sodium and the recombinant hirudin (r-hirudin), lepirudin (see Chap. 14). Here, the treatment of HIT with lepirudin is reviewed.

II. HIRUDIN

A. Chemistry

Hirudin is an antithrombotic substance naturally produced by the salivary glands of the medicinal leech, *Hirudo medicinalis*. It is a 65-amino acid polypeptide (molecular mass, approximately 7000 Da). The NH_2-terminal part of the molecule (residues 1–39) is stabilized by three disulfide bridges integral for its function; the COOH-terminal moiety (residues 40–65) is highly acidic. The three-dimensional structure of hirudin has been resolved (Sukumaran et al., 1987; Clore et al., 1987). Three areas are distinguished: a central core (residues 3–30, 37–46, 56–57); a ''finger'' (residues 31–36); and a loop (residues 47–55).

Hirudin is produced in large quantities by several companies. It is derived from yeast cells using recombinant biotechnology. Currently, the most important r-hirudins are lepirudin (Refludan, HBW 023) and desirudin (Revasc, CGP 39393). These compounds are also called desulfatohirudins because, compared with natural hirudin, they lack a sulfate group at Tyr-63. Also, lepirudin has leucine substituted for isoleucine at its NH_2-terminal end. Although these structural differences result in tenfold reduction in activity, no clinically relevant difference results.

B. Pharmacology

Hirudin is a potent and specific thrombin inhibitor, with an inhibition constant for thrombin in the picomolar range (Stone and Hofsteenge, 1986). Hirudin acts independently of the cofactors antithrombin and heparin cofactor II (Markwardt, 1992). It forms noncovalent, but irreversible, 1 : 1 complexes with thrombin, thus inhibiting all of thrombin's biological activities.

Three amino acids (residues 46–48) near the NH_2-terminus of hirudin bind to the thrombin active site cleft, whereas the core of the hirudin molecule closes off the active site pocket (Fig. 1). The COOH-terminal tail of hirudin interacts with the fibrinogen anion-binding site, blocking thrombin-catalyzed fibrinogen cleavage. Hirudin inhibits by a factor of 10,000 the feedback loop whereby thrombin enhances its own generation through activation of factors Va and VIIIa (Kaiser and Markwardt, 1986; Pieters et al., 1989).

Hirudin also inhibits clot-bound thrombin (Hogg and Jackson, 1989; Weitz et al., 1990) and thrombin bound to fibrin split products (Weitz et al., 1998). In contrast, clot-bound thrombin is protected from inhibition by heparin–antithrombin complexes. This important difference between hirudin and heparin could explain why hirudin enables dissolution of mural thrombi more effectively than does heparin in experimental models (Meyer et al., 1998). Hirudin, therefore, may be particularly useful for anticoagulation in HIT, a disease characterized by

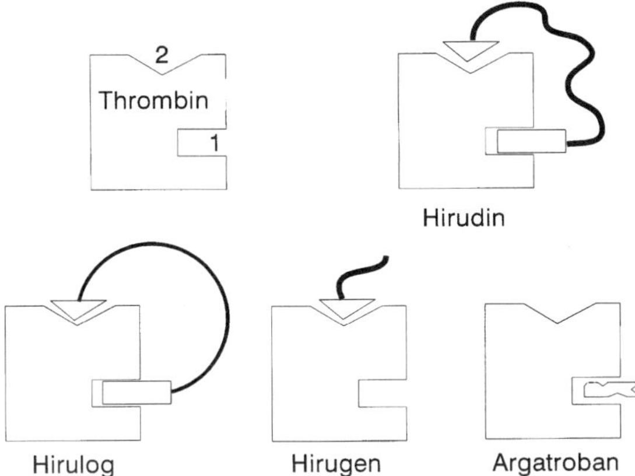

Figure 1 Schematic representation of the thrombin molecule and its inhibition by hirudin, Hirulog, Hirugen, and argatroban: (1) Active-site pocket; (2) fibrinogen-binding site. The active-site pocket catalyzes most of the functions of the thrombin molecule; whereas, the fibrinogen-binding exosite mediates the binding of thrombin to fibrinogen. Hirudin is a 7000-Da protein composed of 65 amino acids, which binds to the active-site pocket and the fibrinogen-binding exosite of thrombin. Hirulog is a synthetic peptide designed to block both active sites of thrombin. Hirugen, a synthetic peptide, mimics the binding site of fibrinogen to thrombin, thereby inhibiting binding of thrombin to fibrinogen and, therefore, fibrinogen cleavage by thrombin. The arginine derivative, argatroban, binds competitively to only the active binding site pocket of thrombin (Adapted from Herrmann et al., 1997.)

in vivo platelet activation and thrombin formation (Chong et al., 1994; Warkentin et al., 1994; Greinacher et al., 1999a).

Hirudin activity is standardized in thrombin inhibitory units (TIU): 1 TIU is the amount of hirudin inhibiting 1 U of thrombin at 37°C. Purified hirudins contain about 10,000–15,000 TIU/mg protein.

C. Pharmacokinetics

After intravenous (iv) administration, r-hirudin is distributed in the extracellular space, and undergoes first-order elimination through the kidneys. Unlike heparin, r-hirudin does not bind to proteins other than thrombin, and is not inactivated by PF4 (Glusa and Markwardt, 1990). Because this extracellular distribution includes the extravascular compartment, r-hirudin levels measured in blood constitute only 15–20% of the total r-hirudin in the body (Glusa, 1998).

The mean terminal half-life of r-hirudin is approximately 1–2 h. Although 90% is eliminated by the kidneys, only about 50% of the drug is excreted intact in urine; the remainder is metabolized by renal tubular cells. Consequently, in patients with renal insufficiency, the half-life is greatly increased. In uremic patients undergoing hemodialysis, the half-life is 48 h; in anephric patients, it approaches 200 h (Nowak et al., 1991). This issue is also relevant to elderly patients, many of whom have renal impairment. Although dosing with r-hirudin is generally stable in a given patient, there may be major differences among individuals; therefore, monitoring of r-hirudin treatment is important.

D. Monitoring

Phase I studies indicated that the activated partial thromboplastin time (aPTT) is an appropriate way to monitor r-hirudin therapy (Verstraete et al., 1993; Marbet et al., 1993). However, the aPTT method is not optimal, because its correlation with plasma r-hirudin levels is only fair (Nurmohamed et al., 1994; Pötzsch et al., 1997); at higher r-hirudin concentrations (aPTT > 70 s), the dose response relation flattens, and correlation becomes poor (Pötzsch et al., 1997). The primary reason for current use of the aPTT to monitor r-hirudin treatment is its wide availability.

A new tool for monitoring r-hirudin treatment is the ecarin-clotting time (ECT). Ecarin is a snake venom enzyme (Nishida et al., 1995) that catalyzes prothrombin to thrombin by cleavage at Arg323–Ile324 (Novoa et al., 1980). Meizothrombin is an intermediate form of thrombin that has substantially less clotting activity. By traces of factor Xa and factor Va, as well as by autocatalysis, meizothrombin is converted to α-thrombin (Boskovic et al., 1990).

The principle of the ECT test is that meizothrombin interacts with r-hirudin the same way thrombin does. As long as there is an excess of r-hirudin, clotting is prevented. When all the r-hirudin in a sample is neutralized by meizothrombin, thrombin is generated and clotting occurs. Therefore, the plasma concentration of r-hirudin correlates with the ECT (Pötzsch et al., 1997). In contrast to the aPTT, the reactions in the ECT do not require calcium, phospholipid surfaces, or γ-carboxyglutamic acid residues on prothrombin; thus, the ECT was first used to evaluate patients with deficiency of vitamin K-dependent coagulation factors (Solano et al., 1990) before Nowak and Bucha (1993) used the test to monitor r-hirudin treatment. Pötzsch and colleagues (1997) have adapted the ECT to measure high r-hirudin concentrations.

The ECT could become the method of choice to monitor r-hirudin treatment once it becomes widely available. Prospective studies show that bleeding complications are the main adverse effect of r-hirudin treatment. It is possible that some bleeding episodes could be prevented by monitoring with the ECT in high-risk situations (e.g., high-dose or perioperative anticoagulation).

E. Reversal of r-Hirudin

The antithrombin potency of r-hirudin means that bleeding is an important, and potentially severe, side effect (Antmann et al., 1994; Neuhaus et al., 1994). Currently, there is no antidote for r-hirudin. In many cases, stopping r-hirudin is sufficient treatment of a bleeding patient, as the concentration falls quickly owing to its short half-life. However, when bleeding is life-threatening, or in patients with renal failure and reduced drug excretion, drug cessation alone may not be adequate. Meizothrombin may prove to be a potentially useful antidote (Nowak and Bucha, 1995), but is not yet available for use in humans. Hemofiltration using cellulose acetate filters with a cutoff point > 50,000 Da appears to eliminate r-hirudin in animal models (Nowak et al., 1992; Riess et al., 1997a), but human data are limited, and hemofiltration is not always a practical option.

Suggested pharmacological means to treat r-hirudin overdosage include: desmopressin (Ibbotson et al., 1991; Bove et al., 1996), factor VII (Butler et al., 1993), von Willebrand factor (vWF) or vWF-containing factor VIII concentrates (Dickneite et al., 1996, 1998). Irami et al. (1995) described a patient in whom r-hirudin–induced bleeding was treated using prothrombin complex concentrates, as shown in animal models (Diehl et al., 1995). However, this approach is dangerous in HIT patients because prothrombin complex concentrates contain heparin.

F. r-Hirudin Derivatives and Synthetic Thrombin Inhibitors

Various other hirudin derivatives and synthetic direct thrombin inhibitors have been developed (Fareed et al., 1998; see Fig. 1). Hirulog (bivalirudin) is a semisynthetic hirudin derivative, in which the COOH-terminal region of hirudin (which blocks fibrinogen cleavage) and the NH_2-terminal region of hirudin (which blocks the active binding site pocket of thrombin) are linked by a spacer. Hirugen is a synthetic peptide that mimics the COOH-terminal region of hirudin; blocking only the fibrinogen-binding site, it has 50 times less potency than hirudin.

Several synthetic thrombin inhibitors, such as argatroban, are now under clinical evaluation (Hermann et al., 1997). Argatroban is an arginine derivative that binds competitively to the active binding site pocket of thrombin. Unlike r-hirudin, its elimination is independent of renal function, but is impaired in patients with hepatic dysfunction (Lewis et al., 1997a,b).

G. Clinical Use of r-Hirudin

Recombinant-hirudin has been investigated in controlled studies of patients with myocardial infarction (Antmann et al., 1994; Neuhaus et al., 1994), unstable angina pectoris (Rupprecht et al., 1995; Organization to Assess Strategies for Ischemic Syndromes [OASIS-2], 1999), and deep venous thrombosis (Parent et al., 1993; Schiele et al., 1997). It has also been tested for prophylaxis of thromboembolism following orthopedic hip surgery (Eriksson et al., 1997) and in patients undergoing extracorporeal circulation (Vanholder et al., 1994; Nowak et al., 1997; see Chaps. 16 and 17). r-Hirudin is an effective anticoagulant in each of these clinical settings.

III. r-HIRUDIN FOR TREATMENT OF HIT

A. Overview of Studies

The pharmacological characteristics of hirudin, and its efficacy in non-HIT patients, suggested that r-hirudin might be safe and effective for parenteral anticoagulation in HIT patients. Our center (Institute for Immunology and Transfusion Medicine, Greifswald) conducted two prospective, multicenter, historically controlled trials, HAT-1 and HAT-2 (Greinacher et al., 1999a,b), using the r-hirudin, lepirudin (Refludan, Hoechst Marion Roussel), for treatment of patients with serologically confirmed HIT. The clinical outcomes of lepirudin-treated patients were compared with a historical control group because the serious natural history of HIT, and the unavailability of approved alternative treatments during the period of these studies (March 1994 to April 1996) made the use of a placebo control unethical.

Study Design

The primary objective of the two studies was to determine whether intravenous lepirudin treatment of patients with confirmed HIT resulted in an increase in the platelet count in thrombocytopenic patients (or maintenance of normal baseline platelet values), while providing effective anticoagulation, defined as a prolongation of the aPTT by 1.5- to 3.0-fold over baseline values. (This range was based on the use of Actin FS or Neothromtin reagents in Europe; with other reagents used in North America, the aPTT target range is a 1.5- to 2.5-fold prolongation.) A secondary objective was the frequency of new arterial or venous TECs, major bleeding, limb amputations, and death.

Patients

Patients were eligible for study if the platelet count fell by more than 50% or to fewer than 100×10^9/L, or new thromboembolytic complications (TECs) had occurred. Laboratory confirmation of the clinical diagnosis of HIT was mandatory before a patient could enter the trial. The heparin-induced platelet activation (HIPA) test was used to detect HIT antibodies (Greinacher et al., 1991; Carlsson et al., 1998; see Chap. 11).

Dosing

Patients received one of the following lepirudin-dosing regimens for 2–10 days, or longer if clinically indicated:

- A1. *Treatment of patients with known TEC*: 0.4 mg/kg* iv bolus followed by 0.15 mg/kg/h* infusion
- A2. *Treatment in conjunction with thrombolysis of patients with known TEC*: 0.2 mg/kg* iv bolus followed by 0.10 mg/kg/h* infusion
- B. *Prophylaxis of patients without thrombosis*: 0.10 mg/kg/hr* infusion
- C. *Cardiopulmonary bypass*: iv bolus or continued iv infusion (see Chap. 17)

Infusion rates were not adjusted if the aPTT ratio was 1.5–3.0 (unless deemed otherwise appropriate because of increased bleeding risk). For confirmed aPTT ratios less than 1.5, the infusion rate, was increased by 20%; for confirmed on-treatment aPTT ratios higher than 3.0, the infusion was discontinued for 2 h, then restarted at a 20% lower rate. Repeat aPTT determinations were required 4–6 h after any dose adjustment.

If patients were switched to oral anticoagulants, the lepirudin dose was reduced to reach an aPTT ratio about 2.0 before beginning oral anticoagulants treatment; lepirudin was discontinued when the international normalized ratio (INR) reached more than 2.0.

Efficacy Measures

Efficacy was measured by laboratory response and prespecified clinical outcomes. Laboratory response was defined as (1) the maintenance of an on-treatment aPTT ratio higher than 1.5 in at least 80% of measurements and requiring no more than two dose increases; and (2) an increase in the platelet count to more than 30% from the nadir, and to more than 100×10^9/L by day 10 of lepirudin treatment (thrombocytopenic patients), or maintenance of normal platelet counts on days 3 and 10 (nonthrombocytopenic patients). Clinical outcomes included death, limb amputation, and new TECs, and included clinical assessment to day 14 after stopping lepirudin treatment. Comparison of clinical outcomes with the historic control group were performed using Kaplan-Meier time-to-event analyses, beginning at laboratory confirmation of HIT for lepirudin-treated patients, and 1 day after laboratory confirmation for controls.

---

* To a maximum body weight of 110 kg; dosage must be adjusted for renal insufficiency (see p. 328, Table 3).

B. HAT-1 Study

Efficacy Outcomes

In the first study, 82 patients with confirmed HIT were treated with lepirudin (Greinacher et al., 1999a). The platelet counts increased to more than 100×10^9/L within 10 days in 55/62 (89%) patients with evaluable platelet counts (Fig. 2), and remained stable in patients with normal platelet counts at baseline. Additionally, the aPTT increased rapidly to between 1.5- and 3.0-times baseline values. The 25–75% aPTT quartiles were within this target range at all time points for regimen A1 and for all but one time point for regimen A2.

Clinical outcomes included six deaths (7.3%, three patients each in groups A1 and B) from heart failure (n = 3), sepsis (n = 2), and multiorgan failure (n = 1). All fatalities were judged to be due to the pretreatment underlying disease, rather than use of the study drug. New TECs occurred in eight (9.8%) patients, four arterial and four venous; however, only two TECs occurred during lepirudin treatment (occlusions of peripheral arterial bypass). Three patients needed limb amputation during lepirudin treatment.

Bleeding Complications

One-third of the patients experienced at least one bleeding event during the study (A1, 33%; A2, 20%; B, 33%, C, 38%). Eleven patients (13%) experienced 15 major bleeding episodes (8 at invasive sites, 7 spontaneous). The frequency of major bleeding was similar among the different treatment regimens. Sixteen patients experienced 27 minor bleeds.

C. HAT-2 Study

Efficacy Outcomes

In the second study, 112 patients with confirmed HIT were enrolled (Greinacher et al., 1999b). Sixty-five patients were assigned to dose regimen A1, 4 patients to regimen A2, and 43 patients to dose regimen B. The median duration of treatment was 11 days (range, 0–104). Platelet response was achieved in 87 of 94 evaluable patients (92.6%), with median platelet counts increasing by about fourfold over the first 10 days. Additionally, anticoagulant response was achieved in 68/94 (72.3%) of patients. Median aPTT ratios reached the target range immediately after initiation of lepirudin treatment, and remained there throughout the treatment course. Complete laboratory response (i.e., meeting both platelet and anticoagulant criteria) was achieved in 69.1% of patients (95% CI, 59.3–78.3%).

Between the time of HIT confirmation until 2 weeks after stopping lepirudin treatment, 11 (9.8%) patients died; cause of death included multiorgan failure (n = 3), sepsis (n = 2), heart failure (n = 2), pulmonary embolism, ventricular

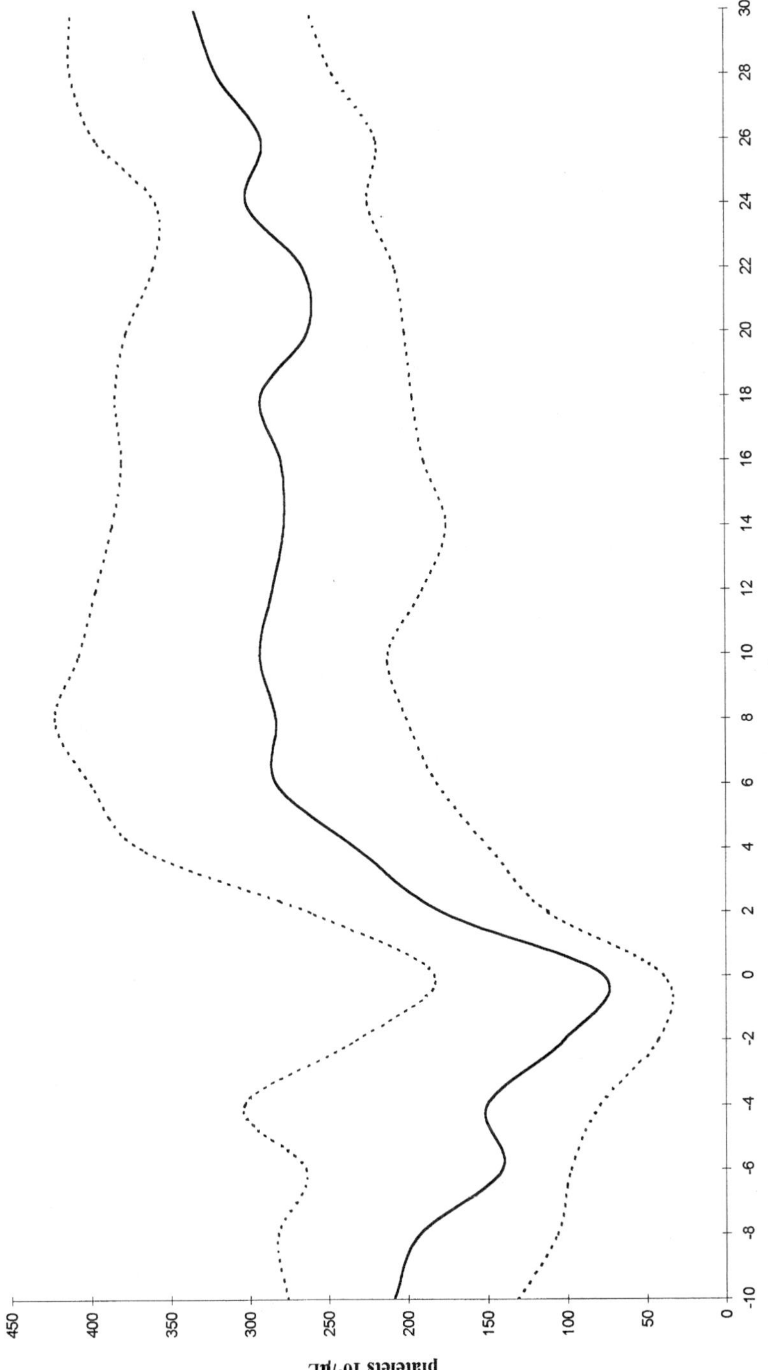

Figure 2 Platelet count summaries of patients in the HAT-1 and HAT-2 trials: The mean (solid line), 25%, and 75% platelet count quartiles (dotted lines) are shown. Following cessation of heparin therapy, and during treatment with lepirudin (beginning on day zero), platelet counts normalized rapidly, even increasing to levels higher than before heparin treatment.

fibrillation, shock, and apnea (n = 1 each). None of the deaths were judged to be related to adverse effects of lepirudin. Ten (8.9%) patients underwent limb amputation, and 20 (17.9%) experienced a new TEC.

To determine the time period during which patients were at highest risk of dying, developing a new TEC, or requiring limb amputation, we assessed the frequency of these clinical events during three time periods: the time between laboratory assay and the start of lepirudin treatment (pretreatment); during active treatment with lepirudin (on-treatment); and during the 14-day observation period following cessation of lepirudin (posttreatment). Nine (8.0%) patients suffered an event during the relatively brief pretreatment period (mean, 1.9 days), 19 (17.0%) patients during the 15.2-day treatment period, and 8 (7.1%) patients in the 13.0-day posttreatment period. Thus, the average combined outcome rate per patient day showed a marked decrease from baseline (5.1%), both during (1.5%) and after (0.6%) lepirudin treatment (Fig. 3).

Bleeding Complications

Bleeding was the most common adverse event: 53 (47.3%) patients experienced at least one bleeding event. Nineteen (17.0%) had a major bleed (9 at invasive sites, 7 spontaneous, 3 both). No intracranial or fatal hemorrhages occurred.

D. Comparison with Historical Control Group

Historical control patients (confirmed by positive HIPA test) received danaparoid (n = 36), oral anticoagulants (e.g., phenprocoumon, n = 27), miscellaneous treatments (e.g., aspirin, thrombolytics, low molecular weight heparin, n = 17), or no anticoagulation (n = 23).

Comparison with HAT-1 Study

Patients in the lepirudin group were an average of 7 years younger than controls, but were more likely to have had multiple TECs before start of treatment. The mean duration of treatment was similar (lepirudin, 15.2 days; controls, 14.9 days). Cumulative frequencies for the combined and individual outcomes are listed in Table 1. The log-rank test showed a significant difference in favor of the lepirudin-treated patients (p = 0.014). The hazards ratio (lepirudin to historical control) adjusted for prespecified prognostic factors was 0.508 (95% CI, 0.290–0.892; p = 0.014).

To avoid bias from misclassification of new TECs, only "hard" endpoints such as death and limb amputation were also analyzed. The combined cumulative frequencies of limb amputations and deaths were consistently lower in the lepirudin group than in the control group (p = 0.043; Fig. 4). Similarly, cumulative frequencies of death and new TECs during treatment were significantly lower in the lepirudin group than in the historical controls (p = 0.02 and p = 0.006, respectively). There was a slightly higher rate of major bleeding in the lepirudin group.

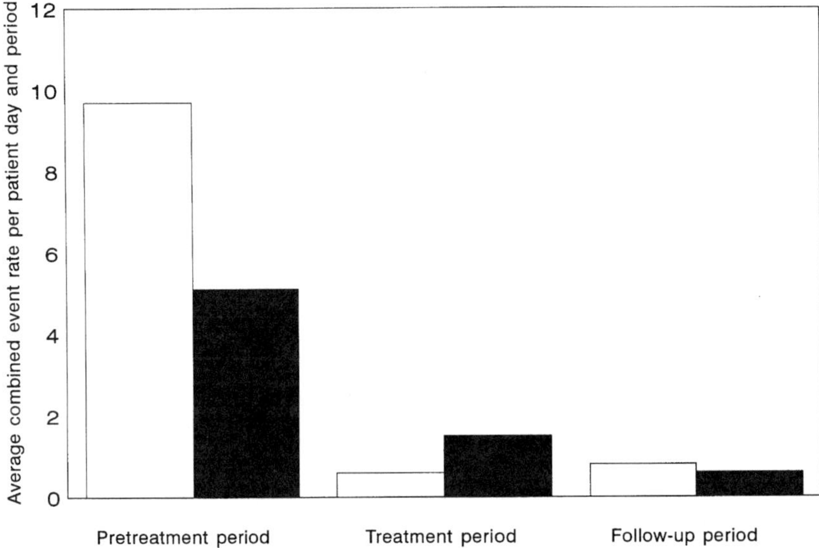

Figure 3 Average combined event rate (death, limb amputation, new TECs) per day, in HAT-1 and HAT-2 studies, according to pretreatment, treatment, and follow-up periods: Confirmation of the clinical diagnosis of HIT by laboratory assay was required as an inclusion criterion in these prospective treatment studies. This caused a time delay during which heparin administration was stopped, but no other anticoagulant administration was started (according to usual practice). The pretreatment period is the time period between laboratory confirmation of HIT and start of lepirudin treatment. Event rates in the HAT-1 study are given as white bars, and in the HAT-2 study as dark bars. The data demonstrate that heparin cessation alone is inadequate in acute HIT, because patients are still at very high risk for developing new complications (initially, as high as 5–10%/day). The number of events per patient day decreased sharply once treatment with lepirudin was started.

Comparison with HAT-2 Study

In this study, at all time points after laboratory confirmation of HIT, the cumulative combined frequencies of death, limb amputation, and new TECs were lower in the lepirudin group than in the control group. At 5 weeks, the frequencies were 31.9% (95% CI, 21.0–40.7%) and 52.1% (95% CI, 40.4–63.9%), respectively. However, differences were not statistically significant in the time-to-event analysis ($p = 0.12$). Lepirudin-treated patients also fared somewhat better than historical control patients at 5 weeks for the individual outcomes of death (10. vs. 22.0%; $p = 0.21$) and new TECs (17.4 vs 32.1%; $p = 0.26$), whereas there was no relevant difference in the frequency of limb amputation (10.0 vs 8.2%); $p = 0.43$). The unadjusted risk ratio for lepirudin-treated patients relative to historical control patients was 0.706 (95% CI, 0.44–1.14; $p = 0.15$).

Table 1 Comparison of Lepirudin-Treated Patients with Historical Controls, HAT-1 Study

		Lepirudin (n = 71)	Historical controls (n = 120)	
Combined endpoint (deaths, new TECs, limb amputations)	Day 7	9.9%		23.0%
	Day 35	25.4%		52.1%
			p = 0.014	
Combined Endpoint (deaths, limb amputations)	Day 7	2.8%		6.9%
	Day 35	11.4%		27.8%
			p = 0.043	
Deaths	Day 7	0.0%		5.2%
	Day 35	8.6%		22.3%
			p = 0.071	
New TECs	Day 7	9.9%		18.0%
	Day 35	18.4%		32.1%
			p = 0.270	
Limb amputations	Day 7	2.8%		1.7%
	Day 35	5.7%		8.2%
			p = 0.783	

TECs, thromboembolic complications.
Source: Greinacher et al., 1999.

There were more bleeding events in the lepirudin-treated group, compared with controls (cumulative frequency at 35 days, 44.6 vs. 27.2%; p = 0.0001 by log-rank test). However, there was no significant difference in the frequency of bleeding requiring transfusion (12.9 vs. 9.1%; p = 0.23). The frequency of serious spontaneous bleeding, such as cerebral hemorrhage (lepirudin, 0 vs. historic control, 2.5%) gastrointestinal hemorrhage (2.1 vs. 5.0%), or lung hemorrhage (2.1 vs. 1.7%), was low and did not significantly differ between the two groups.

E. Discussion of HAT-1 and HAT-2 Trial Results

In both trials, lepirudin allowed rapid normalization of low, or maintained previously normal, platelet counts in 88.7 and 92.6% of patients, respectively, and led to therapeutic prolongation of the aPTT in 77.2 and 72.3% of patients, respectively. Although the aPTT response rates may appear low, this reflects the conservative nature of the treatment protocol, which allowed no more than two dose increases for patients to be considered aPTT responders. Considering that the mean treatment duration was 15.2 days, the aPTT response rate, which is an indirect measure of the intrapatient stability of anticoagulation, appears to be quite high.

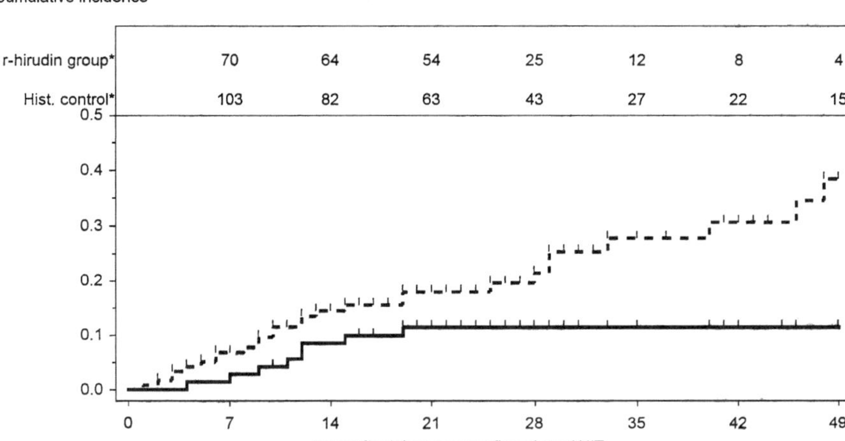

Figure 4 Kaplan-Meier (cumulative incidence) curves of the cumulative incidences of death and limb amputations in patients in the HAT-1 study and in the historical control group. The lepirudin-treated patients are shown as a black line, the historical control group patients as a dotted line. The numbers of patients at risk are given at the top of the figure.

The crude frequencies of death, limb amputation, and new TECs during the two study periods are listed in Table 2. Both studies had similar mortality rates (7.3 and 9.8%); however, limb amputations (3.7 and 8.9%) and new TECs (9.8 and 17.9%) differed more between the studies.

An analysis of the two studies showed that of the 30% of patients who had any adverse clinical outcome, almost half (45%) experienced an event before initiation of lepirudin treatment, even though the pretreatment period accounted

Table 2 Outcomes of the HAT-1 and HAT-2 Studies[a]

	HAT-1 study (n = 82)	HAT-2 study (n = 112)
Number of platelet count responders	88.7%	92.6%
Number of aPTT responders	77.2%	72.3%
Death	7.3%	9.8%
Limb amputation	3.7%	8.9%
New TEC	9.8%	17.9%
Minor bleeding	32.9%	47.3%
Major bleeding	13.4%	17%

[a] Patients may have had more than 1 event.

for only 8.5% (HAT-1) and 6% (HAT-2) of the entire study duration. Thus, the average combined outcome rate per patient day decreased sharply from 9.7 and 5.1% in the pretreatment period, to 0.6 and 1.5% in the treatment period (see Fig. 3). Because the vast majority of these patients did not receive any heparin treatment during the pretreatment period, our findings strongly support the observation of Warkentin and Kelton (1996) that heparin cessation alone is not adequate therapy for HIT.

We observed a significantly lower cumulative frequency of clinical outcomes in the lepirudin-treated group, compared with historical controls, in the HAT-1 study. A trend in favor of lepirudin treatment was also observed for the identical endpoint in the HAT-2 study ($p = 0.12$ for the 35-day time-to-event analysis). Thus, the intratrial data discussed in the foregoing (sharply reduced on-treatment and posttreatment event rates per day, compared with the pretreatment period), as well as the historical control comparisons, strongly support the view that lepirudin is an effective anticoagulant for the treatment of HIT.

A major risk for HIT patients treated with r-hirudin is hemorrhage: in the two studies, major bleeds occurred in 13 and 17% of lepirudin-treated patients. Although these frequencies appear high, they must be interpreted relative to the duration and circumstances of therapy. Usually, bleeds occurred in perioperative settings or at sites of invasive catheters. Spontaneous bleeds generally had underlying explanations (e.g., bleeding into a hepatic cyst during concomitant thrombolytic therapy). No lepirudin-treated patient had intracranial or fatal hemorrhage in either study. These data are comparable with results of other trials of r-hirudin. For example, in the 12,000 patient GUSTO-2B study that compared desirudin with heparin in acute coronary syndromes, 35-day transfusion rates were about 9% in both treatment arms, even though treatment duration was only 72 h (GUSTO investigators, 1996).

A metanalysis (Greinacher et al., 1999c) of the HAT-1 and HAT-2 trials showed that lepirudin-treated patients had a lower incidence of the combined endpoint than did the historical controls ($P = 0.004$, log-rank test), primarily due to a reduced rate of new TECs ($P = 0.005$). Optimal clinical efficacy, with only moderate bleeding risk, was seen when the aPTT ratio was 1.5–2.5; in contrast, suboptimal clinical efficacy was evident when the aPTT ratio was <1.5, and an unacceptably high bleeding rate (without improved efficacy) was observed when the ratio was >2.5.

F. Comparison with Other Treatments for HIT

Little progress has been made in the treatment of HIT, using "classic" approaches that typically have included discontinuation of heparin administration, with or without substitution with oral anticoagulants. Mortality rates have remained essentially unchanged over more than a decade, approximately 20–30% (King and Kelton, 1984; AbuRahma et al., 1991; Warkentin and Kelton, 1996;

Nand et al., 1997). These rates are two to three times higher than observed in the HAT-1 and HAT-2 studies.

Warkentin and Kelton (1996) reported a 51% TEC rate at the time of diagnosis of HIT, similar to the rate we observed in our patients at study entry (52.6%). However, the outcomes of patients in their study were very different. They observed: 47% (10/21) of patients who received warfarin treatment for HIT developed a new TEC; 56% (20/36) of patients with "isolated thrombocytopenia," who received no further anticoagulation, developed a new TEC; mortality in these patient groups was about 20%. These results demonstrate that neither cessation of heparin administration alone, nor switching to vitamin K antagonists, is sufficient to prevent further thrombotic complications in HIT. Other drugs with antithrombin activity (e.g., argatroban) or antifactor Xa activity (e.g., danaparoid) may be appropriate for further parenteral anticoagulation in patients with HIT. Currently, data from a prospective, historically controlled trial of argatroban in HIT patients are pending (Lewis et al., 1997a,b).

Danaparoid has been assessed in a compassionate-use program involving more than 700 patients (Magnani, 1997; Ortel and Chong, 1998; see Chap. 14). The use of danaparoid was judged successful by treating physicians in about 90% of cases. As in the lepirudin studies, platelet counts normalized in nearly 88% of patients. In a few patients (3–5%), however, clinical cross-reactivity of danaparoid with HIT antibodies could not be ruled out. During active danaparoid treatment, 72 patients (10.2%) died, compared with 3.6% during lepirudin treatment. In the danaparoid study, new TECs were reported in 3.1% of the patients vs. 6.2% in the two lepirudin trials. It is noteworthy that the reported frequency of severe bleeding was 7.3% during danaparoid treatment in the compassionate-use protocol, compared with about 15% in the lepirudin studies. However, these results should be interpreted cautiously, because bleeding complications are often under-reported when a patient is not included in a prospective trial.

No direct comparisons between danaparoid and any r-hirudin have yet been performed. Both danaparoid and lepirudin should be considered as options for parenteral anticoagulation of rapid onset in HIT patients. Potentially, the short half-life of lepirudin has advantages in patients who require dose changes (e.g., planned invasive procedures; see Fig. 5), whereas the long half-life of danaparoid may be advantageous in other clinical settings (e.g., subcutaneous prophylaxis and early mobilization of patients; see Fig. 5 in Chap. 3).

IV. r-HIRUDIN TREATMENT OF HIT PATIENTS: SPECIAL CLINICAL CIRCUMSTANCES

A. r-Hirudin for Hemodialysis

Hirudin was the first anticoagulant used for hemodialysis, performed by Haas (1924) at the University of Giessen, Germany. Because native hirudin preparations were rather crude, and adequate supply of leeches problematic, hirudin was quickly replaced by heparin.

r-Hirudin has been used successfully for hemodialysis in humans (see also Chap. 16), but unresolved problems remain:

1. It is unclear which laboratory parameter should be used to monitor r-hirudin. To date, a modified, activated-clotting time (ACT) (Vanholder et al., 1994, 1997), the aPTT (van Wyk et al., 1995), and the ECT (Nowak et al., 1997) have been used successfully.
2. The elimination of r-hirudin is markedly prolonged in renal failure: Nowak et al. (1992) reported elimination half-lives up to 316 h in dialysis patients. Vanholder et al. (1997) found r-hirudin half-life was prolonged by a factor of 31 in hemodialysis patients compared with controls. Moreover, no antidote exists in case of bleeding.
3. There is a correlation between residual creatinine clearance and r-hirudin clearance. We have observed problems in managing intensive care unit (ICU) patients with transient renal failure: substantial dose increases (> 100%) are needed once renal function recovers (Hempel et al., 1998). We use an r-hirudin bolus of 0.1–0.2 mg/kg body weight (b.w.) in stable patients undergoing alternate-day hemodialysis; otherwise, for unstable ICU patients, we prefer a continuous intravenous infusion, starting at 0.005 mg/kg b.w./h, with adjustments according to aPTT.
4. There are scant data on the correlation between the pharmacokinetics of r-hirudin and the type of dialyzer membrane used.

For these reasons, the use of r-hirudin to manage hemodialysis in patients with HIT should be considered experimental.

B. r-Hirudin for Cardiopulmonary Bypass and Vascular Surgery

Data from animal models (Walenga et al., 1991; Riess et al., 1997b) show r-hirudin to be a potential alternative anticoagulant for patients undergoing cardiopulmonary bypass (CPB) surgery (see also Chap. 17). In this situation, neither the ACT nor aPTT are appropriate for monitoring r-hirudin plasma levels. A modified ECT (Pötzsch et al., 1997) must be used. Lepirudin was used to manage CPB patients in the HAT-1 study (Riess et al., 1995, 1996). Experimental and clinical observations suggest that the therapeutic lepirudin level for CPB is between 3.5 and 4.5 μg/mL. Lower levels of r-hirudin may cause clotting in the CPB circuit, and higher intraoperative levels are associated with a higher risk of postoperative bleeding. Table 3 lists a treatment protocol based on ECT monitoring of r-hirudin levels. Clinical data to date (Koster et al., 1998; see Chap. 17) demonstrate that

Table 3 Dosing Schedules for r-Hirudin Treatment of Patients with HIT[a]

	Bolus[c,g]	IV infusion[c,g]	Target aPTT ratio[b]
HIT and TEC	0.4 mg/kg b.w.iv	0.15 mg/kg b.w./h	1.5–2.5
HIT with TEC and concomitant thrombolysis	0.2 mg/kg b.w.iv	0.1 mg/kg b.w./h	1.5–2.5
HIT with isolated thrombocytopenia		0.1 mg/kg b.w./h	1.5–2.0
Thrombosis prophylaxis in patients with a history of HIT	15 mg sc twice daily[d]	0.1 mg/kg b.w./h[e]	1.5–2.0 for iv infusion
Renal dialysis every alternate day	0.1 mg/kg b.w.iv predialysis	—	2.0–2.5
CVVH	—	0.005 mg/kg b.w./h (initial rate)	1.5–2.5
Vascular surgery[h]			
vessel flushes after embolectomy	use up to 250 mL (0.1 mg/mL solution)	—	1.5–2.5
postoperative anticoagulation	—	0.1 mg/kg b.w./h	1.5–2.5
Cardiopulmonary bypass surgery	0.25 mg/kg b.w.iv 0.2 mg/kg b.w. in the priming fluid of the HLM	0.5 mg/min[f]	Monitored by ECT: >2.5 μg/mL before start of HLM; 3.5–4.5 μg/mL during CPB

Abbreviations: aPTT, activated partial thromboplastin time; b.w., body weight; CPB, cardiopulmonary bypass; CVVH, continuous venovenous hemofiltration; ECT, ecarin-clotting time; iv, intravenous; HLM, heart–lung machine; TEC, thromboembolic complication.

Repeat aPTT determinations should be made 4–6 h afters any dose adjustment.

[a] The data were generated with lepirudin unless otherwise indicated.

[b] The ratio is based on comparison with the normal laboratory median aPTT. If Actin FS or Neothromtin reagents are used, the aPTT target range is usually 1.5–3.0.

[c] A maximum body weight 110 kg should be used for dose calculations.

[d] Based on studies evaluating the r-hirudin, desirudin, in patients undergoing hip replacement surgery (Eriksson et al., 1997).

[e] Used in the HAT-1 and HAT-2 trials.

[f] Stop 15 min before end of CPB; put 5 mg into HLM after disconnection to avoid clotting.

[g] Adjustments for renal insufficiency:

Creatinine clearance (mL/min)	Serum creatinine, mg/dL (μmol/L)	Adjusted bolus dose	Adjusted infusion rate (% of original dose)
45–60	1.6–2.0 (141–177)	0.2 mg/kg	50
30–44	2.1–3.0 (178–265)	—	25
15–29	3.1–6.0 (266–530)	—	10
< 15	> 6.0 (> 530)	0.1 mg/kg b.w. on alternate days (only if aPTT ratio < 1.5) without use of infusion	or, 0.005 mg/kg b.w. iv adjusted for aPTT (without bolus doses)

[h] Hach-Wunderle and Hach, 1997.

lepirudin is a suitable alternative for CPB anticoagulation of HIT patients, provided that ECT monitoring is performed. Because no antidote is available, and because high levels are required during CPB, bleeding complications can arise, particularly in patients with impaired renal function. In such patients, hemodialysis can be used to reduce plasma levels of r-hirudin.

For patients requiring vascular surgery, the following strategy has been described (Hach-Wunderle and Hach, 1997): immediately after clamping the artery, or following the surgery itself, a lepirudin infusion is started (0.1 mg/kg b.w./h). If intraoperative flushing of the vessel or graft is needed, up to 250 mL of a 0.1 mg/mL lepirudin-containing flush solution (50 mg in 500 mL saline) can be given.

C. r-Hirudin in Pregnant Women

There is no published experience using r-hirudin in human pregnancy. In rats, r-hirudin crosses the placenta, and there is increased maternal mortality of undetermined cause at a dosage of 30 mg/kg/per day. It is not recommended that r-hirudin be used during pregnancy. Danaparoid may be a better alternative in this situation (see Chap. 14).

D. r-Hirudin for HIT in Children

Except for one study in newborns (Spadone et al., 1992), there are no prospective data on the frequency of HIT in children. However, HIT seems to be rare in children (see Chap. 3). My own observations indicate that HIT antibodies in children (1) occur in the same time frame as in adults; (2) are usually directed against PF4–heparin complexes; (3) are primarily IgG; (4) cause a platelet activation profile similar to that observed using adult HIT sera; and (5) disappear within several weeks of stopping heparin administration. Thus, the immune response leading to HIT in children resembles that observed in adults.

There are case reports describing HIT in children (Oriot et al., 1990; Potter et al., 1992; Murdoch et al., 1993; Klement et al., 1996; Wilhelm et al., 1996). These studies suggest HIT may be more frequent in adolescents than in children younger than 10 years of age. Two children received lepirudin for HIT in the HAT-1 and HAT-2 trials, an 11-year-old girl and 12-year-old boy. The girl was adequately anticoagulated with lepirudin at a dose between 0.15 and 0.22 mg/kg b.w. per hour. The boy's clinical course was as dramatic as observed in many adults (Fig. 5).

Because of the rarity and clinical heterogeneity of children who develop HIT, it is difficult to design a standardized study protocol. Thus, treatment recommendations are based on anecdotal experience. As renal function in children is

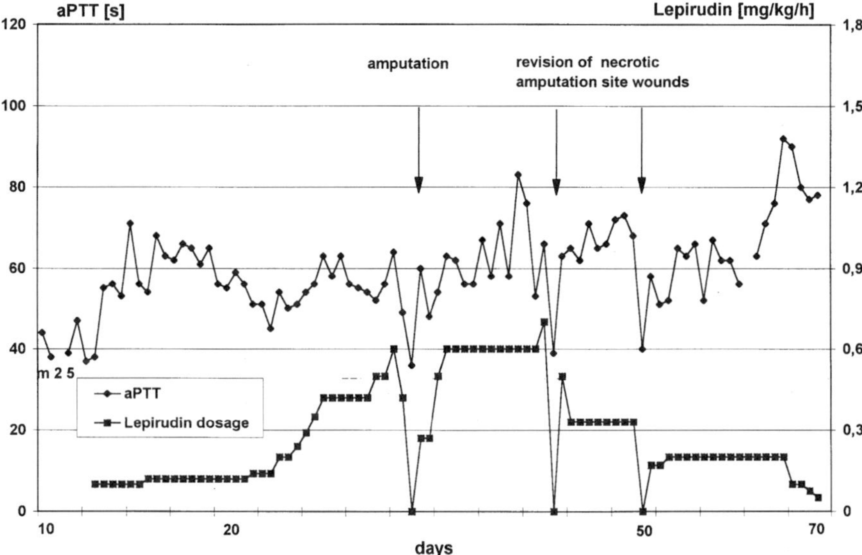

Figure 5 This 12-year-old boy received streptokinase, urokinase, and UFH for idiopathic deep venous thrombosis, but developed HIT, complicated by femoral artery and inferior vena cava thrombosis. Initial danaparoid treatment was stopped after 24 h because of its long half-life and the detection of in vitro cross-reactivity. Lepirudin was substituted, and aggressive treatment, including thrombolytic agents and thromboembolectomy, was performed, but could not prevent forefoot amputation. Discontinuation of lepirudin treatment was rapidly followed by normalization of the aPTT to permit surgical and other invasive procedures. (From Schiffman et al., 1997.)

usually normal, the short half-life of lepirudin is an advantage in case of bleeding complications or need for invasive procedures.

V. ANTIHIRUDIN ANTIBODIES

As a foreign protein, r-hirudin can elicit xenoantibodies. To determine their frequency and clinical importance, we developed an enzyme immunoassay for detecting antihirudin antibodies. Substudies from the HAT-1 and HAT-2 trials showed that about 40% of lepirudin-treated patients developed IgG antihirudin antibodies (Eichler et al., 1997). The antibodies were detectable from day 5 of lepirudin treatment, with peak prevalence at days 9–10. No allergic reactions or other detrimental effects were noted; mortality was actually higher in patients

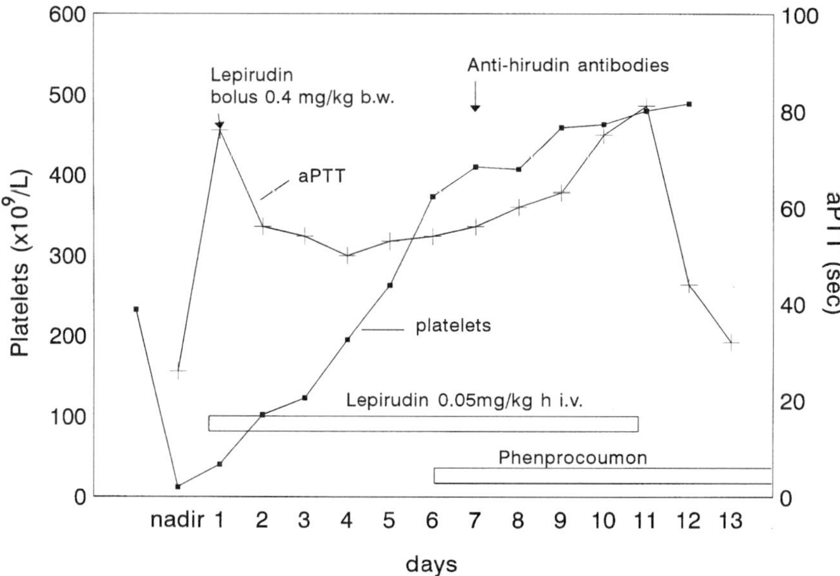

Figure 6 This 53-year-old woman was admitted to the hospital because of an ankle fracture. She received low molecular weight heparin for 10 days, but was switched to unfractionated heparin owing to a distal deep vein thrombosis (DVT). Ten days later she presented with proximal DVT, pulmonary embolism, and a rapid fall in platelet count from more than 200 to 12×10^9/L. She was switched to intravenous (iv) lepirudin (schedule A1). After normalization of platelet counts, she received overlapping oral anticoagulants (phenprocoumon), with lepirudin stopped when the INR reached 2.0. Antihirudin antibodies were first detected on day 7; at the same time, the aPTT increased despite a stable hirudin dosage of 0.05 mg/kg b.w. per hour.

without antihirudin antibodies, without other differences in clinical outcome or in bleeding complications.

Antihirudin antibodies very rarely have an in vivo neutralizing effect on r-hirudin (Eichler et al., 1997). However, in some patients with antihirudin antibodies, the lepirudin dosage had to be decreased by approximately 60% to maintain the aPTT within the target range (Fig. 6). We speculate that this enhanced anticoagulant effect of r-hirudin is caused by decreased renal elimination of the r-hirudin–antihirudin antibody complexes. Although this effect was observed in only a small subset of lepirudin-treated patients (about 2.5% of all patients treated for more than 5 days), daily monitoring of aPTT during r-hirudin treatment is recommended, especially if treatment is for more than 5 days. Our observations on anti-hirudin antibodies were recently confirmed (Huhle et al., 1998).

VI. CONCLUSION

Despite its potential to cause bleeding and xenoantibodies, clinical studies indicate that r-hirudin benefits patients with HIT (Schiele et al., 1995; Schmidt et al., 1997; Olbrich et al., 1998; Greinacher et al., 1999a,b). Lepirudin was approved for treatment of HIT with concomitant thrombosis in the European Community in 1997, and by the U.S. Food and Drug Administration in 1998, and has recently become available in Canada.

Recommended treatment schedules are summarized in Table 3. Data from almost 200 lepirudin-treated patients indicate that the mortality is about 8–10%; approximately 10–15% develop a new TEC. Although I believe that mortality predominantly reflects the underlying disease (and may not be further decreased), it is likely that most HIT-associated thrombosis can be prevented by switching promptly from heparin to lepirudin when HIT is clinically suggested. It remains unknown whether the 15% risk of major hemorrhage can be reduced in the future by routine monitoring using the ECT, rather than the aPTT.

ACKNOWLEDGMENTS

The reported studies were only possible by a close cooperation with the Clinical Research Group of Hoechst Marion Roussel. I am grateful to Drs. H. Völpel, H. Heinrichs, H. Kwasny, and M. Luz for their support and cooperation.

REFERENCES

AbuRahma AF, Boland JP, Witsberger T. Diagnostic and therapeutic strategies of white clot syndrome. Am J Surg 162:175–179, 1991.

Antman EM for the TIMT 9A investigators. Hirudin in acute myocardial infarction: safety report from the thrombolysis and thrombin inhibition in myocardial infarction (TIMI) 9A trial. Circulation 90:1624–1630, 1994.

Boskovic DS, Giles AR, Nesheim ME. Studies of the role of factor Va in the factor Xa-catalyzed activation of prothrombin, fragment 1.2-prethrombin-2, and dansyl-L-glu-amyl-glycyl-L-arginine-meizothrombin in the absence of phospholipid. J Biol Chem 265:10497–10505, 1990.

Bove CM, Casey B, Marder VJ. DDAVP reduces bleeding during continued hirudin administration in the rabbit. Thromb Haemost 75:471–475, 1996.

Butler KD, Dolan SL, Talbot MD, Wallis RB. Factor VII and DDAVP reverse the effect of recombinant desulphatohirudin (CGB 39393) on bleeding in the rat. Blood Coagul Fibrinolysis 4:459–464, 1993.

Carlsson LE, Santoso S, Baurichter G, Kroll H, Papenberg S, Eichler P, Westerdaal NAC, Kiefel V, van de Winkel JGJ, Greinacher A. Heparin-induced thrombocytopenia:

new insights into the impact of the FcγRIIa-R-H131 polymorphism. Blood 92: 1526–1531, 1998.

Chong BH, Murray B, Berndt MC, Dunlop LC, Brighton T, Chesterman CN. Plasma P-selectin is increased in thrombotic consumptive platelet disorders. Blood 83:1535–1541, 1994.

Clore GM, Sukumaran DK, Nilges M, Zarbock J, Gronenborn AG. The conformation of hirudin in solution. A study using nuclear magnetic resonance, distance geometry and restrained molecular dynamics. EMBO J 6:529–537, 1987.

Dickneite G, Friesen HJ, Kumpe G, Reers M. Reduction of rH induced bleeding in pigs by the administration of von Willebrand factor. Platelets 7:283–290, 1996.

Dickneite G, Nicolay U, Friesen HJ, Reers M. Development of an anti-bleeding agent for recombinant hirudin induced skin bleeding in the pig. Thromb Haemost 80:192–198, 1998.

Diehl KH, Römisch J, Hein B, Jessel A, Ronneberger H, Paques EP. Investigation of activated prothrombin complex concentrate as potential hirudin antidote in animal models. Haemostasis 25:182–192, 1995.

Eichler P, Olbrich K, Pötzsch B, Greinacher A. Anti-hirudin antibodies in patients treated with recombinant hirudin for more than five days, a prospective study [abstr]. Thromb Haemost (suppl 98):PS-2014, 1997.

Eriksson BI, Wille-Jörgensen P, Kälebo P, Mouret P, Rosencher N, Bösch P, Baur M, Ekman S, Bach D, Lindbratt S, Close P. A comparison of recombinant hirudin with a low-molecular weight heparin to prevent thromboembolic complications after total hip replacement. N Engl J Med 337:1329–1335, 1997.

Fareed J, Callas D, Hoppensteadt DA, Walenga JM, Bick RL. Antithrombin agents as anticoagulants and antithrombotics. Curr Concepts Thromb 3:569–586, 1998.

Glusa E. Pharmacology and therapeutic applications of hirudin, a new anticoagulant. Kidney Int 53:54–56, 1998.

Glusa E, Markwardt F. Platelet functions in recombinant hirudin-anticoagulated blood. Haemostasis 20:112–118, 1990.

Greinacher A. Antigen generation in heparin-associated thrombocytopenia: the nonimmunologic type and the immunologic type are closely linked in their pathogenesis. Semin Thromb Hemost 21:106–116, 1995.

Greinacher A, Michels I, Kiefel V, Mueller-Eckhardt C. A rapid and sensitive test for diagnosing heparin-associated thrombocytopenia. Thromb Haemost 66:734–736, 1991.

Greinacher A, Völpel H, Janssens U, Hach-Wunderle V, Kemkes-Matthes B, Eichler P, Mueller-Velten HG, Pötzsch B. Recombinant hirudin (lepirudin) provides safe and effective anticoagulation in patients with the immunologic type of heparin-induced thrombocytopenia: a prospective study. Circulation 99:73–80, 1999a.

Greinacher A, Janssens U, Berg G, Böck M, Kwasny H, Kemkes-Matthes B, Eichler P, Völpel H, Pötzsch B, Luz M. Lepirudin (recombinant hirudin) for parenteral anticoagulation in patients with heparin-induced thrombocytopenia. Circulation 100:587–593, 1999b.

Greinacher A, Eichler P, Kwasny H, Luz M. Lepirudin for parenteral anticoagulation of patients with heparin-induced thrombocytopenia (HIT) and thrombosis: meta-analysis of two prospective studies and evaluation of the optimal aPTT range [abstract]. Thromb Haemost 82 (Suppl.):211, 1999c.

GUSTO investigators. A comparison of recombinant hirudin with heparin for the treatment of acute coronary syndromes. The global use of strategies to open occluded coronary arteries (GUSTO) IIb investigators. N Engl J Med 335:775–782, 1996.

Haas G. Über Versuche der Blutauswaschung am Lebenden mit Hilfe der Dialyse. Klin Wochenschr 4:13–14, 1924.

Hach-Wunderle V, Hach W. Hirudin in der Gefäßchirurgie. Gefäßchirurgie 2:218–221, 1997.

Hempel S, Lubenow N, Greinacher A. Nierenersatztherapie unter r-Hirudin (Refludan) bei Heparin-induzierter Thrombozytopenie Typ II [abstr]. Infusionsther Transfusionsmed 25:5/7p, 1998.

Hermann JPR, Kutryk MJV, Serruys PW. Clinical trials of direct thrombin inhibitors during invasive procedures. Thromb Haemost 78:367–376, 1997.

Hogg PJ, Jackson CM. Fibrin monomer protects thrombin from inactivation by heparin-antithrombin III: implications for heparin efficacy. Proc Natl Acad Sci USA 86: 3619–3623, 1989.

Huhle G, Song X, Wang LC, Hoffman U, Harenberg J. Generation and disappearance of antihirudin antibodies during treatment with r-hirudin. Fibrinol Proteol 12 (Suppl 2):91–113, 1998.

Ibbotson SH, Grant PJ, Kerry R, Findlay VS, Prentice CRM. The influence of infusions of 1-desamino-8-arginine vasopressin (DDAVP) in vivo on the anticoagulant effect of r-hirudin. Thromb Haemost 65:64–66, 1991.

Irami MS, Harvey JW, Sexon RG. Reversal of hirudin-induced bleeding diathesis by prothrombin complex concentrate. Am J Cardiol 75:422–423, 1995.

Kaiser B, Markwardt F. Antithrombotic and haemorrhagic effects of synthetic and naturally occurring thrombin inhibitors. Thromb Res 43:613–620, 1986.

King DJ, Kelton JG. Heparin-associated thrombocytopenia. Ann Intern Med 100:535–540, 1984.

Klement D, Rammos S, von Kries R, Kirschke W, Kniemeyer HW, Greinacher A. Heparin as a cause of thrombus progression. Heparin-associated thrombocytopenia is an important differential diagnosis in paediatric patients even with normal platelet counts. Eur J Pediatr 155:11–14, 1996.

Koster A, Kuppe H, Hetzer R, Sodian R, Crystal GJ, Mertzlufft F. Emergent cardiopulmonary bypass in five patients with heparin-induced thrombocytopenia type II employing recombinant hirudin. Anesthesiology 89:777–780, 1998.

Lewis BE, Johnson SA, Grassman ED, Wrona LL. Argatroban as an anticoagulant for coronary procedures in patients with HIT antibody. In: Pifarré R, ed. New Anticoagulants for the Cardiovascular Patient. Philadelphia: Hanley & Belfus, 1997a:301–308.

Lewis BE, Walenga JM, Pifarré R, Fareed J. Argatroban in the management of patients with heparin-induced thrombocytopenia and heparin-induced thrombocytopenia and thrombosis syndrome. In: Pifarré R, ed. New Anticoagulants for the Cardiovascular Patient. Philadelphia: Hanley & Belfus, 1997b:223–229.

Magnani HN. Orgaran (danaparoid sodium) use in the syndrome of heparin-induced thrombocytopenia. Platelets 8:74–81, 1997.

Marbet GA, Verstraete M, Kienast J, Graf P, Hoet B, Tsakiris DA, Silling-Engelhardt G, Close P. Clinical pharmacology of intravenously administered recombinant desulfato-hirudin (CGP 39393) in healthy volunteers. J Cardiovasc Pharmacol 22:364–372, 1993.

Markwardt F. Hirudin: the promising antithrombotic. Cardiovasc Drug Rev 10:211–232, 1992.

Meyer BJ, Badimon JJ, Chesebro JH, Fallon JT, Fuster V, Badimon L. Dissolution of mural thrombus by specific thrombin inhibition with r-hirudin: comparison with heparin and aspirin. Circulation 97:681–685, 1998.

Murdoch IA, Beattie RM, Silver DM. Heparin-induced thrombocytopenia in children. Acta Paediatr 82:495–497, 1993.

Nand S, Wong W, Yuen B, Yetter A, Schmulbach E, Gross Fisher S. Heparin-induced thrombocytopenia with thrombosis: incidence, analysis of risk factors, and clinical outcomes in 108 consecutive patients treated at a single institution. Am J Hematol 56:12–16, 1997.

Neuhaus KL, vEssen R, Tebbe U, Jessel A, Heinrichs H, Mäurer W, Döring W, Harmjanz D, Kötter V, Kalhammer E, Simon H, Horacek T. Safety observation from the pilot phase of the randomized r-hirudin for improvement of thrombolysis (HIT-III) study: a study of the Arbeitsgemeinschaft leitender kariologischer Krankenhausärzte (ALKK). Circulation 90:1638–1642, 1994.

Nishida S, Fujita T, Kohno N, Atoda H, Morita T, Takeya H, Kido I, Paine MJI, Kawabata S-I, Iwanaga S. cDNA cloning and deduced amino acid sequence of prothrombin activator (ecarin) from Kenyan *Echis carinatus* venom. Biochemistry 34:1771–1778, 1995.

Novoa E, Seegers WH. Mechanisms of alpha-thrombin and beta-thrombi-E formation: use of ecarin for isolation of meizothrombin 1. Thromb Res 18:657–668, 1980.

Nowak G, Bucha E. Prothrombin conversion intermediate effectively neutralizes toxic levels of hirudin. Thromb Res 80:317–325, 1995.

Nowak G, Bucha E, Gööck T, Prasa D, Thieler H. Pharmakokinetik von Hirudin bei gestörter Nierenfunktion. Haemostaseologie 11:152–157, 1991.

Nowak G, Bucha E, Gööck T, Thieler H, Markwardt F. Pharmacology of r-hirudin in renal impairment. Thromb Res 66:707–715, 1992.

Nowak G, Bucha E, Brauns I, Czerwinski R. Anticoagulation with r-hirudin in regular haemodialysis with heparin-induced thrombocytopenia (HIT II). The first long term application of r-hirudin in a haemodialysis patient. Wien Klin Wochenschr 109: 354–358, 1997.

Nurmohamed MT, Berckmans RJ, Morrien-Salomons WM, Berends F, Hammes WD, Rijnierse JJMM, Sturk A. Monitoring anticoagulant therapy by activated partial thromboplastin time:hirudin assessment. Thromb Haemost 72:685–692, 1994.

Olbrich K, Wiersbitzky M, Wacke W, Eichler P, Zinke H, Schwock M, Möx B, Kraatz G, Motz W, Greinacher A. Atypical heparin-induced thrombocytopenia complicated by intracardiac thrombus, effectively treated with ultra-low-dose rt-PA lysis and recombinant hirudin (lepirudin). Blood Coagul Fibrinolysis 9:273–277, 1998.

Organization to Assess Strategies for Ischemic Syndromes (OASIS-2) Investigators. Effects of recombinant hirudin (lepirudin) compared with heparin on death, myocardial infarction, refractory angina, and revascularization procedures in patients with acute myocardial ischemia without ST elevation: a randomized trial. Lancet 353: 429–438, 1999.

Oriot D, Wolf M, Wood C, Brun P, Sidi D, Devictor D, Tchernia G, Huault G. Thrombopenie severe induite par l'heparine chez un nourrisson porteur d'une myocardite aigue. Arch Fr Pediatr 47:357–359, 1990.

Ortel TL, Chong BH. New treatment options for heparin-induced thrombocytopenia. Semin Hematol 35(suppl 5):26–34, 1998.

Parent F, Bridey F, Dreyfus M, Musset D, Grimon G, Duroux P, Meyer D, Simonneau G. Treatment of severe thromboembolism with intravenous hirudin (HBW 023): an open pilot study. Thromb Haemost 70:386–388, 1993.

Pieters J, Lindhout T, Hemker HC. In situ-generated thrombin is the only enzyme that effectively activates factor VIII and factor V in thromboplastin-activated plasma. Blood 74:1021–1024, 1989.

Potter C, Gill JC, Scott P, McFarland JG. Heparin-induced thrombocytopenia in a child. J Pediatr 121:135–138, 1992.

Pötzsch B, Madlener K, Seelig C, et al. The whole blood ecarin clotting time assay allows rapid and accurate monitoring of the anticoagulant response of r-hirudin during cardiopulmonary bypass. Thromb Haemost 77:920–925, 1997.

Riess F-C, Löwer C, Seelig C, Bleese N, Kormann J, Müller-Berghaus G, Pötzsch B. Recombinant hirudin as a new anticoagulant during cardiac operations instead of heparin: successful for aortic valve replacement in man. Thorac Cardiovasc Surg 110:265–267, 1995.

Riess FC, Pötzsch B, Jäger K, Bleese N, Schaper W, Müller-Berghaus G. Elimination von rekombinantem Hirudin aus der Blutzirkulation mittels Hämofiltration. Haemostaseologie 17:200–204, 1997a.

Riess FC, Poetzsch B, Mueller-Berghaus G. Recombinant hirudin as an anticoagulant during cardiac surgery. In: Pifarré R, ed. New Anticoagulants for the Cardiovascular Patient. Philadelphia: Hanley & Belfus, 197–222, 1997b.

Riess FC, Pötzsch B, Bader K, Bleese N, Greinacher A, Löwer C, Madlener K, Müller-Berghaus G. A case report on the use of recombinant hirudin as an anticoagulant for cardiopulmonary bypass in open heart surgery. Eur J Cardiothorac Surg 10: 386–388, 1996.

Rupprecht HJ, Terres W, Özbek C, Luz M, Jessel A, Hfner G, vom Dahl J, Kromer EP, Prellwitz W, Meyer J. Recombinant hirudin (HBW 023) prevents troponin release after coronary angioplasty in patients with unstable angina. J Am Coll Cardiol 26: 1637–1642, 1995.

Schiele F, Lindgaerde F, Eriksson H, Bassand J-P, Wallmark A, Hansson P-O, Grollier G, Sjo M, Moia M, Camez A, Smyth V, Walker M, for the International Multicentre Hirudin Study Group. Subcutaneous recombinant hirudin (HBW 023) versus intravenous sodium heparin in treatment of established acute deep vein thrombosis of the legs: a multicentre prospective dose-ranging randomized trial. Thromb Haemost 77:834–838, 1997.

Schiele F, Vuillemenot A, Kramarz P, et al. Use of recombinant hirudin as antithrombotic treatment in patients with heparin-induced thrombocytopenia. Am J Hematol 50: 20–25, 1995.

Schiffmann H, Unterhalt M, Harms K, Figulla HR, Völpel H, Greinacher A. Erfolgreiche Behandlung einer Heparin-induzierten Thrombozytopenie Typ II im Kindesalter mit rekombinantem Hirudin. Monatsschr Kinderheilkd 145:606–612, 1997.

Schmidt OH, Lang W. Heparin-induced thrombocytopenia with thromboembolic arterial occlusion treated with recombinant hirudin. N Engl J Med 337:1389, 1997.

Solano C, Cocroft G, Scott DC. Prediction of vitamin K response using the echis time and echisprothrombin time ratio. Thromb Haemost 64:353–357, 1990.

Spadone D, Clark F, James E, Laster J, Hoch J, Silver D. Heparin-induced thrombocytopenia in the newborn. J Vasc Surg 15:306–312, 1992.

Stone S, Hofsteenge J. The kinetics of the inhibition of thrombin by hirudin. Biochemistry 25:4622–4628, 1986.

Sukumaran DK, Clare GM, Presus A, Zarbock J, Gronenborn AM. Proton nuclear magnetic resonance study of hirudin: resonance assignment and secondary structure. Biochemistry 26:333–338, 1987.

Van Wyk V, Badenhorst PN, Luus HG, Kotzé HF. A comparison between the use of recombinant hirudin and heparin during hemodialysis. Kidney Int 48:1338–1343, 1995.

Vanholder R, Camez A, Veys N, Soria J, Mirshahi MC, Soria C, Ringoir S. Recombinant hirudin. A specific thrombin-inhibiting anticoagulant for haemodialysis. Kidney Int 45:1754–1759, 1994.

Vanholder RC, Camez A, Veys N, Van Loo A, Dhondt AM, Ringoir S. Pharmacokinetics of recombinant hirudin in hemodialyzed end-stage renal failure patients. Thromb Haemost 77:650–655, 1997.

Verstraete M, Nurmohamed M, Kienast J, Siebeck M, Silling-Engelhardt G, Büller H, Hoet B, Bichler J, Close P. Biological effects of recombinant hirudin (CGP 39393) in human volunteers. J Am Coll Cardiol 22:1080–1088, 1993.

Walenga JM, Bakhos M, Messmore HL, Koza M, Wallock M, Orfei E, Fareed J, Pifarre R. Comparison of recombinant hirudin and heparin as an anticoagulant in a cardiopulmonary bypass model. Blood Coagul Fibrinolysis 2:105–111, 1991.

Warkentin TE. Limitations of conventional treatment options for heparin-induced thrombocytopenia. Semin Hematol 35(suppl 5):17–25, 1998.

Warkentin TE, Kelton JG. A 14-years study of heparin-induced thrombocytopenia. Am J Med 101:502–507, 1996.

Warkentin TE, Hayward CPM, Boshkov LK, Santos AV, Sheppard JI, Bode AP, Kelton JG. Sera from patients with heparin-induced thrombocytopenia generate platelet-derived microparticles with procoagulant activity: an explanation for the thrombotic complications of heparin-induced thrombocytopenia. Blood 84:3691–3699, 1994.

Warkentin TE, Chong BH, Greinacher A. Heparin-induced thrombocytopenia:towards consensus. Thromb Haemost 79:1–7, 1998.

Weitz JI, Hudoba M, Massel D, Marganore J, Hirsh J. Clot bound thrombin is protected from inhibition by heparin–antithrombin III but is susceptible to inactivation by antithrombin III-independent inhibitors. J Clin Invest 86:385–391, 1990.

Weitz JI, Leslie B, Hudoba M. Thrombin binds to soluble fibrin degradation products where it is protected from inhibition by heparin–antithrombin but susceptible to inactivation by antithrombin-independent inhibitors. Circulation 97:544–552, 1998.

Wilhelm MJ, Schmid C, Kececioglu D, Möllhoff T, Ostermann H, Scheld HH. Cardiopulmonary bypass in patients with heparin-induced thrombocytopenia using Org 10172. Ann Thorac Surg 61:920–924, 1996.

16
Hemodialysis in Heparin-Induced Thrombocytopenia

Karl-Georg Fischer
University Hospital Freiburg, Freiburg, Germany

I. HEPARIN-INDUCED THROMBOCYTOPENIA IN HEMODIALYSIS PATIENTS

Because unfractionated heparin (UFH) is the major anticoagulant in hemodialysis (HD), it is important to define the potential role of heparin-induced thrombocytopenia (HIT) in contributing to morbidity and mortality in patients with chronic renal failure. In a recent study, 154 consecutive patients newly treated with HD were investigated for the development of HIT (Yamamoto et al., 1996). Six patients (3.9%) were clinically suspected of having developed HIT because of a fall in the platelet count accompanied by clotting of the dialyzer and extracorporeal circuit. The clinical diagnosis was confirmed by the detection of HIT antibodies in all but one patient. Only one patient developed organ damage from thrombosis (myocardial infarction and stroke). All six patients were switched to an alternative anticoagulant, and did not suffer from thromboembolic events in the follow-up period. Compared with the incidence of HIT of 2.7% found in 332 hip surgery patients treated with UFH (Warkentin et al., 1995), the incidence of HIT in hemodialysis patients thus appears to be similar, regardless of the underlying cause of renal dysfunction (Finazzi and Remuzzi, 1996).

Greinacher and colleagues (1996) performed a cross-sectional study of 165 patients undergoing hemodialysis using UFH, and identified 7 (4.2%) patients as having HIT antibodies using a sensitive activation assay for HIT; however, there was no difference in the incidence of thromboembolic events in HIT antibody-positive patients, when compared with HIT antibody-negative patients. They considered alternative anticoagulants to be justified only if clinical symptoms of HIT occurred.

Similar findings were reported that used an antigen assay for HIT antibodies (platelet factor 4 (PF4)–heparin enzyme immunoassay; EIA) in three other cross-sectional studies of HD patients. In patients undergoing HD using UFH, the frequency of HIT IgG antibodies varied from 0% (0/45; de Sancho et al., 1996), to 2.3% (3/128; Boon et al., 1996), to 6% (3/50, Luzzatto et al., 1998); for patients undergoing HD using LMWH, the frequency in one study was 0.3% (1/133; Boon et al., 1996). Thrombocytopenia was usually not observed in patients who formed HIT antibodies, and none of the patients developed bleeding or thrombosis.

Tentative conclusions suggested by these studies are that only a few patients who form HIT antibodies in association with HD develop clinical events, and that these are more likely to be clotting of the dialyzer and extracorporeal circuit than symptomatic thrombosis affecting the patient. It is also possible that the risk of clinical HIT is higher in patients undergoing short-term HD (the population studied by Yamamoto et al.) than in patients in the long-term phase of HD (as per the remaining studies). Anecdotal case reports of HIT complicating HD also seem frequently to include patients undergoing short-term HD (Matsuo et al., 1989; Hall et al., 1992; Nowak et al., 1997; Gupta et al., 1998).

II. CLINICAL PRESENTATION OF HIT IN HEMODIALYSIS PATIENTS

The diagnosis of HIT and respective management decisions should be primarily based on clinical criteria (Lewis et al., 1997). A further consideration in HD patients is that the procedure of HD itself is associated with a relative decrease in platelet count, even when so-called biocompatible dialyzer membranes are used (Beijering et al., 1997; Schmitt et al., 1987). Furthermore, the fall in platelet count in HD patients developing HIT may be only moderate (Matsuo et al., 1997).

The occurrence of fibrin formation, or even frank clotting of the extracorporeal circuit, despite apparent sufficient anticoagulation, should lead to a strong suggestion of possible HIT (Koide et al., 1995). One of the most serious complications, occlusion of vascular access (the "Achilles heel" of HD), may also indicate HIT, and it has been described both for native fistulae as well as prosthetic grafts (Hall et al., 1992; Laster et al., 1989). Severe skin necrosis, even in the presence of normal platelet count, has been reported in association with the presence of HIT antibodies in patients after both short- and long-term HD (Bredlich et al., 1997; Leblanc et al., 1994).

Rarely, patients can develop HIT after years of regular long-term maintenance HD. Tholl et al. (1997) reported on a patient developing HIT following surgery after 9 years of long-term intermittent HD performed with UFH. In this patient, an anaphylactic reaction to heparin, accompanied by a platelet count fall, led to the diagnosis of HIT. It is possible that the surgery itself contributed to HIT antibody formation, as the highest reported rates of HIT are in postoperative patients receiving UFH (see Chap. 4).

Unfortunately, HD complications associated with HIT are not very specific. Thus, the clinician must consider other factors that could compromise patency of the extracorporeal circuit (e.g., low blood flow, high ultrafiltration rate, excess turbulence within the circuit, or foam formation in the drip chambers). The quality of the vascular access plays a crucial role in this. Other patient-related factors include low arterial blood pressure, high hematocrit, and the need for intradialytic blood transfusion or lipid infusion (Caruana and Keep, 1994). In addition to insufficient anticoagulation, these factors should be ruled out first as the underlying causes of clotting within the extracorporeal circuit, before HIT is considered in the differential diagnosis.

III. MANAGEMENT OF HEMODIALYSIS IN HIT PATIENTS

A. Discontinuation of Heparin Treatment

As HIT is frequently associated with potentially life-threatening thrombotic events (Warkentin et al., 1995; Warkentin and Kelton, 1996), discontinuation of heparin treatment and initiation of adequate alternative anticoagulation is generally considered mandatory (Warkentin et al., 1998). Thus, heparin must not be added to any flushing solution, and no heparin-coated systems can be used.

B. Unsuitable Approaches

Low Molecular Weight Heparin

Low molecular weight heparin is not recommended as alternative anticoagulant. In vitro tests for HIT antibodies show a high degree of cross-reactivity between UFH and LMWH (Greinacher et al., 1992b; Vun et al., 1996). Furthermore, in vivo cross-reactivity manifesting as persistent or recurrent thrombocytopenia or thrombosis during LMWH treatment of HIT appears to be common (Greinacher et al., 1992a; Horellou et al., 1984; Roussi et al., 1984). Because nonheparin anticoagulants are available, LMWH should not be used even if in vitro cross-reactivity is reported to be negative.

Regional Heparinization

Regional heparinization is defined as application of heparin at the inlet of the extracorporeal circuit and its neutralization by protamine at the outlet of the circuit. However, its use in HIT is problematic because of the potential for heparin ''contamination'' of the patient, as well as for heparin ''rebound anticoagulation'' (recurrence of heparin anticoagulation owing to shorter half-life of protamine compared with heparin) (Blaufox et al., 1966). Moreover, direct injurious effects of protamine on the clotting cascade can occur. Consequently, this regimen is not recommended for HD of patients with HIT.

Aspirin

Acetylsalicylic acid has been used as an antiplatelet agent together with continued anticoagulation with UFH for HD of patients with HIT (Hall et al., 1992; Janson et al., 1983; Matsuo et al., 1989). This approach is not recommended for several reasons: (1) protection against heparin-induced platelet activation may be incomplete or absent, as aspirin's effects on blocking the thromboxane-dependent pathway of platelet activation does not reliably inhibit platelet activation by HIT antibodies (Kappa et al., 1987; Polgár et al., 1998); (2) the bleeding risk of uremic patients is increased; and (3) theoretically, it may lead to induction of persistently high levels of HIT antibodies.

Hemodialysis Without Anticoagulant

Hemodialysis without an anticoagulant (Romao Jr. et al., 1997) is not adequate for maintenance HD. Without anticoagulation, the artificial surfaces become coated, first by plasma proteins, followed by adhesion and activation of platelets, with accompanying activation of the coagulation cascade. This will markedly reduce dialysis quality in removal of fluid and solutes long before clotting of the circuit is visible. Moreover, this approach may aggravate HIT. However, in patients at high risk of bleeding (e.g., owing to hepatic disorders or multiorgan failure, or those requiring surgery), temporary hemodialysis without anticoagulant may be useful.

C. Adequate Anticoagulants for Hemodialysis in HIT Patients

Patients with renal failure show plasma hypercoagulability as well as uremic platelet defects, both of which can be worsened by HD (Ambühl et al., 1997; Sreedhara et al., 1995; Vecino et al., 1998). Therefore, selection of an appropriate anticoagulant in HD patients who also suffer from HIT is difficult.

Reports on specific anticoagulant strategies in HIT are anecdotal. Large studies, especially those comparing different anticoagulant regimens, are lacking. Therefore, no treatment recommendations based on level A or B evidence can be provided. Furthermore, because UFH is the routine anticoagulant in use for HD, considerable additional time, effort, and costs are usually required to manage a new anticoagulant for HD, especially during initial use. Ideally, therefore, a center should try to gain experience with a single appropriate alternative anticoagulant for management of these difficult patients. Fear of inducing bleeding should not be used to justify underanticoagulation, with the potential risk for thrombotic complications.

Danaparoid Sodium

Danaparoid sodium (Orgaran, formerly known as Org 10172) is the alternative anticoagulant most widely used for management of HD in patients with HIT (Chong and Magnani, 1992; Greinacher et al., 1992a, 1993; Henny et al., 1983; Magnani, 1993; Ortel et al., 1992; Tholl et al., 1997; Wilde and Markham, 1997). Some of its characteristics require specific attention:

1. The anticoagulant activity of danaparoid can be monitored only by measurement of antifactor Xa levels based on a danaparoid calibration curve; however, many laboratories do not routinely perform these assays. Except for an emergency situation, such as when HIT is strongly suspected and danaparoid is the only available alternative, HD should not be performed without monitoring the antifactor Xa activity to evaluate the dose required for adequate anticoagulation. Once the optimal dose is identified, it can often be used without alteration for several subsequent HD sessions, provided no bleeding or inappropriate clotting occurs, and no surgical intervention is scheduled. Periodic measurement of antifactor Xa activity to validate the appropriate dosage of danaparoid is recommended. For maintenance HD without complications, single determination of pre-HD antifactor Xa activity probably suffices. If there are concerns about adequate or excess anticoagulation, then monitoring of levels at three time points is appropriate (e.g., 30–60 min pre-HD, 30 min after beginning HD, and just before completion).

2. Relative to the pharmacokinetics of danaparoid, it must be emphasized that the elimination half-life of its antifactor Xa activity, which is about 24 h even in healthy individuals (Danhof et al., 1992), is prolonged far more in patients with impaired renal function, and may reach up to 4 days. Thus, significant antifactor Xa levels can be detected in patients undergoing HD with danaparoid even during the interdialytic interval. Whether this yields clinical benefit, such as decreased risk of thrombosis or greater maintenance of vascular access, is unknown. An increase in interdialytic bleeding episodes has not been reported.

3. HIT antibodies potentially cross-react with danaparoid. Although the respective clinical risk has been claimed to be less than 5% (Warkentin et al., 1998), individual patients, nevertheless, may be severely threatened if this condition occurs. This may be especially true for maintenance HD patients, who would be exposed to danaparoid repeatedly. As positive in vitro cross-reactivity is of uncertain clinical significance (Warkentin, 1996; Wilde and Markham, 1997;

Newman et al., 1998), attention should focus on platelet count monitoring. A further fall in platelet count, or new fibrin deposits and clot formation within the extracorporeal circuit after application of danaparoid, may indicate clinically relevant cross-reactivity. To differentiate in vivo cross-reactivity from "under-anticoagulation" owing to insufficient dosage, determination of antifactor Xa levels and HIT antibody cross-reactivity studies are needed.

Table 1 lists dose recommendations for use of danaparoid for HD. The recommendations should be considered as guidelines, and not followed uncritically in any individual patient. If applied with appropriate care, danaparoid provides adequate anticoagulation for HD of HIT patients with a favorable benefit/risk ratio, even during long-term use.

Recombinant Hirudin (r-Hirudin)

Native hirudin was the first anticoagulant used for HD over 75 years ago (Haas, 1925). Recently, interest in its use for HD has redeveloped because of the availability of recombinant preparations, as well as the clinical need for managing patients with HIT. A preparation of r-hirudin, lepirudin (Refludan or HBW 023), has been successfully used in humans for single HD sessions (Nowak et al., 1992; Vanholder et al., 1994; Van Wyk et al., 1995). Clot formation was prevented, and bleeding complications did not occur. Only one patient has been reported to have received lepirudin for regular HD for more than 50 HD sessions without major side effects (Nowak et al., 1997).

For regular HD, some aspects should be specifically addressed:

1. As there is repetitive exposure to r-hirudin when used in regular HD, its immunogenicity is of particular interest. Initially, r-hirudin appeared to be a weak immunogen (Bichler et al., 1991). Recently, it was found that more than 40% of patients receiving lepirudin for more than 5 days developed antihirudin antibodies (Eichler et al., 1997). A patient with proved hirudin allergy after reexposure to r-hirudin was reported (Huhle et al., 1998). With increasing use of r-hirudin, this adverse reaction may become increasingly important.

2. There is evidence that antihirudin antibodies reduce renal clearance of lepirudin in a minority of patients (Eichler et al., 1997), without an effect on its thrombin inhibition. However, this should not be an issue in chronic renal failure patients undergoing HD.

3. It is unclear which laboratory parameter is best-suited for monitoring r-hirudin treatment. According to Vanholder and colleagues (1994, 1997), a modified activated clotting time (ACT) correlated better with the occurrence of clots in the extracorporeal circuit than did the activated partial thromboplastin time (aPTT). By contrast, van Wyk et al. (1995) found the aPTT to be a reliable parameter for monitoring. Nowak et al. (1997) used the ecarin clotting time (ECT; Nowak and Bucha, 1996) for monitoring r-hirudin treatment (see Chap. 17).

4. The elimination of r-hirudin is markedly prolonged in renal impairment. Nowak et al. (1992) reported elimination half-lives of up to 316 h in dialysis patients. Vanholder et al. (1997) found a prolongation of hirudin half-life by a factor of 31 in HD patients, compared with healthy controls. Both studies showed a correlation between the residual creatinine clearance and the r-hirudin clearance in that a minor increase in creatinine clearance resulted in a shorter elimination half-life of r-hirudin. As is true with HD patients treated with danaparoid, r-hirudin-treated patients are anticoagulated into the interdialytic interval (Nowak et al., 1997). Because various organs metabolize hirudin (Grötsch and Hropot, 1991), other factors contributing to its metabolic clearance are possibly also inhibited in patients with end-stage renal failure.

5. Pharmacokinetics of r-hirudin are also influenced by the type of dialyzer used. Although this issue is far from being resolved, there are apparent differences (e.g., between cellulose-based and polysulfone-based dialyzers) relative to the dose of hirudin required for sufficient anticoagulation (Vanholder et al., 1997; Van Wyk et al., 1995). Whereas a high permeability of hemophan low-flux dialyzers for r-hirudin has been reported (Nowak et al., 1997), polysulfone high-flux dialyzers, with a cutoff point of approximately 50 kDa, did not clear r-hirudin with its molecular weight of approximately 7 kDa from circulation. Vanholder et al. (1997) suggested protein–tissue binding or the electrostatic charge of hirudin could explain this finding.

In case of overdosage or drug accumulation leading to adverse effects, r-hirudin can be rapidly cleared from circulation by hemofiltration (Riess et al., 1997). A future treatment option for this situation may be the use of enzymatically modified nonactive thrombin analogues with high affinity for hirudin (Brüggener et al., 1989). In conclusion, r-hirudin seems to be a promising alternative anticoagulant for HD procedures in HIT patients, but owing to lack of broader experience in this setting it should be used with caution and monitored carefully.

Argatroban

Argatroban (Novastan, MD-805) is a potent arginine-derived synthetic catalytic site-directed thrombin inhibitor that lacks antiplatelet and antifibrinolytic activities (Koide et al., 1995; Matsuo et al., 1992). It does not cross-react with HIT antibodies. Apart from an even better relative ability to inhibit fibrin-bound versus soluble thrombin (Berry et al., 1996; Lunven et al., 1996), the principal advantages of argatroban over heparin are similar to r-hirudin (Markwardt, 1991; Matsuo et al., 1992). However, argatroban is metabolized primarily by the liver, and its half-life is only moderately extended in patients with renal insufficiency.

After argatroban proved to be a valuable anticoagulant in HD (Matsuo et al., 1986), it was applied successfully to HIT patients undergoing this procedure (Koide et al., 1995; Matsuo et al., 1992). Whether anticoagulation with argatroban

Table 1 Alternative Anticoagulation for Hemodialysis and Hemofiltration of Patients with HIT

Agent	Dialysis procedure			Bolus	Continuous infusion	Monitoring parameter[a]	Target range
Danaparoid sodium (Org 10172; Orgaran)	Intermittent HD (every 2nd day)	1st HD		3750 (2500)[b,c]	—	Anti-Xa activity	0.5–0.8[d,e]
		2nd HD		3750 (2000)[b,c]	—		
		Subsequent HD	*Pre*dialytic anti-Xa activity (U/mL)[f]				
			< 0.3	3000 (2000)[b,c]	—		
			0.3–0.35	2500 (1500)[b,c]	—		
			0.35–0.4	2000 (1500)[b,c]	—		
			> 0.4	0[g]	—		
	Intermittent HD (daily)	1st HD		3750 (2500)[b,c]	—	Anti-Xa activity	0.5–0.8[d,e]
		2nd HD		2500 (2000)[b,c]	—		
		Subsequent HD		See above	—		
	Continuous HD/HF			2500 (2000)[b,c]			
			First 4 h		600 (600)[c,h]	Anti-Xa activity	0.5–1.0[d,i]
			Next 4 h		400 (400)[c,h]		
			Subsequently		200–600[g,h,j] (150–400)[c,g,h,j]		
Lepirudin (HBW 023; Refludan)	Intermittent HD (every 2nd day)			0.08–0.15[k,l,m]	—	aPTT ratio[n,o] Hirudin conc.[q]	2–3[e,p] 500–1200[e,r]
	Continuous HD[s,t]		At start	0.01[k,l,m,u]	—	aPTT ratio[n,o]	1.5–2.5[v,w]
			Subsequently	0.005–0.01[k,l,m,u]	—		
			Alternatively	—	0.005–0.01[u,x,y]		
Argatroban (MD-805; Novastan)	Intermittent HD[s] (every 2nd day)			0.1[k]	0.1–0.2[y]	aPTT ratio[n]	1.5–3.0[p]

Many of the approaches discussed in this chapter have not been formally studied, none has yet been approved. Treatment examples are given based on a limited number of cases successfully treated with the respective regimen. The different anticoagulants thus cannot be uncritically applied in the dosage given here. The choice of anticoagulant should depend on the experience of the center and the anticoagulant monitoring available.

Abbreviations: HD, hemodialysis; HF, hemofiltration; conc., concentration; aPTT, activated partial thromboplastin time; anti-Xa, antifactor Xa.

[a] Monitoring the condition of the dialyzer after a HD session as well as the time required for termination of bleeding of the fistula should also be included.

[b] Dosage given in anti-Xa units (bolus).

[c] Dosage in parentheses for patients with body weight < 55 kg.

[d] Target range given in U/mL.

[e] Peak activity determined after about 30 min of HD; this level is not required throughout the whole HD session.

[f] Determination 30–60 min before start of the respective HD session.

[g] If fibrin deposition in the dialyzer or clots in the extracorporeal circuit occur, addition of 1500 anti-Xa U as a single bolus.

[h] Dosage given in anti-Xa U/h (infusion).

[i] To achieve the same anti-Xa activity, smaller doses may be required in hemodialysis as compared with hemofiltration.

[j] Maintenance dosage dependent on actual anti-Xa activity; determination every 12 h (provided that no bleeding or clotting occurs).

[k] Dosage given in mg/kg body weight for hemodialysis performed with high-flux hemodialyzers.

[l] The dosage required to reach the target range may vary, for example, owing to residual renal function or the type of dialyzer used (see text).

[m] If larger doses are needed to achieve the target range or to avoid clotting of the extracorporeal circuit, changing to another type of dialyzer may be helpful.

[n] The aPTT ratio is determined relative to the median of the laboratory normal range; according to the literature, alternative tests such as ecarin-clotting time or activated-clotting time also appear suitable for monitoring.

[o] It is unclear which test is best-suited to monitor anticoagulation with r-hirudin, as no test has yet been prospectively evaluated in HD patients.

[p] A peak aPTT of 100 s should not be exceeded.

[q] Determination in plasma by chromogenic assays.

[r] Target range given in ng/mL.

[s] The agent has not yet been formally studied in continuous hemodialysis procedures.

[t] This approach has been successfully performed in several patients in our center without adverse events.

[u] Dosage given for anuric patients; in case of polyuria a higher dosage may be required; the daily dosage may significantly vary between patients.

[v] As patients requiring continuous procedures often are at an increased risk of bleeding, a lower aPTT is to be preferred (50–70 s).

[w] To be initially controlled every 4–6 h to avoid overdosage, especially in patients at risk of bleeding.

[x] In our experience a continuous infusion is more often associated with bleeding events; however, this aspect has not yet been prospectively studied.

[y] Dosage given in mg/kg body weight/h.

alone is always sufficient to prevent clotting in the extracorporeal circuit is unclear: in one HD patient treated with argatroban, marked spontaneous platelet aggregation occurred, perhaps because of HIT together with additional platelet activation known to occur in HD (Koide et al., 1995). Because platelet aggregation could not be suppressed by argatroban alone in this patient, aspirin was added to achieve patency of the extracorporeal circuit.

As nonspecific inactivation of argatroban may occur in blood, periodic monitoring of its anticoagulant activity is recommended (Matsuo et al., 1992), for example, by measuring the aPTT (Koide et al., 1995; Matsuo et al., 1992) or the ECT (Berry et al., 1998). Argatroban appears to be at least as well-suited as r-hirudin for anticoagulation of HIT patients requiring HD, but its precise role in this setting still needs to be defined.

Oral Anticoagulation

For HIT patients requiring long-term anticoagulation, orally active agents are usually given. Although coumarins interfere with the clotting cascade, fibrin formation within the extracorporeal circuit is not always sufficiently blocked. In these cases, additional low-dose intravenous anticoagulation with UFH is usually given for regular maintenance HD. However, in HIT patients requiring HD, alternative low-dose anticoagulation has not been formally studied. The need for additional intravenous anticoagulation depends on the increase of the INR, which should be checked regularly before HD. Priming of the extracorporeal circuit by addition of a compatible anticoagulant to the filling solution with subsequent washout before start of the respective HD session may be of value in diminishing the risk of ''overanticoagulation.''

D. Other Approaches

Dermatan Sulfate

Dermatan sulfate is a natural glycosaminoglycan that selectively inhibits both soluble and fibrin-bound thrombin through potentiation of endogenous heparin cofactor II. It does not interfere with platelet function. Dermatan sulfate has been used successfully to anticoagulate patients with HIT (Agnelli et al., 1994), and has also been applied successfully as an anticoagulant for HD (Boccardo et al., 1997).

Nafamostat Mesilate

Nafamostat mesilate (FUT-175), a synthetic nonspecific serine protease inhibitor with a short half-life, has been evaluated for regional hemodialysis in patients at risk of bleeding (Akizawa et al., 1993). It has also been applied occasionally to HIT patients on HD (Koide et al., 1995). However, owing to significant clot formation at the dialyzer outlet, despite a twofold prolongation of aPTT, reported both in HIT and non-HIT patients (Koide et al., 1995; Matsuo et al., 1993), this anticoagulant cannot currently be recommended for HD of HIT patients.

Prostacyclin

Prostacyclin (PGI_2, epoprostenol), a potent antiplatelet agent with a short half-life, has been evaluated both as a substitute for, and as an adjunct to, standard heparin for HD of patients with acute or chronic renal insufficiency (Samuelsson et al., 1995; Smith et al., 1982; Turney et al., 1980). Adverse effects, such as nausea, vomiting, and hypotension, can be avoided by dose reduction, use of bicarbonate- instead of acetate-containing dialysate, or infusion of the drug at the inlet of the extracorporeal circuit. Because of its mode of action, prostacyclin cannot inhibit activation of coagulation during HD (Novacek et al., 1997; Rylance et al., 1985). Moreover, in a HIT patient receiving continuous venovenous HD, prostacyclin was unable to suppress platelet consumption effectively after heparin had been reinstituted, owing to a false-negative platelet aggregation assay (Samuelsson et al., 1995). Prostacyclin does not seem to be a suitable antithrombotic agent for HD in HIT. Whether it may be a useful adjunct in selected cases remains to be clarified.

Regional Citrate Anticoagulation

Anticoagulation by regional citrate is based on the concept of inhibition of clotting by chelation of ionized calcium, and it was first developed as an alternative anticoagulant regimen in HD patients at risk of bleeding (Pinnick et al., 1983). Metabolic alkalosis, hypernatremia, alterations in calcium homeostasis, and hyperalbuminemia are reported side effects that are generally manageable (Flanigan et al., 1996; Janssen et al., 1996; Ward and Mechta, 1993). Regional citrate anticoagulation is a valuable approach in experienced centers. Regional citrate HD has not yet been described as a regimen in the treatment of HIT patients receiving HD, but it may be a treatment option for those patients who do not require systemic anticoagulation in the interdialytic periods.

IV. SUMMARY

An alternative anticoagulant is required for HD in patients with HIT. Appropriate agents would appear to be danaparoid sodium; r-hirudin derivatives, such as lepirudin; or argatroban, as these appear to be able to suppress clot formation without substantially increasing the bleeding risk. As these results are based on experience with a limited number of patients, larger prospective trials are needed to define the best treatment options in this setting. Even today, though, HIT should no longer be a life-threatening problem for patients requiring dialysis.

REFERENCES

Agnelli G, Iorio A, De Angelis V, Nenci GG. Dermatan sulphate in heparin-induced thrombocytopenia [letter]. Lancet 344:1295–1296, 1994.

Akizawa T, Koshikawa S, Ota K, Kazama M, Mimura N, Hirasawa Y. Nafamostat mesilate: a regional anticoagulant for hemodialysis in patients at high risk for bleeding. Nephron 64:376–381, 1993.

Ambühl PM, Wüthrich RP, Korte W, Schmid L, Krapf R. Plasma hypercoagulability in haemodialysis patients: impact of dialysis and anticoagulation. Nephrol Dial Transplant 12:2355–2364, 1997.

Beijering RJR, ten Cate H, Nurmohamed MT, ten Cate JW. Anticoagulants and extracorporeal circuits. Semin Thromb Hemost 23:225–233, 1997.

Berry CN, Girardot C, Lecoffre C, Lunven C. Effects of the synthetic thrombin inhibitor argatroban on fibrin- or clot-incorporated thrombin: comparison with heparin and recombinant hirudin. Thromb Haemost 72:381–386, 1996.

Berry CN, Lunven C, Girardot C, Lechaire I, Girard D, Charles MC, Ferrari P, O'Brien DP. Ecarin clotting time: a predictive coagulation assay for the antithrombotic activity of argatroban in the rat. Thromb Haemost 79:228–233, 1998.

Bichler J, Gemmerli R, Fritz H. Studies for revealing a possible sensitization to hirudin after repeated intravenous injections in baboons. Thromb Res 61:39–51, 1991.

Blaufox MD, Hampers CL, Merrill JP. Rebound anticoagulation occurring after regional heparinization for hemodialysis. ASAIO Trans 12:207–209, 1966.

Boccardo P, Melacini D, Rota S, Mecca G, Boletta A, Casiraghi F, Gianese F. Individualized anticoagulation with dermatan sulphate for haemodialysis in chronic renal failure. Nephrol Dial Transplant 12:2349–2354, 1997.

Boon DMS, van Vliet HHDM, Zietse R, Kappers-Klunne MC. The presence of antibodies against a PF4–heparin complex in patients on haemodialysis. Thromb Haemost 76: 480, 1996.

Bredlich RO, Stracke S, Gall H, Proebstle TM. Heparin-associated platelet aggregation syndrome with skin necrosis during haemodialysis. Dtsch Med Wochenschr 122: 328–332, 1997.

Brüggener E, Walsmann P, Markwardt F. Neutralization of hirudin anticoagulant action by DIP-thrombin. Pharmazie 44:720–721, 1989.

Caruana RJ, Keep DM. Anticoagulation. In: Daugirdas JT, Ing TS, eds. Handbook of Dialysis. 2nd ed. Boston: Little, Brown, 1994:121–136.

Chong BH, Magnani HN. Orgaran in heparin-induced thrombocytopenia. Haemostasis 22: 85–91, 1992.

Danhof M, De Boer A, Magnani HN, Stiekema JC. Pharmacokinetic considerations of Orgaran (Org 10172) therapy. Haemostasis 22:73–84, 1992.

De Sancho M, Lema MG, Amiral J, Rand J. Frequency of antibodies directed against heparin–platelet factor 4 in patients exposed to heparin through chronic hemodialysis [letter]. Thromb Haemost 75:695–696, 1996.

Eichler P, Olbrich K, Pötzsch B, Greinacher A. Anti-hirudin antibodies in patients treated with recombinant hirudin for more than five days, a prospective study [abstr]. Thromb Haemost (suppl.);PS 2014, June 1997.

Finazzi G, Remuzzi G. Heparin-induced thrombocytopenia—background and implications for haemodialysis. Nephrol Dial Transplant 11:2120–2122, 1996.

Flanigan MJ, Pillsbury L, Sadewasser G, Lim VS. Regional hemodialysis anticoagulation: hypertonic tri-sodium citrate or anticoagulant citrate dextrose-A. Am J Kidney Dis 27:519–524, 1996.

Greinacher A, Drost W, Michels I, Leitl J, Gottsmann M, Kohl HJ, Glaser M, Mueller-Eckhardt C. Heparin-associated thrombocytopenia: successful therapy with the heparinoid Org 10172 in a patient showing cross-reaction to LMW heparins. Ann Hematol 64:40–42, 1992a.

Greinacher A, Michels I, Mueller-Eckhardt C. Heparin-associated thrombocytopenia: the antibody is not heparin specific. Thromb Haemostas 67:545–549, 1992b.

Greinacher A, Philippen KH, Kemkes-Matthes B, Möckl M, Mueller-Eckhardt C, Schaefer K. Heparin-associated thrombocytopenia type II in a patient with end-stage renal disease: successful anticoagulation with the low-molecular-weight heparinoid Org 10172 during haemodialysis. Nephrol Dial Transplant 8:1176–1177, 1993.

Greinacher A, Zinn S, Wizemann U, Birk W. Heparin-induced antibodies as a risk factor for thromboembolism and haemorrhage in patients undergoing chronic haemodialysis. Lancet 348:764, 1996.

Grötsch H, Hropot M. Degradation of rDNA hirudin and α-human thrombin hirudin complex in liver and kidney homogenates from rat. Thromb Res 64:763–767, 1991.

Gupta AK, Kovacs MJ, Sauder DN. Heparin-induced thrombocytopenia. Ann Pharmacother 32:55–59, 1998.

Haas G. Versuche der Blutauswaschung am Lebenden mit Hilfe der Dialyse. Klin Wochenschr 4:13–14, 1925.

Hall AV, Clark WF, Parbtani A. Heparin-induced thrombocytopenia in renal failure. Clin Nephrol 38:86–89, 1992.

Henny CP, ten Cate H, ten Cate JW, Surachno S, Van Bronswijk H, Wilmink JM, Ockelford PA. Use of a new heparinoid as anticoagulant during acute haemodialysis of patients with bleeding complications. Lancet 1:890–893, 1983.

Horellou MH, Conard J, Lecrubier C, Samama M, Roque-D'Orbcastel O, de Fenoyl O, Di Maria G, Bernadou A. Persistent heparin induced thrombocytopenia despite therapy with low molecular weight heparin [letter]. Thromb Haemost 51:134, 1984.

Huhle G, Hoffmann U, Wang L, Bayerl C, Harenberg J. Allergy and positive IgG in a patient reexposed to r-hirudin [abstr]. Ann Hematol 76(suppl 1):A97, 1998.

Janson PA, Moake JL, Carpinito G. Aspirin prevents heparin-induced platelet aggregation in vivo [letter]. Br J Haematol 53:166–168, 1983.

Janssen MJFM, Deegens JK, Kapinga TH, Beukhof JR, Huijgens PC, Van Loenen AC, Van der Meulen J. Citrate compared to low molecular weight heparin anticoagulation in chronic hemodialysis patients. Kidney Int 49:806–813, 1996.

Kappa JR, Fisher CA, Berkowitz HD, Cottrel ED, Addonizio VP. Heparin-induced platelet activation in sixteen surgical patients: diagnosis and management. J Vasc Surg 5: 101–109, 1987.

Koide M, Yamamoto S, Matsuo M, Suzuki S, Arima N, Matsuo T. Anticoagulation for heparin-induced thrombocytopenia with spontaneous platelet aggregation in a patient requiring haemodialysis. Nephrol Dial Transplant 10:2137–2140, 1995.

Laster J, Elfrink R, Silver D. Reexposure to heparin of patients with heparin-associated antibodies. J Vasc Surg 9:677–682, 1989.

Leblanc M, Roy LF, Legault L, Dufresne LR, Morin C, Thuot C. Severe skin necrosis associated with heparin in hemodialysis. Nephron 68:133–137, 1994.

Lewis BE, Walenga JM, Wallis DE. Anticoagulation with Novastan (argatroban) in patients with heparin-induced thrombocytopenia and heparin-induced thrombocytopenia and thrombosis syndrome. Semin Thromb Hemost 23:197–202, 1997.

Lunven C, Gauffeny C, Lecoffre C, O'Brien DP, Roome NO, Berry CN. Inhibition by argatroban, a specific thrombin inhibitor, of platelet activation by fibrin clot-associated thrombin. Thromb Haemost 75:154–160, 1996.

Luzzatto G, Bertoli M, Cella G, Fabris F, Zaia B, Girolami A. Platelet count, anti-heparin/platelet factor 4 antibodies and tissue factor pathway inhibitor plasma antigen level in chronic dialysis. Thromb Res 89:115–122, 1998.

Magnani HN. Heparin-induced thrombocytopenia (HIT): an overview of 230 patients treated with Orgaran (Org 10172). Thromb Haemost 70:554–561, 1993.

Markwardt F. Past, present and future of hirudin. Haemostasis 21:11–26, 1991.

Matsuo T, Nakao K, Yamada T, Matsuo O. Effect of a new anticoagulant (MD 805) on platelet activation in the hemodialysis circuit. Thromb Res 41:33–41, 1986.

Matsuo T, Yamada T, Chikahira Y, Kadowaki S. Effect of aspirin on heparin-induced thrombocytopenia (HIT) in a patient requiring hemodialysis. Blut 59:393–395, 1989.

Matsuo T, Kario K, Kodama K, Okamoto S. Clinical application of the synthetic thrombin inhibitor, argatroban (MD-805). Semin Thromb Hemost 18:155–160, 1992.

Matsuo T, Kario K, Nakao K, Yamada T, Matsuo M. Anticoagulation with nafamostat mesilate, a synthetic protease inhibitor, in hemodialysis patients with a bleeding risk. Haemostasis 23:135–141, 1993.

Matsuo T, Koide M, Kario K. Application of argatroban, a direct thrombin inhibitor, in heparin-intolerant patients requiring extracorporeal circulation. Artif Organs 21: 1035–1038, 1997.

Newman PM, Swanson RL, Chong BH. IgG binding to PF4–heparin complexes in the fluid phase and cross-reactivity with low molecular weight heparin and heparinoid. Thromb Haemost 80:292–297, 1998.

Novacek G, Kapiotis S, Jilma B, Quehenberger P, Michitsch A, Traindl O, Speiser W. Enhanced blood coagulation and enhanced fibrinolysis during hemodialysis with prostacyclin. Thromb Res 88:283–290, 1997.

Nowak G, Bucha E. Quantitative determination of hirudin in blood and body fluids. Semin Thromb Hemost 22:197–202, 1996.

Nowak G, Bucha E, Gööck T, Thieler H, Markwardt F. Pharmacology of r-hirudin in renal impairment. Thromb Res 66:707–715, 1992.

Nowak G, Bucha E, Brauns I, Czerwinski R. Anticoagulation with r-hirudin in regular haemodialysis with heparin-induced thrombocytopenia (HIT II). The first long term application of r-hirudin in a haemodialysis patient. Wien Klin Wochenschr 109: 354–358, 1997.

Ortel TL, Gockermann JP, Califf RM, McCann RL, O'Connor CM, Metzler DM, Greenberg CS. Parenteral anticoagulation with the heparinoid Lomoparan (Org 10172) in patients with heparin-induced thrombocytopenia and thrombosis. Thromb Haemost 67:292–296, 1992.

Pinnick RV, Wiegmann TB, Diederich DA. Regional citrate anticoagulation for hemodialysis in the patient at high risk for bleeding. N Engl J Med 308:258–261, 1983.

Polgár J, Eichler P, Greinacher A, Clemetson KJ. Adenosine diphosphate (ADP) and ADP receptor play a major role in platelet activation/aggregation induced by sera from heparin-induced thrombocytopenia patients. Blood 91:549–554, 1998.

Riess F-C, Pötzsch B, Jäger K, Bleese N, Schaper W, Müller-Berghaus G. Elimination von rekombinantem Hirudin aus der Blutzirkulation mittels Hämofiltration. Untersuchungen im Schweinemodell. Hämostaseologie 17:200–204, 1997.

Romao JE Jr, Fadil MA, Sabbaga E, Marcondes M. Haemodialysis without anticoagulant: haemostasis parameters, fibrinogen kinetic, and dialysis efficiency. Nephrol Dial Transplant 12:106–110, 1997.

Roussi JH, Houbouyan LL, Goguel AF. Use of low-molecular-weight heparin in heparin-induced thrombocytopenia with thrombotic complications [letter]. Lancet 1:1183, 1984.

Rylance PB, Gordge MP, Ireland H, Lane DA, Weston MJ. Haemodialysis with prostacyclin (epoprostenol) alone. Proc Eur Dial Transplant Assoc Eur Renal Assoc 21: 281–286, 1985.

Samuelsson O, Amiral J, Attman P-O, Bennegård K, Björck S, Larsson G, Tengborn L. Heparin-induced thrombocytopenia during continuous haemofiltration. Nephrol Dial Transplant 10:1768–1771, 1995.

Schmitt GW, Moake JL, Rudy CK, Vicks SL, Hamburger RJ. Alterations in hemostatic parameters during hemodialysis with dialyzers of different membrane composition and flow design. Platelet activation and factor VIII-related von Willebrand factor during hemodialysis. Am J Med 83:411–418, 1987.

Smith MC, Danviriyasup K, Crow JW, Cato AE, Park GD, Hassid A, Dunn MJ. Prostacyclin substitution for heparin in long-term hemodialysis. Am J Med 73:669–678, 1982.

Sreedhara R, Itagaki I, Lynn B, Hakim RM. Defective platelet aggregation in uremia is transiently worsened by hemodialysis. Am J Kidney Dis 25:555–563, 1995.

Tholl U, Greinacher A, Overdick K, Anlauf M. Life-threatening anaphylactic reaction following parathyroidectomy in a dialysis patient with heparin-induced thrombocytopenia. Nephrol Dial Transplant 12:2750–2755, 1997.

Turney JH, Williams LC, Fewell MR, Parsons V, Weston MJ. Platelet protection and heparin sparing with prostacyclin during regular dialysis therapy. Lancet 2:219–222, 1980.

Vanholder RC, Camez AA, Veys NM, Soria J, Mirshahi M, Soria C, Ringoir S. Recombinant hirudin: a specific thrombin inhibiting anticoagulant for hemodialysis. Kidney Int 45:1754–1759, 1994.

Vanholder R, Camez A, Veys N, van Loo A, Dhondt AM, Ringoir S. Pharmacokinetics of recombinant hirudin in hemodialyzed end-stage renal failure patients. Thromb Haemost 77:650–655, 1997.

Van Wyk V, Badenhorst PN, Luus HG, Kotzé HF. A comparison between the use of recombinant hirudin and heparin during hemodialysis. Kidney Int 48:1338–1343, 1995.

Vecino A, Navarro-Antolin J, Teruel J, Navarro J, Cesar J. Lipid composition of platelets in paticnts with uremia. Nephron 78:271–273, 1998.

Vun CM, Evans S, Chong BH. Cross-reactivity study of low molecular weight heparins and heparinoid in heparin-induced thrombocytopenia. Thromb Res 81:525–532, 1996.

Ward DM, Mehta, RL. Extracorporeal management of acute renal failure patients at high risk of bleeding. Kidney Int 43:S-237-S-244, 1993.

Warkentin TE. Danaparoid (Orgaran) for the treatment of heparin-induced thrombocytopenia (HIT) and thrombosis: effects on in vivo thrombin and cross-linked fibrin generation, and evaluation of the clinical significance of in vitro cross-reactivity (XR) of danaparoid for HIT–IgG [abstr]. Blood 88:626a, 1996.

Warkentin TE, Kelton JG. A 14-year study of heparin-induced thrombocytopenia. Am J Med 101:502–507, 1996.

Warkentin TE, Chong BH, Greinacher A. Heparin-induced thrombocytopenia: towards consensus. Thromb Haemost 79:1–7, 1998.

Warkentin TE, Levine MN, Hirsh J, Horsewood P, Roberts RS, Gent M, Kelton JG. Heparin-induced thrombocytopenia in patients treated with low-molecular-weight heparin or unfractionated heparin. N Engl J Med 332:1330–1335, 1995.

Wilde MI, Markham A. Danaparoid. A review of its pharmacology and clinical use in the management of heparin-induced thrombocytopenia. Drugs 54:903–924, 1997.

Yamamoto S, Koide M, Matsuo M, Suzuki S, Ohtaka M, Saika S, Matsuo T. Heparin-induced thrombocytopenia in hemodialysis patients. Am J Kidney Dis 28:82–85, 1996.

17

Management of Cardiopulmonary Bypass Anticoagulation in Patients with Heparin-Induced Thrombocytopenia

Bernd Poetzsch
Rheinische Friedrich-Wilhelms-University Bonn, Bonn, Germany

Katharina Madlener
Kerckhoff-Klinik, Bad Nauheim, Germany

I. INTRODUCTION

Immediate cessation of, and avoidance of reexposure to, heparin are important principles underlying the management of patients with immune-mediated heparin-induced thrombocytopenia (HIT) (Chong and Berndt, 1989; Warkentin et al., 1998). Because further antithrombotic therapy is often necessary for these patients, several alternative anticoagulant strategies have been developed (see Chaps. 13–15). However, patients with HIT who require cardiac surgery present special problems. Considerable activation of the hemostatic system results when blood is exposed to the artificial surfaces of the cardiopulmonary bypass (CPB) pump used for most heart surgery (Edmunds, 1993; Slaughter et al., 1994). Heparin is the current anticoagulant of choice for CPB, and there is relatively little experience with other forms of anticoagulation in this patient setting. Moreover, any alternative anticoagulant considered for HIT patients should ideally meet certain requirements. First, the agent should be effective in minimizing activation of coagulation during CPB. Second, a rapid and simple method of monitoring its anticoagulating effects should be available to avoid inappropriate under- or overanticoagulation. Finally, rapid and complete reversibility of the anticoagulating effects is important to minimize postoperative bleeding complications. Unfortunately, no existing agent meets all of these requirements.

II. ALTERNATIVE STRATEGIES FOR CPB ANTICOAGULATION

A variety of approaches to perform CPB anticoagulation in HIT patients has been reported, including the use of danaparoid sodium, the thrombin inhibitors hirudin and argatroban, the defibrinogenating enzyme ancrod, and antiplatelet agents, such as aspirin and iloprost. We will review the advantages and disadvantages of these various strategies for the CPB setting in patients with acute or previously documented HIT. The possibility of a brief reexposure to heparin in a patient with previous HIT who subsequently has no detectable HIT antibodies will also be discussed.

A. Danaparoid Sodium

The efficacy of danaparoid sodium for CPB anticoagulation was first shown in a dog model (Henny et al., 1985). Subsequently, this agent was used for patients with HIT who needed heart surgery (Doherty et al., 1990; Magnani, 1993; Wilhelm et al., 1996). Recently, Magnani and co-workers (1997) summarized the experience in 53 patients with HIT who underwent CPB using danaparoid for anticoagulation. The patients included in this study generally received an intravenous (iv) bolus of 8750 U of danaparoid after thoracotomy. The CPB circuit was primed with 7500 U. During CPB, booster intravenous injections (1500 U) were to be administered up to once hourly if there was visually apparent clot or fibrin formation. Plasma levels of antifactor Xa (anti-Xa) activity generally were not monitored during CPB.

With this fixed-dosing schedule, ''clots'' in the operative field, as an indicator of inadequate anticoagulation, were observed in 18 (34%) patients. One patient, reported elsewhere, developed near-fatal thrombosis of the CPB circuit during weaning from bypass (Grocott et al., 1997). Severe postoperative bleeding, defined as more than 20 U of blood transfused, was noted in 11 (20%) patients. As a result of these data, the authors recommended a modified treatment regimen that included a priming dose of 3 U/mL, a weight-adjusted postthoracotomy iv bolus dose of 125 U/kg body weight (b.w.), and a constant intravenous infusion of 7 U/kg b.w. per hour started immediately after institution of the CPB, and stopped 45 min before the expected end of CPB. Thus, for a 70-kg person undergoing an operation with a CPB time of 2 h and a priming volume of 1500 mL, a total dose of approximately 13,860 U danaparoid, or 198 U/kg, is recommended by the authors.

However, this revised protocol was developed empirically, with adjustments made based on some of the complications observed using the fixed-dose protocol (Grocott et al., 1997). Even though the revised protocol means that many patients would receive a lower dose of danaparoid than with the earlier fixed-dose regimen, this might not lead to reduced bleeding outcomes. Paradoxically, less effective anticoagulation during CPB could lead to more thrombin generation during the procedure potentially leading to even greater postoperative bleeding because of secondary hyperfibrinolysis, even if the postoperative danaparoid levels are not high. Indeed, Insler and colleagues (1997) reported a patient receiving danaparoid for CPB who first developed clots in the operative field and arterial filter of the CPB, followed by severe postoperative bleeding requiring surgical reexploration. Regardless of the explanation for excessive bleeding, even a weight-modified treatment regimen bears the risk of under- or overanticoagulation, if the anticoagulant effect is not monitored.

Therefore, we developed a danaparoid-dosing schedule for CPB with dose adjustments made, according to the results of anti-Xa measurements (Table 1). Unfortunately, although both the activated clotting time (ACT) and the activated partial thromboplastin time (aPTT) are prolonged by the higher plasma levels of

Table 1 Modified Treatment Protocol for CPB Anticoagulation with Danaparoid Sodium[a]

Initial danaparoid dosing (pre-CPB)	
Initial intravenous (iv) danaparoid bolus[b]:	100 U/kg body weight
Danaparoid added to priming solution:	3000 U
Initial target antifactor Xa level:	> 1.5 U/mL before start of CPB
Additional danaparoid dosing if pre-CPB plasma anti-Xa level < 1.5 U/mL	
Anti-Xa level	Dosing modification
< 1.2 U/mL	Check measurement; if confirmed, give extra 1500 U bolus
1.2–1.5 U/mL	Give additional 750 U bolus
Dosing and monitoring while on CPB	
Danaparoid infusion rate at start of CPB:	200 U/h
Frequency of anti-Xa level monitoring:	Every 15 min
Intraoperative dose adjustments, based on plasma anti-Xa levels:	
Anti-Xa level	Dosing modification
> 1.8 U/mL	Stop infusion until anti-Xa level < 1.5 U/mL
1.2–1.8 U/mL	No change in infusion rate
< 1.2 U/mL	Increase infusion rate to 300 U/h
< 1.0 U/mL	Administer additional iv bolus of 3000 U
Special steps toward end of CPB	
Stop danaparoid infusion 30 min before anticipated end of CPB	

[a] This protocol, developed by the authors, is based on the availability of rapid-turnaround plasma anti-Xa levels obtained intraoperatively. Another protocol that is not based on intraoperative anti-Xa monitoring, and that results in somewhat higher danaparoid dosing, is given in Chap. 14.

[b] The initial intravenous danaparoid bolus should be given 15–20 min before start of CPB (generally at the time the surgeon opens the sternum).

danaparoid used during CPB, there is no acceptable linear correlation (Gitlin et al., 1998). Because only the plasma anti-Xa levels correlate linearly with the plasma levels of danaparoid, we based our schedule on anti-Xa levels. Similar to the protocol recommended by Magnani and co-workers (1997), the intravenous bolus and priming dose are adjusted to body weight and priming volume, respectively. After beginning CPB, plasma anti-Xa levels should be maintained at 1.5 ± 0.3 U/mL. The continuous infusion is stopped 30 min before the expected end of bypass. However, in our experience, even if such an anti-Xa-adjusted danaparoid treatment regimen is used, increased postoperative bleeding is a problem. Possible explanations for the increased postoperative bleeding include an ongoing anticoagulant effect of danaparoid (half-life, approximately 17 h) for which there is no pharmacological antagonist (Meuleman, 1992), as well as the incomplete inhibition of thrombin generation during CPB, potentially leading to increased postoperative hyperfibrinolysis.

In all, CPB anticoagulation with danaparoid can lead to successful outcomes. About three-quarters (36 of 47; 77%) of the patients reported by Magnani and co-workers (1997) were alive 6 weeks after cardiac surgery with danaparoid. Nevertheless, the disadvantages of danaparoid, including its long-lasting anticoagulant activity that cannot be neutralized, and the significant difficulties in monitoring its anticoagulant effects in an operating room setting, render danaparoid a ''second-choice'' anticoagulant in HIT patients requiring cardiac surgery.

B. Recombinant Hirudin

Various forms of recombinant hirudin (r-hirudin), an anticoagulant naturally produced by the salivary gland of the leech (*Hirudo medicinalis*), are now available in North America and Europe for clinical use. Hirudin is a single-chain polypeptide of 65 amino acids (7000 Da) that forms a tight 1 : 1 stoichiometric complex with thrombin, thereby occupying the putative fibrinogen-binding site and blocking the catalytic site of thrombin. As a result, all of the thrombin-catalyzed procoagulant reactions, such as conversion of fibrinogen to fibrin, activation of coagulation factors V, VIII, and XIII, and thrombin-induced platelet activation, are inhibited.

Because of its potent anticoagulant effect, r-hirudin has been studied as an anticoagulant for use in open heart surgery, both in dogs (Walenga et al., 1991) and pigs (Riess et al., 1997). In both animal models, effective CPB anticoagulation could be achieved by administration of r-hirudin as a bolus injection (1 mg/kg b.w.) followed by a continuous infusion of 1 mg/kg b.w., started after initiation of CPB, and continuing until end of CPB. In humans, however, recovery of hirudin in the plasma following body weight-adjusted dosing shows a high interindividual variability (Koza et al., 1993). Therefore, a fixed-dose protocol for r-hirudin in the CPB setting bears the risk of both inadequate anticoagulation and overdosing. Although the latter is complicated by excessive and potentially fatal postoperative bleeds, the former may result in the occurrence of thromboembolic complications while on pump, including catastrophic total pump occlusion.

To establish a treatment schedule that is adjusted to the individual's response to hirudin, we investigated different monitoring systems for hirudin plasma levels. Several in vitro and in vivo experiments demonstrated that the ACT and aPTT were not sufficiently sensitive to monitor hirudin plasma levels (Pötzsch et al., 1997). However, reliable results were obtained by using the whole blood ecarin clotting time (Pötzsch et al., 1997).

Ecarin is a prothrombin-activating enzyme, derived from the venom of the snake *Echis carinatus*, that activates prothrombin to an intermediate product, meizothrombin (Nishida et al., 1995). Meizothrombin expresses only moderate clotting activity, but is fully reactive toward, and thus inhibited by, hirudin. As a result, in r-hirudin-containing plasma, meizothrombin forms stable 1:1 complexes with r-hirudin. Only when hirudin is neutralized does clotting become initiated, either by meizothrombin or subsequently generated thrombin. Ecarin is available from commercial sources.

Table 2 outlines the whole blood ecarin clotting time method, which we perform using the KC10a coagulometer (Pötzsch et al., 1997). The method is easily adaptable to any other coagulometer. A calibration curve is constructed by using citrate-anticoagulated whole blood spiked with r-hirudin to achieve final concentrations of 0.5, 1.0, 1.5, 2.0, 3.0, and 4.0 μg/mL. Critical levels of r-hirudin during the CPB operation were established in an in vitro CPB setting, and in a first series of HIT patients undergoing cardiac surgery (Pötzsch et al., 1993; Riess et al., 1995, 1996). Clot formation in the CPB apparatus was seen at levels of r-hirudin below 1.8 μg/mL, and increasing levels of fibrinopeptide A (an indicator of thrombin-mediated fibrinogen cleavage) occurred at r-hirudin plasma levels less than 2.0 μg/mL. Based on these results, the therapeutic level of r-hirudin during CPB was set between 3.5 and 4.5 μg/mL. Higher intraoperative levels of r-hirudin could be complicated by a higher postoperative bleeding risk, especially because no antidote is available.

A treatment protocol based upon the ECT-monitoring of hirudin levels is

Table 2 Whole Blood Ecarin Clotting Time

	50 μL citrate-anticoagulated whole blood to be analyzed
+	50 μL standard normal human plasma
	Incubate for 1 min at 37°C
+	50 μL ecarin solution (20 U/mL) containing 0.025 M calcium chloride
	Determination of the clotting time

Table 3 Treatment Protocol for r-Hirudin Anticoagulation During CPB

Initial lepirudin dosing (pre-CPB)	
Initial intravenous lepirudin bolus:	0.25 mg/kg body weight
Lepirudin added to priming solution:	0.2 mg/kg body weight
Control of lepirudin plasma levels:	> 2.5 μg/mL at start of CPB If < 2.5 μg/mL, give additional bolus (10 mg)
Lepirudin dosing and monitoring while on CPB	
Continuous iv infusion[a] at start of CPB:	30 mL/h (0.5 mg/min.)
Frequency of lepirudin level monitoring:	every 15 min using ECT
Intraoperative dose adjustments, based on ECT:	
Lepirudin plasma level	Dosing modification
> 4.5 μg/mL	Reduce infusion rate by 10 mL/h
3.5–4.5 μg/mL	No change in infusion rate
< 3.5 μg/mL	Increase infusion rate by 10 mL/h
Special steps toward end of CPB	
Stop lepirudin infusion 15 min before anticipated end of CPB.	
After disconnection of CPB, administer 5 mg hirudin to the heart–lung machine to avoid clot formation.	

CPB, cardiopulmonary; iv, intravenous.
[a] 50 mg of lepirudin are dissolved in 50 mL 0.9% sodium chloride

given in Table 3. The data obtained from ten patients with HIT, treated with r-hirudin for heart surgery, demonstrated that stable r-hirudin plasma levels in the range from 3.5 to 5.0 μg/mL could be obtained using the ECT-adjusted treatment schedule (Fig. 1a). Because of the relatively short half-life of r-hirudin of approximately 1 h, plasma levels of r hirudin declined rapidly after stopping its infusion (Fig. 1b). However, in renally impaired patients, r-hirudin can accumulate, leading to postoperative bleeding.

To date, the clinical data demonstrate that r-hirudin is a suitable alternative for anticoagulation of CPB in HIT patients. The ECT provides adequate monitoring and allows an adjusted treatment schedule with apparently minimal risk for thrombotic problems on pump. Because of the relatively short half-life, plasma levels of r hirudin decline rapidly after stopping its infusion. As hirudin is almost completely eliminated by the kidney in humans, patients with impaired renal function may require hemofiltration to reduce plasma levels of r-hirudin.

C. Platelet Inhibition as a Strategy to Permit Heparinization for CPB

Another approach described to manage CPB in a patient with HIT is to combine full heparinization with one or more antiplatelet agents. Several groups of investi-

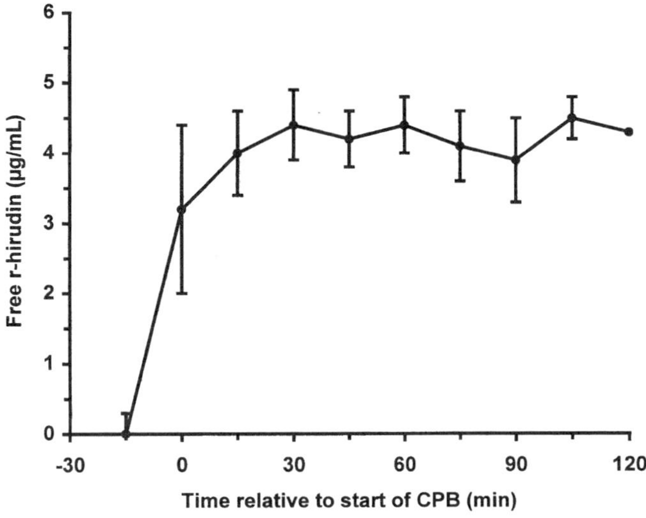

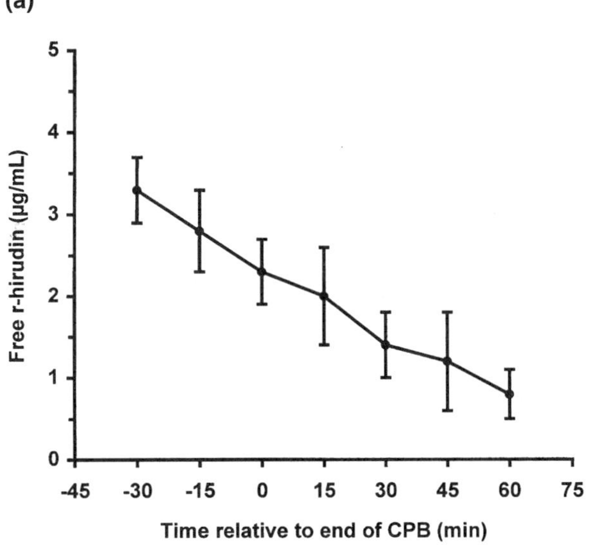

Figure 1 Course of free r-hirudin concentrations in HIT patients ($n = 10$) treated with hirudin before, (a) during, and (b) after CPB. Free r-hirudin was measured using a chromogenic thrombin-based assay as described. (From Pötzsch et al., 1997.)

gators have used iloprost for this situation (Kappa et al., 1985; Long, 1985; Palmer Smith et al., 1985; Addonizio et al., 1987; Kraenzler and Starr, 1988), following the original observation by Olinger and colleagues (1984) that iloprost inhibited heparin-dependent platelet activation in the presence of HIT serum. Iloprost is a stable analogue of prostacyclin; thus, it stimulates adenylate cyclase, resulting in increased platelet cAMP levels, which prevents platelet activation by various platelet agonists, including HIT antibodies.

Since iloprost acts immediately on infusion, treatment can be started shortly before heparin use. Nevertheless, in the treatment protocols described, iloprost infusion was generally begun 0.5–1 h before heparinization, to permit demonstration ex vivo that the patient's platelets would not be aggregated by heparin. Doses between 10 and 30 ng/kg min^{-1} were needed to achieve complete inhibition of heparin-induced platelet aggregation. Iloprost is generally continued until 15 min before protamine administration.

Because of its short elimination half-life of 15–30 min, platelet reactivity returns approximately 3 h after its cessation. Increased postoperative bleeding is generally not a problem in iloprost-treated patients. Its major drawback is its effects on vasomotor tone, particularly the marked vasodilation and severe hypotension that can result. Although Addonizio and colleagues (1987) reported that hypotension was manageable, Kraenzler and co-workers (1988) reported severe hypotension resistant to relatively large doses of phenylephrine in iloprost-treated HIT patients.

Pretreatment of patients with more conventional antiplatelet agents, such as aspirin and dipyridamole, followed by heparin use, has been used successfully in patients with a documented previous history of HIT (Makhoul et al., 1987). However, such an approach is controversial for a patient with acute HIT, because in vitro activation of platelets by HIT antibodies is not reliably inhibited by these relatively weak antiplatelet agents (Kappa et al., 1987).

D. Other Anticoagulant Strategies

Ancrod

The thrombin-like snake venom, ancrod (Arvin), is a defibrinogenating agent that cleaves fibrinopeptide A, but not fibrinopeptide B, from fibrinogen. This results in formation of fibrinogen–fibrin polymers into an unstable configuration that is susceptible to rapid degradation by plasmin. Ancrod has been used as a treatment for HIT (Demers et al., 1991; Cole and Bormanis, 1988), including as an alternative anticoagulant for cardiac surgery requiring CPB (Zulys et al., 1989; Teasdale et al., 1989). The recommended initial dose is usually 70 U in normal saline, administered slowly, over at least 6–12 h.

There are some important disadvantages of using ancrod for cardiac surgery. First, ancrod must be given slowly, because a very rapid infusion can lead to life-threatening intravascular fibrin deposition. Thus, it is not appropriate for emergency situations. Second, it is difficult to determine accurately the fibrinogen level at the recommended target fibrinogen range (0.2–0.5 g/L). Furthermore, it is uncertain what fibrinogen level is required, if any, to prevent clinically important fibrin formation during CPB. Third, reversal of ''anticoagulation'' requires a blood product, fibrinogen concentrates (Europe) or cryoprecipitate (North America), to replace fibrinogen. Finally, ancrod does not inhibit thrombin generation, and has even been associated with increased thrombin generation in some clinical settings, such as acute HIT (Warkentin, 1998). It is possible that this could lead to thrombotic or post-CPB hemorrhagic complications when used for the management of acute HIT. All of the considerations suggest that ancrod is not a suitable alternative to heparin in the setting of CPB surgery.

Argatroban

Argatroban (Novastan) is a specific thrombin inhibitor derived from L-arginine. It is a small molecule (532 Da) that binds reversibly to thrombin. It has a half-life of about 30 min in normal humans. The potential of argatroban to be an effective anticoagulant in patients with HIT has been recently investigated (Lewis et al., 1997a). Although argatroban has been a successful anticoagulant in a CPB model, there is only limited information available on its use in humans (for review see Lewis et al., 1997b).

III. USE OF HEPARIN FOR CPB IN PATIENTS WITH A REMOTE HISTORY OF HIT

An intriguing option for patients with a history of HIT, but in whom persisting HIT antibodies can no longer be detected, is to consider reexposure to heparin for CPB, and to avoid heparin completely both before surgery (e.g., at heart catheterization) and in the postoperative period. This approach has been used successfully by some physicians (Makhoul et al., 1987; Warkentin and Kelton, 1998), and it is based on the following rationale. First, HIT antibodies are transient, and they usually are not detectable after 100 days following an episode of HIT (see Chap. 3). Thus, no immediate problems would be expected in a patient without residual HIT antibodies whose previous episode of HIT was ''remote'' (i.e., more than several months before the need for heart surgery). Second, it appears that a minimum of 5 days are required before clinically significant levels of HIT antibodies are generated following any episode of heparin treatment (Warkentin and Kelton, 1998). Although the literature has raised the issue of an even more rapid ''anamnestic'' immune response in HIT, there is evidence that these episodes represent acute-onset HIT in a patient who has residual circulating HIT antibodies resulting from a recent episode of HIT, rather than a rapid recurrence of HIT antibodies because of immune memory caused by a remote exposure to heparin.

Testing for HIT antibodies in patients with a history of HIT before anticipated heparin reexposure at heart surgery should be performed using one or more sensitive tests (see Chap. 11) if this approach is to be considered. Particularly in cardiac surgical centers where there is limited experience with nonheparin anticoagulation for CPB, risk–benefit considerations favor a brief use of heparin for these patients. For example, a patient who developed near-fatal CPB circuit thrombosis during danaparoid anticoagulation had had HIT 11 years earlier, and had no detectable HIT antibodies at the time danaparoid was used (Grocott et al., 1997).

IV. ACUTE HIT BEFORE AND AFTER HEART SURGERY

There are several reasons why a patient with HIT might require urgent heart surgery, including the result of life-threatening thrombotic complications of HIT

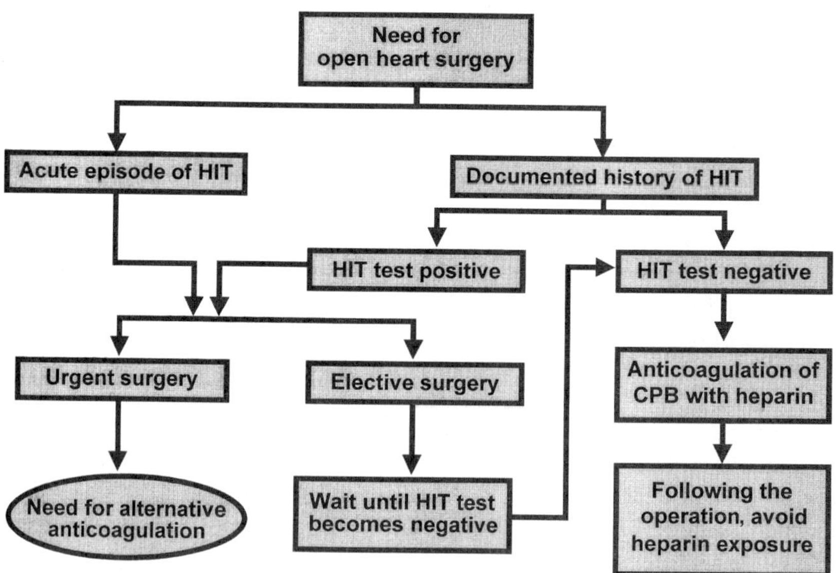

Figure 2 Algorithm for decision making for alternative anticoagulation in HIT patients.

affecting the heart (e.g., acute coronary insufficiency or myocardial infarction; removal of intracardiac thrombus), or because HIT has complicated the course of a critically ill patient receiving heparin before anticipated heart surgery (e.g., while awaiting a heart for cardiac transplantation, or during use of an intra-aortic balloon pump). The latter group of patients appear to have a relatively high risk of developing HIT (Walls et al., 1992).

Studies of the frequency of HIT antibody formation (Bauer et al., 1997; Visentin et al., 1996; Warkentin et al., 1999) following heart surgery suggest that as many as 15–50% of patients form HIT antibodies, using an enzyme immunoassay that detects IgG antibodies that recognize platelet factor 4–heparin complexes (see Chap. 4). With the washed platelet serotonin-release assay, HIT antibodies are detected in 13–20% of patients (Bauer et al., 1997; Warkentin et al., 1999). However, despite this high rate of seroconversion, only about 1–2% of patients who receive further postoperative anticoagulation with unfractionated heparin develop HIT. Currently, there is no convincing evidence that patients who form HIT antibodies in the absence of thrombocytopenia are at increased risk for thrombosis (Bauer et al., 1997; Trossaërt et al., 1998; Warkentin et al., 1999).

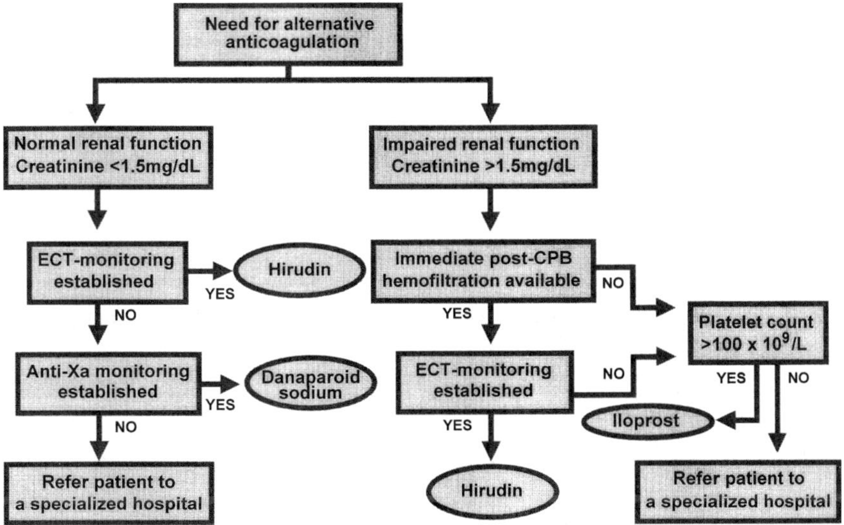

Figure 3 Treatment strategies for HIT patients requiring alternative CPB anticoagulation: The estimated risk of bleeding is highest for azotemic patients receiving r-hirudin, intermediate for patients receiving danaparoid, and lowest for patients with normal renal function receiving r-hirudin.

However, postoperative cardiac surgical patients who develop HIT appear to be at increased risk for both venous and arterial thrombotic events (Walls et al., 1990; van Dyck et al., 1996).

V. DECISION MAKING FOR ANTICOAGULATION IN HIT PATIENTS

Given these data and clinical experience, an algorithm has been developed to assist in determining the need for alternative anticoagulation for CPB in HIT patients (Fig. 2). After the decision to avoid use of heparin in the CPB setting, the important remaining question is, which strategy should be chosen? Because each of the different approaches described here provides specific advantages and limitations, it is not possible to recommend one treatment regimen that is applicable for each patient. The algorithm shown in Figure 3 considers typical clinical settings in HIT patients and is constructed to support the decision in finding which of the different approaches is best suited for the individual patient.

REFERENCES

Addonizio VP Jr, Fisher CA, Kappa JR, Ellison N. Prevention of heparin-induced thrombocytopenia during open heart surgery with iloprost (ZK36374). Surgery 102:796–807, 1987.

Bauer TL, Arepally G, Konkle BA, Mestichelli B, Shapiro SS, Cines DB, Poncz M, McNulty S, Amiral J, Hauck WW, Edie RN, Mannion JD. Prevalence of heparin-associated antibodies without thrombosis in patients undergoing cardiopulmonary bypass surgery. Circulation 95:1242–1246, 1997.

Chong BH, Berndt MC. Heparin-induced thrombocytopenia. Blut 58:53–57, 1989.

Cole CW, Bormanis J. Ancrod: a practical alternative to heparin. J Vasc Surg 8:59–63, 1988.

Demers C, Ginsberg JS, Brill-Edwards P, Panju A, Warkentin TE, Anderson DR, Turner C, Kelton JG. Rapid anticoagulation using ancrod for heparin-induced thrombocytopenia. Blood 78:2194–2197, 1991.

Doherty DC, Ortel TL, De Bruijn N, Greenberg CS, Van Trigt P Ill. ''Heparin free'' cardiopulmonary bypass: first reported use of heparinoid (Org 10172) to provide anticoagulation for cardiopulmonary bypass. Anesthesiology 73:562–565, 1990.

Edmunds LH Jr. Blood-surface interactions during cardiopulmonary bypass. J Cardiovasc Surg 8:404–410, 1993.

Gitlin SD, Deeb GM, Yann C, Schmaier AH. Intraoperative monitoring of danaparoid sodium anticoagulation during cardiovascular operations. J Vasc Surg 27:568–575, 1998.

Grocott HP, Root J, Berkowitz SD, deBruijn N, Landolfo K. Coagulation complicating cardiopulmonary bypass in a patient with heparin-induced thrombocytopenia receiving the heparinoid, danaparoid sodium. J Cardiothorac Vasc Anesth 11:875–877, 1997.

Henny CP, ten Cate H, ten Cate JW, Moulijn AC, Sie TH, Warren P, Büller HR. A randomized blind study comparing standard heparin and a new low molecular weight heparinoid in cardiopulmonary bypass in dogs. J Lab Clin Med 106:187–196, 1985.

Insler SR, Kraenzler EJ, Bartholomew JR, Kottke-Marchant K, Lytle B, Starr NJ. Thrombosis during use of the heparinoid Organon 10172 in a patient with heparin-induced thrombocytopenia. Anesthesiology 86:495–498, 1997.

Kappa JR, Horn D, McIntosh CL, Fisher CA, Ellison N, Addonizio VP. Iloprost (ZK36374), a new prostacyclin analogue, permits open cardiac surgery in patients with heparin-induced thrombocytopenia. Surg Forum 36:285–286, 1985.

Kappa JR, Cottrell ED, Berkowitz HD, Fisher CA, Sobel M, Ellison N, Addonizio VP Jr. Carotid endarterectomy in patients with heparin-induced platelet activation: comparative efficacy of aspirin and iloprost (ZK36374). J Vasc Surg 5:693–701, 1987.

Koza MJ, Walenga JM, Fareed J, Pifarre R. A new approach in monitoring recombinant hirudin during cardiopulmonary bypass. Semin Thromb Hemost 19:90–96, 1993.

Kraenzler EJ, Starr NJ. Heparin-associated thrombocytopenia: management of patients for open heart surgery. Case reports describing the use of iloprost. Anesthesiology 69: 964–967, 1988.

Lewis BE, Johnson SA, Grassman ED, Wrona LL. Argatroban as an anticoagulant for coronary procedures in patients with HIT antibody. In: Pifarré R, ed. New Anticoagulants for the Cardiovascular Patient. Philadelphia: Hanley & Belfus, 1997a:301–308.

Lewis BE, Walenga JM, Pifarré R, Fareed J. Argatroban in the management of patients with heparin-induced thrombocytopenia and heparin-induced thrombocytopenia and thrombosis syndrome. In: Pifarré R, ed. New Anticoagulants for the Cardiovascular Patient. Philadelphia: Hanley & Belfus, 1997b:223–229.

Long RW. Management of patients with heparin-induced thrombocytopenia requiring cardiopulmonary bypass. J Thorac Cardiovasc Surg 89:950–951, 1985.

Magnani HN. Heparin-induced thrombocytopenia (HIT): an overview of 230 patients treated with Orgaran (Org 10172). Thromb Haemost 70:554–561, 1993.

Magnani HN, Beijering RJR, ten Cate JW, Chong BH. Orgaran anticoagulation for cardiopulmonary bypass in patients with heparin-induced thrombocytopenia. In: Pifarré R, ed. New Anticoagulants for the Cardiovascular Patient. Philadelphia: Hanley & Belfus, 1997:487–500.

Makhoul RG, McCann RL, Austin EH, Greenberg CS, Lowe JE. Management of patients with heparin-associated thrombocytopenia and thrombosis requiring cardiac surgery. Ann Thorac Surg 43:617–621, 1987.

Meuleman DG. Orgaran (Org 10172): its pharmacological profile in experimental models. Haemostasis 22:58–64, 1992.

Nishida S, Fujita T, Kohno N, Atoda H, Morita T, Takeya H, Kido I, Paine MJI, Kawabata S, Iwanaga S. cDNA cloning and deduced amino acid sequence of prothrombin activator (ecarin) from Kenyan *Echis carinatus* venom. Biochemistry 34:1771–1778, 1995.

Olinger GN, Hussey CV, Olive JA, Malik MI. Cardiopulmonary bypass for patients with previously documented heparin-induced platelet aggregation. J Thorac Cardiovasc Surg 87:673–677, 1984.

Palmer Smith J, Walls JT, Muscato MS, Scott McCord E, Worth ER, Curtis JJ, Silver D. Extracorporeal circulation in a patient with heparin-induced thrombocytopenia. Anesthesiology 62:363–365, 1985.

Pötzsch B, Iversen S, Riess FC, Tzanova N, Seelig C, Nowak G, Müller-Berghaus G. Recombinant hirudin as an anticoagulant in open-heart surgery: a case report [abstr]. Ann Hematol 68(suppl 2):A46, 1993.

Pötzsch B, Madlener K, Seelig C, Riess CF, Greinacher A, Müller-Berghaus G. Monitoring of r-hirudin anticoagulation during cardiopulmonary bypass—assessment of the whole blood ecarin clotting time. Thromb Haemost 77:920–925, 1997.

Riess FC, Löwer C, Seelig C, Bleese N, Kormann J, Müller-Berghaus G, Pötzsch B. Recombinant hirudin as a new anticoagulant during cardiac operations instead of heparin: successful for aortic valve replacement in man. Thorac Cardiovasc Surg 110: 265–267, 1995.

Riess FC, Pötzsch B, Bader K, Bleese N, Greinacher A, Löwer C, Madlener K, Müller-Berghaus G. A case report on the use of recombinant hirudin as an anticoagulant for cardiopulmonary bypass in open heart surgery. Eur J Cardiothorac Surg 10: 386–388, 1996.

Riess FC, Poetzsch B, Mueller-Berghaus G. Recombinant hirudin as an anticoagulant during cardiac surgery. In: Pifarré R, ed. New Anticoagulants for the Cardiovascular Patient. Philadelphia: Hanley & Belfus, 1997:197–222.

Slaughter TF, LeBleu TH, Douglas JM Jr, Leslie JB, Parker JK, Greenberg CS. Characterization of prothrombin activation during cardiac surgery by hemostatic molecular markers. Anesthesiology 80:520–526, 1994.

Teasdale SJ, Zulys VJ, Mycyk T, Baird RJ, Glynn MFX. Ancrod anticoagulation for cardiopulmonary bypass in heparin-induced thrombocytopenia and thrombosis. Ann Thorac Surg 48:712–713, 1989.

Trossaërt M, Gaillard A, Commin PL, Amiral J, Vissac AM, Fressinaud E. High incidence of anti-heparin/platelet factor 4 antibodies after cardiopulmonary bypass surgery. Br J Haematol 101:653–655, 1998.

Van Dyck MJ, Lavenne-Pardonge E, Azerad M-A, Matta AG, Moriau M, Comunale ME. Thrombosis after the use of heparin-coated cardiopulmonary bypass circuit in a patient with heparin-induced thrombocytopenia. J Cardiothorac Vasc Anesth 10: 809–815, 1996.

Visentin GP, Malik M, Cyganiak KA, Aster RH. Patients treated with unfractionated heparin during open heart surgery are at high risk to form antibodies reactive with heparin: platelet factor 4 complexes. J Lab Clin Med 128:376–383, 1996.

Walenga JM, Bakhos M, Messmore HL, Koza M, Wallock M, Orfei E, Fareed J, Pifarre R. Comparison of recombinant hirudin and heparin as an anticoagulant in a cardiopulmonary bypass model. Blood Coagul Fibrinolysis 2:105–111, 1991.

Walls JT, Curtis JJ, Silver D, Boley TM. Heparin-induced thrombocytopenia in patients who undergo open heart surgery. Surgery 108:686–693, 1990.

Walls JT, Boley TM, Curtis JJ, Silver D. Heparin-induced thrombocytopenia in patients undergoing intra-aortic balloon pumping after open heart surgery. ASAIO J 38: M574–M576, 1992.

Warkentin TE. Limitations of conventional treatment options for heparin-induced thrombocytopenia. Semin Hematol 35(suppl 5):17–25, 1998.

Warkentin TE, Kelton JG. Timing of heparin-induced thrombocytopenia (HIT) in relation to previous heparin use: absence of an anamnestic immune response, and implications for repeat heparin use in patients with a history of HIT [abstr]. Blood 92(suppl 1):182a, 1998a.

Warkentin TE, Chong BH, Greinacher A. Heparin-induced thrombocytopenia: towards consensus. Thromb Haemost 79:1–7, 1998b.

Warkentin TE, Simpson PJ, Sheppard JI, Moore JC, Horsewood P, Kelton JG. Importance of patient population in the frequency of HIT: a comparison of activation and antigen assays [abstr]. Thromb Haemost 82(suppl):363–364, 1999.

Wilhelm MJ, Schmid C, Kececioglu D, Möllhoff T, Ostermann H, Scheld HH. Cardiopulmonary bypass in patients with heparin-induced thrombocytopenia using Org 10172. Ann Thorac Surg 61:920–924, 1996.

Zulys VJ, Teasdale SJ, Michel ER, Skala RA, Keating SE, Viger JR, Glynn MFX. Ancrod (Arvin) as an alternative to heparin anticoagulation for cardiopulmonary bypass. Anesthiology 71:870–877, 1989.

18

Legal Aspects of Heparin-Induced Thrombocytopenia

Klaus Ulsenheimer
University of Munich, Munich, Germany

I. RISK–BENEFIT ASSESSMENT FOR ANTITHROMBOTIC PROPHYLAXIS

Antithrombotic prophylaxis has become virtually routine in certain perioperative settings, especially for hospital inpatients judged to be at medium or high risk for thrombosis. In low-risk situations, such as minor operations in healthy outpatients, the need for antithrombotic prophylaxis is not uniformly well established. According to the German Society of Surgeons:

> All discussants were of the opinion that in patients with a medium, and especially those with a high risk of thrombosis, a pharmacologic prophylaxis is indicated, along with other measures such as physiotherapy and early mobilisation. Peri- and postoperative intermittent calf compression has also been described as useful. There is not enough evidence for a general recommendation of pharmacologic prophylaxis in patients at low risk of thrombosis. Here, an intervention must be based on a risk versus benefit consideration for each individual patient (Mitt Dtsch Ges Chire, 1997)

Prophylaxis against thrombosis thus involves a medical decision involving risk–benefit assessment for an individual patient.

II. CHOICE OF ANTITHROMBOTIC PROPHYLAXIS

The choice of an antithrombotic prophylactic agent leads to the principle of freedom of choice of therapy, meaning that it is primarily the right of the physician to decide on the treatment (Bundesgerichtshof, 1982). This right is limited by the duty to choose the treatment that, benefit being equal, carries the lowest risk for the patient. Choosing a higher-risk agent has to be justified by special circumstances in individual cases or a higher chance of successful treatment (Bundesgerichtshof, 1987). Thus, the doctor violates his duty of care if choice of prophylaxis increases patient risk without medical justification.

These considerations have implications for choice of prophylaxis for heparin-induced thrombocytopenia (HIT): If serious side-effects, such as HIT, are very rare and associated complications usually not serious, then use of heparin prophylaxis is certainly indicated. (This also applies to the more common entity known as nonimmune heparin-associated thrombocytopenia, which is a benign event without adverse consequences.) Under these circumstances, effective pharmacological prophylaxis using heparin can be justified to decrease the risk to immobilized patients even in an otherwise low-risk category.

However, if the frequency of HIT is greater, even as high as 0.5–5% in certain clinical settings (Greinacher, 1996a; Warkentin et al., 1998; see Chap. 4), the risk–benefit assessment leads to a different conclusion: prophylaxis with heparin entails significant risk, and may no longer be less dangerous than no prophylaxis. Whether there are alternate antithrombotic maneuvers available that are as effective as UFH, but cause HIT less frequently, has to be defined by the medical community.

The decision for or against prophylaxis thus depends on the overall risk/benefit ratio, including the frequency and clinical effect of HIT in a particular patient population, compared with the expected benefit of the heparin in reducing thrombotic events. If, as current opinion suggests, the benefits of a particular heparin preparation outweigh the low risk of HIT, then prophylaxis using heparin may be justified, even in patients at relatively low risk for thrombosis. The relative frequencies of HIT in different clinical settings are discussed in Chap. 4.

According to the *Stufenplanverfahren des Bundesinstituts für Arzneimittel und Medizinprodukte* [Official measurements to reduce drug-associated risks of the German Federal Institute for Drugs and Medicinal Products], it is necessary to monitor the platelet count in every patient treated with heparin. However, there is no medical consensus about the details of the monitoring. The usual recommendation is one platelet count measurement before commencing the heparin therapy, followed by three measurements a week from day 5 and one weekly count from day 20 (Greinacher, 1996b). However, as new information on the different risks of developing HIT among patient populations emerge from clinical studies, an individualized approach to platelet monitoring taking into account the particular degree of risk may be appropriate (see Chap. 4).

III. THE INFORMED PATIENT

Another important legal aspect is the duty of the physician to inform the patient about the actual risk of thrombosis, including the possible risks and expected benefits of prophylaxis. This information is divided into two parts: procedure-related and therapy-related. One example is the current discussion on pharmacological prophylaxis of thrombosis in outpatients. The Bundesgerichtshof (Federal state court, 1996a, b) is of the opinion that the current discussion in medical science about the danger of thrombosis and the means of pharmacological prophylaxis in outpatients justify a duty to provide information. In these cases, ''patient autonomy demands information about possible dangers of treatment and the means available to avoid or alleviate such undesired effects.''

Information about prophylaxis against thrombosis must include hemorrhage; allergic reactions, including HIT and its possible complications; the need for platelet count monitoring; and, for long-term prophylaxis, osteoporosis. Even if the risk of HIT is very low, information about it must be provided. Furthermore, information about certain life-threatening consequences of HIT, such as permanent organ damage and even death, as well as possible countermeasures against these outcomes, must be communicated. Statistical probabilities in mathematical terms are not of major importance: they are, according to the Bundesgerichtshof (1994a), of ''minor importance only.'' Critical, however, is whether the complications are relatively specific for the treatment intervention in question. Thus, even extremely rare risks need to be mentioned if they are known to be associated specifically with an intervention, and if their occurrence would have noticeable influence on the patient's life and occupation (Bundesgerichtshof 1994b, 1996a; Oberlandesgericht Hamm, 1995). Consequently, there can be no doubt over the duty to inform about the risks associated with HIT, as these complications are known to be caused by heparin and, therefore, are specific for this intervention.

If a doctor recommends using heparin in a low-risk patient outside an approved indication, the patient must also be informed about this. This is because in legal terms, approval of a drug is ''like a seal of quality, that—independent of the actual quality or safety—can be decisive for the patients decision-making in the area where the pharmaceutical law is applicable, so he has to be informed'' (Bundesgerichtshof, 1996b).

Physicians are allowed to use drugs to treat diseases for which they have not been approved, provided the medical necessity arises and there is a rationale or precedence for its benefit and reasonable safety in the clinical context (Oberlandesgericht Köln, 1991). The regulatory approval of a drug merely creates a state of confidence; that is, the doctor can rely on the fact ''that the risk versus benefit ratio is considered favorable in the light of the evidence provided by the manufacturer and the examination of the Bundesinstitut für Arzneimittel und Medizinprodukte'' (Weißauer, 1994).

On the other hand, for a doctor using a nonapproved drug or an approved drug outside its approved indication, this state of confidence does not cover him or her in the event of damaging side effects. The physician may then be required to justify the treatment, for example, by showing that the drug has been used with a favorable side effect profile, that reputable specialists recommend its use, and that there are no alternative treatments available. This is not an uncommon situation in the management of complications of HIT itself, where an alternative anticoagulant, danaparoid sodium, is often used outside its approved indication (i.e., antithrombotic prophylaxis following orthopedic surgery), or even without any approval in some countries, for the treatment or prevention of thrombosis associated with HIT.

The physician must inform the patient about reasonable precautions in optimizing the safety of a prescribed treatment. This includes educating outpatients about typical signs and symptoms of therapeutic complications. For example, informing patients about the possibility and significance of skin reactions at heparin injection sites as an early manifestation of HIT is appropriate. The main content of the information given to the patient should be documented in writing by the physician, as legal protection in the event of a subsequent adverse event occurring. It is especially prudent to document the informed consent process if practice outside of usual medical care is contemplated, or if the patient refuses recommended treatment, such as antithrombotic prophylaxis. Incomplete or lacking documentation can lead to a reversal of the burden of proof in favor of the patient, if in the event of a pulmonary embolism or deep vein thrombosis, the doctor has to prove that he had informed the patient.

IV. THE HARMED PATIENT

The mere violation of approved medical practice, or failure in the duty to obtain informed consent, by themselves do not constitute a punishable offence nor justify claims for compensation. For the physician's mistake in treating or informing the patient to become punishable, it must be proved that the patient was harmed.

If it can be demonstrated that a patient who was not informed about the risks of HIT would nevertheless have chosen this prophylactic treatment despite its potential risks, then violation of the duty to obtain informed consent becomes irrelevant. This is no longer true if the patient who suffered HIT or any other complication can prove that having known about the risks, he or she would have refused the treatment. In this context, the frequency of HIT among various patient populations could be a factor determining the likelihood that a patient would have given informed consent. For example, a court may determine that a reasonable patient might not have given informed consent to receive unfractionated heparin if the frequency of HIT is shown to be about 5% (e.g., postoperative orthopedic patients), particularly if other therapeutic options exist (e.g., low molecular weight heparin or warfarin).

In case of a treatment error, such as omission to provide antithrombotic prophylaxis, proof is needed that adequate prophylaxis against thrombosis would have prevented the damage. In civil cases of alleged malpractice, the burden of proof required by the plaintiff is relatively low, such as prima facie evidence. In cases of gross negligence, the burden of proof even is reversed: if, for example, there has not been any prophylaxis despite constitutional risk factors and immobilization of a patient, the physician would have the difficult task to prove that the pulmonary embolism or deep vein thrombosis would have occurred even with prophylaxis.

This required burden of proof in a civil litigation is substantially less than in a criminal case. In criminal law, one of the basic tenets is, the benefit of doubt goes in favor of the accused. This means that negligent treatment, or lack of treatment when indicated, can only be proved to be causative in a criminal case if the "correct" treatment (e.g., prophylaxis against thrombosis) would have prevented death or damage to the patient with a "probability bordering on certainty." This legal term cannot be defined in precise statistical terms (e.g., 95 or 99%). Rather, by raising a "reasonable doubt," even a "high" or "very high" probability that an omitted treatment might otherwise have prevented death or disability would not be sufficient to prove the causality of a violation of duty in a criminal court (Bundesgerichtshof, 1988). "Probability bordering on certainty" means the exclusion of reasonable doubts, i.e., doubts which are based upon concrete facts. Given the level of uncertainty in medical knowledge, the required "probability bordering on certainty" in a criminal case (e.g., when the physician is accused to have omitted prophylaxis against thrombosis as a breach of the duty of care) cannot be postulated.

V. COST OF ANTITHROMBOTIC PROPHYLAXIS

Cost is not an argument against indicated prophylaxis. The less expensive, but equally effective drug, should be used, but social law's duty to work economically does not legitimize lowering the standard of medical care. Medical duty for care and the duty to work economically are not mutually exclusive, as social law acknowledges the need for approved treatment. However, economic considerations and price have to give way to aspects of effectiveness of a drug and its indication. So, if there is an appropriate indication for prophylaxis for an individual patient's health, insurance must bear the cost.

REFERENCES

Bundesgerichtshof. Neue Juristische Wochenschr 35:2121–2122, 1982.
Bundesgerichtshof. Neue Juristische Wochenschr 40:2927, 1987.
Bundesgerichtshof. Monatsschrift für Deutsches Recht 42:100, 1988.
Bundesgerichtshof. Neue Juristische Wochenschr 47:3012, 1994a.
Bundesgerichtshof. Neue Juristische Wochenschr 47:793 and 3012–3014, 1994b.
Bundesgerichtshof. Neue Juristische Wochenschr 49:776–777, 1996a.
Bundesgerichtshof. Monatsschr Dtsch Rechts 50:1015–1016, 1996b.
Bundesgerichtshof. Neue Zeitschrift für Strafrecht 16:34, 1996c.
Dtsch Ges Chire: Supplement to the Mitt Dtsch Ges Chir Heft 5/1997, G 79.
Greinacher A. Heparin-induzierte Thrombozytopenien. Internist 37:S1172–S1178, 1996a.
Greinacher A. Heparin-induzierte Thrombozytopenie (HIT): Wie kann das Risiko einer postoperativen Thrombose oder Lungenembolie reduziert werden? Orthopaede 25: 379–384, 1996b.
Oberlandesgericht Hamm. Versicherungsrecht 46:47–48, 1995.
Oberlandesgericht Köln. Versicherungsrecht 42:186–188, 1991.
Warkentin TE, Chong BH, Greinacher A. Heparin-induced thrombocytopenia: towards consensus. Thromb Haemost 79:1–7, 1998.
Weißauer W. Anaesthesiol Intensivmed 35:204–205, 1994.

APPENDIX 1. TEN CLINICAL "RULES" FOR DIAGNOSING HIT

Rule 1: A thrombocytopenic patient whose platelet count fall began between days 5 and 10 of heparin treatment (inclusive) should be considered to have HIT unless proved otherwise (first day of heparin use is considered "day 0").

Rule 2: A rapid fall in the platelet count soon after starting heparin is unlikely to represent HIT unless the patient has received heparin in the recent past, usually within the past 100 days.

Rule 3: A platelet count fall of more than 50% from the postoperative peak between days 5 and 14 after surgery associated with heparin treatment can indicate HIT even if the platelet count remains higher than 150×10^9/L.

Rule 4: Petechiae and other signs of spontaneous bleeding are not clinical features of HIT, even in patients with very severe thrombocytopenia.

Rule 5: HIT is associated with a high frequency of thrombosis despite discontinuation of heparin with or without substitution by coumarin: the initial rate of thrombosis is about 5–10% per day over the first 1–2 days; the 30-day cumulative risk is about 50%.

Rule 6: Localization of thrombosis in patients with HIT is strongly influenced by independent acute and chronic clinical factors, such as the postoperative state, atherosclerosis, or the location of intravascular catheters in central veins or arteries.

Rule 7: In patients receiving heparin, the more unusual or severe a subsequent thrombotic event, the more likely the thrombosis is caused by HIT.

Rule 8: Venous limb gangrene is characterized by (1) in vivo thrombin generation associated with acute HIT; (2) active deep vein thrombosis in the limb(s) affected by venous gangrene; and (3) a supratherapeutic international normalized ratio (INR) during coumarin anticoagulation. This syndrome can be prevented by delaying coumarin use in acute HIT until therapeutic anticoagulation is achieved with an agent that reduces thrombin generation (e.g., danaparoid) or that inhibits thrombin directly (e.g., lepirudin).

Rule 9: Erythematous or necrotizing skin lesions at heparin injection sites should be considered dermal manifestations of the HIT syndrome, irrespective of the platelet count, unless proved otherwise. Patients who develop thrombocytopenia in association with heparin-induced skin lesions are at increased risk for venous and, especially, arterial thrombosis.

Rule 10: Any inflammatory, cardiopulmonary, or other unexpected acute event that begins 5–30 min after an intravenous heparin bolus should be considered acute HIT unless proved otherwise. The postbolus platelet count should be measured promptly, and compared with prebolus levels, because the platelet count fall is abrupt and often transient.

Disclaimer: The preceding ten clinical ''rules'' have been formulated primarily for didactic purposes, and are not intended necessarily to imply any standard of care in relation to their clinical application.

APPENDIX 2. TREATMENT RECOMMENDATIONS*

Nonimmune Heparin-Induced Thrombocytopenia

Recommendation. Heparin should not be discontinued in patients clinically suspected of having nonimmune heparin-associated thrombocytopenia (grade C-2).

Immune Heparin-Induced Thrombocytopenia

Discontinuation of Heparin for Clinically Suspected HIT

Recommendation. All heparin administration should be discontinued in patients clinically suspected of having (immune) HIT (grade C-1).
Recommendation. A clearly visible note should be placed above the patient's bed stating ''NO HEPARIN: HIT'' (grade C-2).
Recommendation. Heparin can be safely restarted in patients proved not to have HIT antibodies by sensitive activation or antigen assay (grade C-1).

Anticoagulation of the HIT Patient with Thrombosis

Recommendation. Therapeutic-dose anticoagulation with a rapidly acting anticoagulant, e.g., danaparoid or lepirudin, should be given to a patient with thrombosis complicating acute HIT. Treatment should not be delayed for laboratory confirmation in a patient strongly suspected of having HIT (grade C-1).

Anticoagulation of the HIT Patient Without Thrombosis

Recommendation. Alternative anticoagulation with an appropriate anticoagulant, such as danaparoid or lepirudin, should be considered in patients with clinically suspected HIT even in the absence of symptomatic thrombosis. Anticoagulation should be continued at least until recovery of the platelet counts to a stable plateau. Patients should be carefully assessed for lower limb DVT, especially those at highest risk for venous thromboembolism, such as postoperative patients (grade C-2).

Longer-Term Anticoagulant Management of the HIT Patient with Thrombosis

Recommendation. The drug of choice for longer-term anticoagulation of HIT patients is an oral anticoagulant of the coumarin class (e.g., warfarin or phenprocoumon). However, in a patient with acute HIT, oral anticoagulant therapy should

---

* The grades of recommendation are from Cook et al. (1995) and Guyatt et al. (1998), and are described on pp 261–262 of Chap. 13.

be delayed until the patient is adequately anticoagulated with a rapidly acting parenteral anticoagulant, and ideally not until there has been substantial platelet count recovery (grade C-1).

Recommendation. Prothrombin complex concentrates should not be used to "reverse" coumarin anticoagulation in a patient with acute or recent HIT unless bleeding is otherwise unmanageable (grade C-2).

Reexposure of the HIT Patient to Heparin

Heparin Reexposure of the Patient with Acute or Recent HIT

Recommendation. Deliberate reexposure to heparin of a patient with acute or recent HIT for diagnostic purposes is not recommended. Rather, the diagnosis should be confirmed by testing acute patient serum or plasma for HIT antibodies using a sensitive activation or antigen assay (grade A-1).

Heparin Reexposure of the Patient with a History of Remote HIT

Recommendation. Heparin should not be used for antithrombotic prophylaxis or therapy in a patient with a previous history of HIT, except under special circumstances (e.g., cardiac or vascular surgery) (grade C-2).

Cardiopulmonary Bypass or Vascular Surgery

Management of the Patient with Acute or Recent HIT

Recommendation. Heparin should not be used for heart or vascular surgery in a patient with acute or recent HIT with detectable HIT antibodies. Either danaparoid or lepirudin are appropriate alternatives for intraoperative anticoagulation, provided that rapid-turnaround laboratory monitoring and blood product support to manage potentially severe bleeding complications are available (grade C-2).

Management of the Patient Following Disappearance of HIT Antibodies

Recommendation. In a patient with a previous history of HIT, heart or vascular surgery can be performed using heparin, provided that HIT antibodies are absent (by sensitive assay), and heparin use is restricted to the surgical procedure itself (grade C-1).

HIT During Pregnancy

Recommendation. Danaparoid is preferred for parenteral anticoagulation of pregnant patients with HIT or those who have a previous history of HIT (grade C-2).

Adjunctive Therapies for HIT

Medical Thrombolysis

Recommendation. Regional or systemic pharmacological thrombolysis should be considered as a treatment adjunct in selected patients with limb-threatening thrombosis or pulmonary embolism with severe cardiovascular compromise (grade C-2).

Surgical Thromboembolectomy

Recommendation. Surgical thromboembolectomy is an appropriate adjunctive treatment for selected patients with limb-threatening large-vessel arterial thromboembolism. Thrombocytopenia is not a contraindication to surgery. An alternative anticoagulant to heparin should be used for intraoperative anticoagulation (grade C-1).

Intravenous Gammaglobulin

Recommendation. ivIgG is a possible adjunctive treatment in selected patients requiring rapid blockade of the Fc receptor-dependent platelet-activating effects of HIT antibodies (e.g., management of patients with sinus vein thrombosis, severe limb ischemia, or very severe thrombocytopenia) (grade C-2).

Plasmapheresis

Recommendation. Plasmapheresis, using plasma as replacement fluid, may be a useful adjunctive therapy in selected patients with acute HIT and life- or limb-threatening thrombosis who are suspected or proved to have acquired deficiency of one or more natural anticoagulant proteins (grade C-2).

Dextran

Recommendation. Dextran should not be used as primary therapy for acute HIT complicated by thrombosis (grade C-1).

Acetylsalicylic Acid and Dipyridamole

Recommendation. Antiplatelet agents such as aspirin may be used as adjuncts to anticoagulant therapy of HIT, particularly in selected patients at high risk for arterial thromboembolism. The possible benefit in preventing arterial thrombosis should be weighed against the potential for increased bleeding (grade C-2).

Platelet Glycoprotein IIb/IIIa Inhibitors

Recommendation. GP IIb/IIIa inhibitors should be considered as experimental treatment in HIT and used with extreme caution if combined with anticoagulant drugs (grade C-2).

Caveats for the Treatment of HIT

Low Molecular Weight Heparin (LMWH)

Recommendation. LMWH should not be used to treat patients with acute HIT (grade C-1).

Oral Anticoagulants (Vitamin K Antagonists)

Recommendation. Oral anticoagulants are contraindicated in patients with acute HIT, unless combined with an agent that reduces thrombin generation (grade C-1).

Ancrod

Recommendation. Ancrod should not be used to treat patients with HIT (grade C-1).

Platelet Transfusions

Recommendation. Prophylactic platelet transfusions are contraindicated in patients with HIT (grade C-2).

Disclaimer. The listed recommendations represent the general views of the editors (as of December 1999), and are intended primarily as an educational guide for physicians who must treat patients with clinically suspected, or serologically proven, HIT. The editors wish to emphasize that these recommendations cannot be applied indiscriminately to all clinical situations, for reasons that can include concomitant clinical factors, diagnostic uncertainty, availability of alternative anticoagulant options, and the availability and turnaround times for HIT antibody and anticoagulant monitoring assays.

APPENDIX 3. DANAPAROID DOSING SCHEDULES

Clinical indication	Danaparoid dosing schedule
Venous thromboembolism: prophylaxis	750 U sc b.i.d. or t.i.d.
Venous thromboembolism: treatment	2250 U iv bolus,[a] followed by 400 U/h for 4 h, 300 U/h for 4 h, then 150–200 U/h for $\geq$ 5 days, aiming for a plasma anti-Xa level of 0.5–0.8 U/mL *Subcutaneous administration schedule*: 1500–2250 U sc b.i.d. (bioavailability is almost 100% when given by sc injections; thus, 2250 U sc b.i.d. is approximately equal to an iv infusion rate of 200 U/h (4500 U/24 h vs. 4800 U/24 h, respectively)
Arterial thromboembolism: treatment	See venous thromboembolism treatment schedule
Embolectomy or other peripheral vascular surgery	*Preoperative*: 2250 U iv bolus;[a] *intraoperative flushes*: 750 U in 250 mL saline, using up to 50 mL (see p. 277); *postoperative*: 750 U sc t.i.d. (low-risk patients) or 150–200 U/h (high-risk patients) beginning at least 6 h after surgery
Hemodialysis (on alternate days)	3750 U iv before 1st and 2nd dialyses; 3000 U for 3rd dialysis; then 2250 U for subsequent dialyses, aiming for plasma anti-Xa level of < 0.3 U/mL before each dialysis and 0.5–0.8 U/mL during dialysis (see also Chap. 16).
Hemofiltration	2250 U iv bolus, followed by 600 U/h for 4 h, then 400 U/h for 4 h, then 200–400 U/h aiming for a plasma anti-Xa level of 0.5–1.0 U/mL (see also Chap. 16)
Cardiopulmonary bypass surgery (CPB)	125 U/kg iv bolus after thoracotomy; 3 U/mL in priming fluid of CPB apparatus; 7 U/kg/h iv infusion commencing after bypass hookup, and continued until 45 min before expectation of stopping bypass (see also Chap. 17)
Cardiac catheterization,	*Preprocedure*: 2250 U iv bolus (3000 U if 75–90 kg and 3750 U if > 90 kg)
Percutaneous transluminal coronary angioplasty (PTCA) or intra-aortic balloon pump	*Preprocedure*: bolus as per above; *postprocedure*: 150–200 U/h for 1–2 days after PTCA (or until removal of balloon pump)
Catheter patency	750 U in 50 mL saline, then 5–10 mL per port, or as required
Pediatric dosage considerations	*Prophylaxis*: 10 U/kg sc b.i.d. *Treatment*: 30 U/kg b.w. iv bolus, then 1.2–2.0 U/kg b.w. per hour (depending upon severity of thrombosis)

Abbreviations: b.w., body weight; b.i.d., twice daily; iv, intravenous; t.i.d., three times daily.

[a] Adjust iv danaparoid bolus for body weight: < 60 kg, 1500 U; 60–75 kg, 2250 U; 75–90 kg, 3000 U; > 90 kg, 3750 U.

Compatibility with intravenous solutions: Danaparoid is compatible for dilution with any of the following solutions: saline, dextrose, dextrose/saline, Ringer's, lactated Ringer's, 10% mannitol.

Preparation of solution for infusion: There are several options. One approach used by the author is to add four ampules containing 3000 U (i.e., 750 anti-Xa U per 0.6 mL ampule) of danaparoid to 300 mL of intravenous solution (i.e., a solution comprised of 10 U danaparoid per milliliter of intravenous solution); thus, an infusion rate of 40 mL/h corresponds to a dose of 400 U/h, 20 mL/h to an infusion rate of 200 U/h, and so on.

APPENDIX 4. DOSING SCHEDULES FOR r-HIRUDIN TREATMENT OF PATIENTS WITH HIT[a]

	Bolus[c,g]	IV infusion[c,g]	Target aPTT ratio[b]
HIT and TEC	0.4 mg/kg b.w.iv	0.15 mg/kg b.w./h	1.5–2.5
HIT with TEC and concomitant thrombolysis	0.2 mg/kg b.w.iv	0.1 mg/kg b.w./h	1.5–2.5
HIT with isolated thrombocytopenia		0.1 mg/kg b.w./h	1.5–2.0
Thrombosis prophylaxis in patients with a history of HIT	15 mg sc twice daily[d]	0.1 mg/kg b.w./h[e]	1.5–2.0 for iv infusion
Renal dialysis every alternate day	0.1 mg/kg b.w.iv predialysis	—	2.0–2.5
CVVH	—	0.005 mg/kg b.w./h (initial rate)	1.5–2.5
Vascular surgery[h]			
vessel flushes after embolectomy	use up to 250 mL (0.1 mg/mL solution)	—	1.5–2.5
postoperative anticoagulation	—	0.1 mg/kg b.w./h	1.5–2.5
Cardiopulmonary bypass surgery	0.25 mg/kg b.w.iv 0.2 mg/kg b.w. in the priming fluid of the HLM	0.5 mg/min[f]	Monitored by ECT: >2.5 μg/mL before start of HLM; 3.5–4.5 μg/mL during CPB

Abbreviations: aPTT, activated partial thromboplastin time; b.w., body weight; CPB, cardiopulmonary bypass; CVVH, continuous venovenous hemofiltration; ECT, ecarin-clotting time; iv, intravenous; HLM, heart–lung machine; TEC, thromboembolic complication.

Repeat aPTT determinations should be made 4–6 h afters any dose adjustment.

[a] The data were generated with lepirudin unless otherwise indicated.

[b] The ratio is based on comparison with the normal laboratory median aPTT. If Actin FS or Neothromtin reagents are used, the aPTT target range is usually 1.5–3.0.

[c] A maximum body weight 110 kg should be used for dose calculations.

[d] Based on studies evaluating the r-hirudin, desirudin, in patients undergoing hip replacement surgery (Eriksson et al., 1997).

[e] Used in the HAT-1 and HAT-2 trials.

[f] Stop 15 min before end of CPB; put 5 mg into HLM after disconnection to avoid clotting.

[g] Adjustments for renal insufficiency:

Creatinine clearance (mL/min)	Serum creatinine, mg/dL (μmol/L)	Adjusted bolus dose	Adjusted infusion rate (% of original dose)
45–60	1.6–2.0 (141–177)	0.2 mg/kg	50
30–44	2.1–3.0 (178–265)	—	25
15–29	3.1–6.0 (266–530)	—	10
< 15	> 6.0 (> 530)	0.1 mg/kg b.w. on alternate days (only if aPTT ratio < 1.5) without use of infusion	or, 0.005 mg/kg b.w. iv adjusted for aPTT (without bolus doses)

[h] Hach-Wunderle and Hach, 1997.

Index

D

E

F

G

H

M

N

O

P

R

S

T

V

W

About the Editors

THEODORE E. WARKENTIN is an Associate Professor in the Department of Pathology and Molecular Medicine as well as the Department of Medicine at McMaster University, Hamilton, Ontario, Canada, and Associate Head of Transfusion Medicine at the Hamilton Regional Laboratory Medicine Program of the Hamilton Health Sciences Corporation, Hamilton. The author or coauthor of more than 100 journal articles and book chapters, he is a Fellow of the Royal College of Physicians and Surgeons of Canada and the American College of Physicians. Dr. Warkentin was awarded the 1996 Jean Julliard Prize from the International Society of Blood Transfusion for his research into heparin-induced thrombocytopenia. He received the M.D. degree (1983) from the University of Manitoba, Winnipeg.

ANDREAS GREINACHER is a Professor in the Department of Immunology and Transfusion Medicine and Head of Transfusion Medicine at Ernst-Moritz-Arndt University, Greifswald, Germany. The author of more than 80 journal articles and book chapters, he serves as a consultant to the German Federal Institute of Drugs and Medical Products. Dr. Greinacher received the M.D. degree (1988) from the Julius Maximilian University, Würzburg, Germany, and his training in immunology and transfusion medicine at the Justus-Liebig University, Giessen, Germany.